SUFFERING AND MORAL RESPONSIBILITY

OXFORD ETHICS SERIES

Series Editor: Derek Parfit, All Souls College, Oxford

SUFFERING
AND MORAL
RESPONSIBILITY

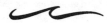

Jamie Mayerfeld

New York   Oxford

Oxford University Press

1999

Oxford University Press

Oxford   New York
Athens   Auckland   Bangkok   Bogotá   Buenos Aires   Calcutta
Cape Town   Chennai   Dar es Salaam   Delhi   Florence   Hong Kong   Istanbul
Karachi   Kuala Lumpur   Madrid   Melbourne   Mexico City   Mumbai
Nairobi   Paris   São Paulo   Singapore   Taipei   Tokyo   Toronto   Warsaw

and associated companies in
Berlin   Ibadan

Library of Congress Cataloging-in-Publication Data
Mayerfeld, Jamie.
Suffering and moral responsibility / Jamie Mayerfeld.
p.   cm. — (Oxford ethics series)
Includes bibliographical references.
ISBN 0-19-511599-6
1. Suffering—Moral and ethical aspects.   2. Responsibility.
I. Title.   II. Series.
BJ1409.M28   1999
179—dc21   98-19813

1 3 5 7 9 8 6 4 2

Printed in the United States of America
on acid-free paper

For my parents,
Ernest Mayerfeld and Marilyn Mayerfeld,
and my friend,
Morris Jackson

Preface

The world knows an immense amount of suffering, much of it humanly inflicted and much of it humanly preventable. My book seeks to shed light on the moral dimensions of this fact. Ultimately, it aims to clarify the nature of the duty to relieve suffering, and to encourage reflection on the kinds of changes that would be necessary to bring our lives into adequate compliance with this duty.

I have brooded on these matters for a long time. From an early age I enjoyed many wide-ranging and eye-opening conversations with Morris Jackson, who greeted my views with good-natured skepticism and subjected them to steady critique. My parents, with whom I began to share my thoughts around the same time, reacted with something closer to alarm. I have learned much from their protests, and I owe more than I can say to their unceasing love, encouragement, and support. To them and to Morris, I dedicate this book.

I thank the professors at Oberlin College who introduced me to moral and political philosophy. In my sophomore year, I wrote on my own initiative what I fancied to be a definitive discussion of the duty to relieve suffering. Norman Care read it, gave me detailed comments, and suggested that I might benefit from actually studying philosophy. His course on "Philosophy and Values" was a revelation. I also learned from the superlative teaching of Alfred MacKay, who wisely devoted a course to Sidgwick's *Methods of Ethics*, and Harlan Wilson, who did his best to teach me some political theory.

This work first took shape as a doctoral dissertation in politics at Princeton University. I owe an enormous debt to my advisors, Alan Ryan and George Kateb, for expert guidance at the start, middle, and end of the dissertation project. Both were sympathetic to the undertaking, but warned me to abandon some of my more foolish ideas. I heeded their advice in some instances, and may come to regret that

I did not do so in others. Their wisdom, learning, and generosity are a continuing source of inspiration.

My greatest debt is to Derek Parfit. Derek took an early interest in my manuscript, and treated draft after draft to wonderfully detailed and penetrating comments. Reading Derek's comments was an education in itself, and it is hard to convey the pleasure I felt in absorbing a wealth of insights into the very issues that had so long occupied my attention. The pleasure was not unmixed with fear, since I was sure I could never meet the challenges Derek continually threw in my direction. I never did meet them adequately, but I tried my best, and the effort led to a greatly improved manuscript. Derek encouraged me to think I could fulfill his high expectations, and for this I shall always be grateful.

Jeff McMahan and Larry S. Temkin, who reviewed the manuscript for Oxford University Press, saved me from many errors, and their suggestions for recasting the discussion proved extremely helpful. Jeff went far beyond the call of duty by supplying a second round of detailed comments on a subsequent draft.

To Amy Gutmann I am grateful for early advice and encouragement. To Dennis McKerlie I am indebted for an invaluable conversation over e-mail on the moral asymmetry of happiness and suffering, and to Clancy Bailey for a similarly beneficial e-mail conversation on the role of intuitions in moral reasoning. Amy, Dennis, and Clancy all gave me valuable feedback on the manuscript at different stages of its completion. At the University of Washington, I have enjoyed the continuing guidance of my colleague from the Department of Philosophy, Bill Talbott. Bill lavished careful comments on repeated drafts, and has greatly enhanced my understanding of the methods and limits of moral philosophy.

For enlightening discussions on pain and pain measurement, I am indebted to Dr. Mark Jensen, Dr. John Loeser, and Dr. Mark Sullivan, all members of the world-famous research community on pain relief at the University of Washington.

Several other people generously set aside time to comment on full or partial drafts of my book, or to discuss specific issues with me in person, or both. The results of their criticisms, suggestions, insights, and questions appear in innumerable places, and I am profoundly grateful to them. They include Brom Anderson, Randolph Clarke, Christine Di Stefano, Stephen E. Hanson, Richard Hare, Greg Hill, Thomas Hurka, Frank Jackson, John Goldberg, Frances Kamm, Elizabeth Kiss, Cliff Landesman, Margaret Mack, Michael McCann, Jean Roberts, Paul Sigmund, Peter Singer, Martin Tweedale, Mark van Roojen, Paul Vogt, and Alan Wertheimer. I thank any others who belong on this list and whose names I unintentionally omit.

I am fortunate to have received able assistance from the many talented people at Oxford University Press. Matthew Diamond came to my rescue by correcting the page proofs with remarkable care and skill.

I thank the support of my departmental colleagues, especially Christine Di Stefano, Nancy Hartsock, Michael McCann, and Michael Taylor. I also thank successive department chairs—Donald McCrone, Lance Bennett, and Michael McCann—for help in arranging research time.

RTPREFACE ix

For their unflagging support, cheerful encouragement, and indispensable advice over many years, I thank my sister and brother-in-law, Diane Mayerfeld and Michael Bell, and my friends Luis Corteguera, Patrick Dobel, Morris B. Kaplan, Donna Kerr, and Cynthia Steele. I thank my partner, Peter Mack, for all these things, and also for the unexpected gift of happiness.

Parts of the following discussion appeared in "The Moral Asymmetry of Happiness and Suffering," *The Southern Journal of Philosophy* 34 (1996): 317–38.

Contents

SUFFERING AND MORAL RESPONSIBILITY

ONE

Introduction

THIS BOOK IS ABOUT THE DUTY TO relieve suffering. It asks what the content of this duty is, and what it implies for how we should live our lives.

Most people underestimate the strength of this duty. There are different reasons for this, some of which are discussed later. But one reason is that most people aren't very clear what the duty to relieve suffering is. There is widespread confusion about the meaning and measurement of suffering, which in turn breeds confusion about its moral relevance. I hope to clear away some of this confusion. Understanding the content of the duty to relieve suffering is the first step toward grasping its importance.

Among philosophers, attention to suffering has been a casualty of a long series of attacks on hedonistic utilitarianism—the doctrine that people are morally required to maximize the total surplus of happiness over suffering. I believe that hedonistic utilitarianism *should* be rejected, but that most philosophers have made too wholesale a rejection and have thus lost sight of the moral significance of suffering. The following account differs from hedonistic utilitarianism in two respects: first, I do not claim that all of morality can be reduced to the requirement to promote happiness and reduce suffering; and second, I argue that the relief of suffering is morally more important than the promotion of happiness.

In this book I employ a particular conception of suffering. I follow the usage of hedonistic thinkers—such as Epicurus, Jeremy Bentham, and Henry Sidgwick—for whom suffering refers to an affliction of feeling. Suffering can also be given a broader meaning, to include other sorts of afflictions. One could write a book about the duty to relieve suffering in this larger sense. I believe we have a great need for such a book, but it is not the book I have written. I employ the narrower, hedonistic conception of suffering, not because I think it is the only correct one, but because

3

I think it carries enormous moral significance in its own right and therefore requires a separate discussion.

The organization of this book is fairly straightforward. Chapter 2 discusses what suffering means and chapter 3 how it ought to be measured. Chapter 4 examines the moral significance of suffering in its own right and in comparison to other values. Chapter 5 discusses some basic features of the duty to relieve suffering. Chapter 6 defends the view that the alleviation of suffering is morally more important than the promotion of happiness, while chapter 7 examines the proper resolution of trade-offs internal to the duty to relieve suffering: for example, What should we do when we can eliminate the suffering of one group of people or another group of people, but not both? The final chapter addresses the question of how to identify those occasions when the relief of suffering is not morally required or is indeed wrong.

In the remainder of this chapter I discuss the nature of moral reasoning. I end with some remarks about moral terminology.

I am interested in the relevance of suffering to morality. My goal is to contribute to our understanding of how we ought to behave—or, as I prefer to put it, how we ought not to behave. The aim is to improve our identification of wrong conduct. This subject is of overriding importance. Suppose you go out and shoot your neighbor dead. An act as wrong as this is something you desperately want to avoid. And you want to avoid it if for no other reason than that it is wrong (in this case extremely wrong).

Here some of my readers may breathe easily, knowing that they are not about to shoot their neighbor. But they shouldn't breathe too easily. It is possible that we already engage in behavior that is very wrong. We may not think of it as wrong, but our beliefs may be in error.

It helps to think about the false moral beliefs of people in the past. Many people have been gravely mistaken about morality; this includes highly intelligent people who have earnestly desired not to do wrong and have been judged morally upright by their contemporaries. Throughout much of history, for example, torture was considered an acceptable practice. It was legally recognized and regularly carried out for specified purposes: as a method of, or accompaniment to, capital punishment; as a technique of judicial prosecution; and as a discipline for recalcitrant slaves. Its use in the courts persisted in most of Europe until laws abolishing it were passed in the eighteenth century. In ancient Greek and Roman law, it was considered necessary to elicit reliable evidence from slaves. Furthermore, harsh corporal punishment, often bearing the character of torture, has always been seen as a necessary last resort—though it need not be resorted to last—for getting slaves to perform hard or loathsome work that otherwise they would not do.[1] Throughout these cen-

1. On the history of torture, see Edward Peters, *Torture* (New York: Basil Blackwell, 1985); Malise Ruthven, *Torture: The Grand Conspiracy* (London: Weidenfeld and Nicolson, 1978); and M. I. Finley, *Ancient Slavery and Modern Ideology* (New York: Viking, 1980).

turies there were few people who criticized the practice of torture, and those who did usually attacked it on pragmatic, not moral, grounds.[2]

Roman slave owners and medieval judges who used torture did not think they were doing anything wrong. Nevertheless, what they did was extremely wrong. We need to consider that we might be in the same situation. We might be engaged in practices that are wrong, or extremely wrong, though we mistakenly believe they are innocent. Perhaps the truth is that we have escaped danger—that those behaviors which we believe are permissible are in fact permissible. But this thesis, if we subscribe to it, must be defended against possible doubts. If the doubts prove justified, then we must learn which behaviors, currently judged to be innocent, are in fact wrong, and end them forthwith.

How do we correctly identify what kinds of behavior are wrong? How do we arrive at a correct set of moral beliefs? I concur with a growing number of philosophers that the truth about morality cannot be revealed by means of some proof—at least, no persuasive proof has yet been discovered. Some philosophers say that in the absence of a moral proof we should be guided by the basic moral principles that underlie the communities or cultures in which we live. Perhaps these principles are not strictly *undeniable* (the thinking runs), yet they still seem capable of commanding our belief, and anyway it may be futile to look for something more basic than the moral heritage of our communities.

My objection to this approach is that it doesn't pay sufficient mind to the possibility that community values may be mistaken—even those that are revealed by careful interpretation, and that emerge after an effort to render them mutually consistent. Torture within prescribed limits was accepted practice in several ancient civilizations and in late medieval Europe, and (with the possible exception of Christian Europe) appears to have been fully compatible with the underlying moral codes of those communities, on any plausible interpretation. But it is difficult to believe that people who inflicted torture in such communities did nothing wrong. Rather, it appears that the communities themselves were deeply mistaken about the morality of torture. It seems that the values of one's community can be a misleading moral guide.

Morality is too important to leave to the jurisdiction of community values. To learn the truth about morality, you should ask yourself what *you* believe. But at the same time you should keep in mind that your current beliefs may not be the correct ones. You should test your current beliefs for trustworthiness and be on the lookout for other more trustworthy beliefs.

The most trustworthy moral beliefs are those that emerge after critical reflection. By critical reflection, I mean asking yourself whether you clearly understand the content of a particular belief and still believe it; whether you have foreseen and can approve all its implications; whether it contradicts another belief of yours, demonstrating that one of them, at least, must be false; and whether it expresses a stable and deeply felt belief, and not merely a passing impulse or social norm that you

2. Peters, *Torture*, pp. 21, 34–36.

repeat by rote without independent conviction. To test for the last feature—authenticity of belief—you should also try to learn how you came to hold your present moral views, for you may find that your confidence in them will not survive the discovery of their psychological origins. Finally, you should carefully consider the ethical views of other people, in case you discover moral hypotheses that you had not succeeded in formulating to yourself before but that convince you of their truth immediately upon acquaintance, or win your assent at a later stage of critical reflection.[3]

Critical reflection, in other words, involves a number of tests of the validity of your beliefs: clarity and intelligibility, acceptability of implications, mutual consistency, authentic conviction, and impartial consideration of alternative beliefs. A complete list may need to include other tests as well. I should note that discussion with people holding different views from your own is an essential part of this process, not only because it exposes you to moral propositions you hadn't thought of before, but also because it assists in the application of the other tests as well. People who disagree with you will press for ever more rigorous applications of those tests as they try to change your mind.[4]

The application of the tests that together constitute the method of critical reflection requires great intellectual labor and is never at an end. It occupies the full-time efforts of professional moral philosophers. Its results are not negligible, for it can lead people to alter their beliefs, sometimes radically. When critical reflection changes our moral beliefs, we think that our new beliefs rest on stronger grounds than the ones we held before.

Some readers may be impatient with a method that places so much weight on moral intuition. I would share this impatience if I knew of a method that supplied moral judgments with a stronger foundation. Many such methods have been suggested, but I have yet to see one that is persuasive. The reasons why they fail to persuade vary from case to case. Many of these methods, though claiming to dispense with moral intuition, appeal to it covertly. This book is not the place for the comprehensive survey needed to defend this assessment. It is, however, an assessment shared by many moral theorists today.

Critical reflection does not promise infallibility. One proof of this is the distressing fact that two people may apply the method with equal thoroughness to the question of whether some form of behavior is morally permissible and still disagree whether it is. They may disagree about the content of the relevant moral principle,

3. My account of critical reflection is based on and inspired by Henry Sidgwick's discussion of the necessary conditions of a trustworthy moral belief, though I do not follow Sidgwick on all particulars. See Sidgwick, *The Methods of Ethics* (London: Macmillan, 1907), pp. 338–42. Readers may recognize resemblances to what John Rawls calls the search for reflective equilibrium. See Rawls, *A Theory of Justice* (Cambridge, Mass.: Harvard University Press, 1971), pp. 19–20.

4. Compare Amy Gutmann: "We can potentially learn more about political morality from listening and responding to reasonable arguments with which we disagree than from thinking on our own." "The Challenge of Multiculturalism in Political Ethics," *Philosophy and Public Affairs* 22 (1993): 171–206, p. 202.

and not just about the proper application of that moral principle to the case at hand. Such disagreement is distressing because it proves that one of these people is morally mistaken.

Since critical reflection does not guarantee a correct answer, and since there is no better method, it may be suggested that we should decline to have moral beliefs at all. But there is, I believe, no principled reason to adopt this policy. If we want to avoid acting wrongly, both agnosticism and belief carry dangers. The danger of trusting our beliefs is that they may be mistaken and may lead us to act wrongly. The danger of not trusting our beliefs is that they may be correct and our disregarding them may lead us to act wrongly. There is no reason to suppose that the first of these dangers generally outweighs the second, especially when the beliefs in question are those that emerge from extended critical reflection. Because of this, it is not unreasonable to trust beliefs that survive critical reflection.

Complete agnosticism seems to me a mistake. But so does the opposite extreme of trusting every moral intuition to which one is susceptible. At some point one should hold each intuition at arm's length, as it were, and ask, "Is it telling me the truth?" In some cases one may find oneself doubting an intuition even though it preserves a hold on one's feelings. I believe this possibility is permanently kept alive for those who take seriously the danger of moral error. We want true moral beliefs, but only the true ones.

The ultimate test of one's moral judgments is not, What do I feel? but What do I believe? (Or: What should I believe?) Belief is a higher judge than feeling. Admittedly, these are often hard to separate. Our moral beliefs are nourished by moral feelings (what we "feel" to be true). But sometimes they diverge. Consider the example of retributivism—the attitude that a criminal should be made to suffer for his crime whether or not deterrence or reform is thereby achieved. Some of us (I include myself) are often subject to powerful retributivist feelings, feelings that are morally colored, and yet we think that at least some of these feelings ought not to be trusted. We think that they require a reason, and that a good enough reason has not been found. Although we are susceptible to these feelings, we do not believe what they say. I think the same may hold true for other moral feelings. We need to beware both of believing too little and believing too much. Moral progress requires a careful balance between skepticism and belief.

Skepticism need not imply greater moral leeway. There are two kinds of moral belief—the belief that X is wrong, and the belief that X is permitted. One may be skeptical both about moral requirements and moral permissions. Therefore, we cannot say in advance whether a partial skepticism lessens or increases the scope of moral obligation.

I include these remarks to make evident my views about the nature and purpose of moral reasoning. We need moral inquiry to identify wrong kinds of behavior so that we can avoid them. The ultimate test of a moral claim is whether you believe it, and the most trustworthy beliefs are those that emerge from critical reflection. One can think of moral reasoning as a kind of accelerated natural selection in which only the most believable of beliefs survive, and critical reflection sorts out those that are most believable. Underlying this approach is the faith (it can be no more than that) that the effort to know the truth will bring us closer to it.

This book is intended as a contribution to the task of critical moral reflection. I shall present for the consideration of my readers the claim that we have a strong duty to prevent suffering, and I shall try to spell out as clearly as I can what this duty means. My hypothesis is that belief in a strong duty to relieve suffering will tend to emerge from a process of extended critical moral reflection. I make no pretense of conducting a thorough application of the tests previously described to the question of suffering and its relevance to morality. (To a large extent those tests are better gone over in the reader's mind than on the written page.) My ambition is not to complete, but rather to assist, the task of critical moral reflection.

Before proceeding, I shall make a few remarks about moral terminology. First, I assume that the concept of wrong encompasses failures to act as well as actions. Here our language has a tendency to lead us astray. The useful word *wrongdoing* seems to imply that wrong behavior must be a doing or action of some kind. But a moment's reflection reminds us that this is not so. We know that it is wicked to watch a small child drown when we could save him without serious risk to ourselves. This example shows that one can *do wrong* by *doing nothing*.[5] Because I want a category that includes both actions and non-actions as objects of moral judgment, I sometimes speak of "behaviors" to refer to both.

On some people's view, the claim that an agent has behaved wrongly implies that it is appropriate to apply a negative sanction of some kind: the agent ought to feel guilty, or other people ought to rebuke, punish, or condemn the agent. I assume, however, that the question, Which behaviors are wrong? is distinct from the question, Which behaviors ought to receive negative sanctions? To call a behavior wrong is simply to declare that it must not be done. So it is possible that a behavior could be wrong, yet no negative sanction would be appropriate. I discuss this point briefly in chapter 5.

I often refer to the duty to relieve suffering. But, unless I specify otherwise, I usually mean a prima facie duty to relieve suffering. The term "prima facie duty" was coined by W. D. Ross, and has now entered the philosophical vocabulary, although, as Ross recognized, it is not an ideal term for what it is meant to describe.[6] A prima facie duty is a genuine duty, not merely something that appears to be so, as its name might suggest. The contrast to a prima facie duty is not a genuine duty, but an all-things-considered duty. A prima facie duty to do X gives me a genuine

---

5. It is harder than one might think to explain the difference between "doing" and "not doing." Jonathan Bennett offers one account in *The Act Itself* (Oxford: Clarendon Press, 1995). He argues that the distinction lacks intrinsic moral significance.

6. Ross, *The Right and the Good* (Oxford: Oxford University Press, 1930), pp. 19–20. Shelly Kagan emphasizes the shortcomings of the term and substitutes the phrase "pro tanto reason." See Kagan, *The Limits of Morality* (Oxford: Clarendon Press, 1989), p. 17.

reason to do X, and, in the absence of countervailing moral considerations, implies that I must do X. However, rival moral considerations may succeed in overriding the prima facie duty to do X, in which case my prima facie duty to do X is no longer my duty, all things considered.

Rival moral considerations may take the form either of conflicting prima facie duties or conflicting prima facie permissions. A prima facie duty establishes a presumption (which may be overridden by rival moral considerations) that a certain class of behaviors is wrong (all those that do not fit the description of the required behavior). A prima facie permission establishes a presumption (which may be overridden by rival moral considerations) that any of a certain class of behaviors is *not* wrong, or that *at least one* of a certain class of behaviors is not wrong.[7]

The prima facie duty to relieve suffering is sometimes overridden by such considerations. For example, it is sometimes overridden by the prima facie duty not to kill. There could be situations in which one could relieve suffering by killing someone painlessly. (Imagine that the rest of the person's life would have been miserable and that killing the person wouldn't be attended by any of the usual pain or inconvenience to others or yourself.) Nevertheless, in many of these situations, it would still be wrong to kill the person. This is because, in these situations, the prima facie duty not to kill outweighs or defeats the prima facie duty to relieve suffering.

And it may be the case, though I reserve judgment for now whether it really is, that the prima facie duty to relieve suffering is sometimes overridden by prima facie permissions. There is plausibility in the notion that we enjoy a prima facie permission not to incur grave sacrifices, and that this sometimes excuses us from complying with the demands of the prima facie duty to relieve suffering. To take a dramatic example, imagine that by allowing myself to be tortured I could save another person from being tortured more severely. The prima facie duty to relieve suffering asks that I make this sacrifice because the suffering I thereby prevent is cumulatively worse than the suffering I incur; nevertheless, it may be suggested that I am not duty bound to comply, because the sacrifice demanded of me is too great.

Much of this book is taken up with defending the claim that we are subject to a prima facie duty to relieve suffering and with clarifying the content of that duty. But because our underlying interest is the avoidance of wrong, we cannot leave matters there. We need to know when the prima facie duty to relieve suffering is overridden by other moral considerations. Therefore, at the end of the book, I inquire into the limits of the duty to relieve suffering. This is a large and difficult question, and unfortunately I can do little more than broach the topic.

To my regret, I have had to bracket an all-important question: What kind of obligation do we have to prevent the suffering of non-human animals? My own view, for what it is worth, is that the suffering of non-human animals is no less evil from a moral point of view than the suffering of human beings when equivalent in

7. In *The Right and the Good*, Ross overlooked the possibility of prima facie permissions—an omission later criticized by Bernard Williams in *Ethics and the Limits of Philosophy* (Cambridge, Mass.: Harvard University Press, 1985), pp. 180–82.

intensity and duration, and that consequently our duty to prevent animal suffering is just as strong as our duty to prevent human suffering.[8] I believe, therefore, that many of the principles defended below ought to be applied to the entire sentient creation, and in chapter 5 I touch briefly on what this could imply. However, I do not attempt to defend this view. The moral puzzles raised by human suffering are formidable in their own right; to address animal suffering would have required a major expansion of an already complex discussion. In most of my discussion I simply refer to the suffering of people, though I sometimes use the expandable term "individuals" so as not to beg the question against animals. Though I set aside the issue of the proper treatment of animals, it remains an urgent moral question demanding our immediate attention.

8. For a powerful defense of this position, with a review of the relevant literature, see David De-Grazia, *Taking Animals Seriously* (Cambridge: Cambridge University Press, 1996).

TWO

The Meaning of Suffering

Why did I not die at birth,
   come forth from the womb and expire?
Why did the knees receive me?
   Or why the breasts, that I should suck?
For then I should have lain down and been quiet;
   I should have slept; then I should have been at rest.
                                                —Job 3.11–13

1. Psychological Versus Objectivist Understandings of Suffering

People tend to use the word *suffering* in either of two ways: in a psychological sense, or in what I will call, for want of a better word, an "objectivist" sense. In the "objectivist" sense, suffering is roughly synonymous with calamity or misfortune. In this sense, the precise meaning of suffering remains partly to be filled in, because what counts as calamity or misfortune is somewhat vague and partly subject to dispute. But often enough, calamity is unmistakable. One is murdered; one's relatives are massacred; one's house of a lifetime is swept away by a flood; one loses one's job and is turned onto the street; one is malnourished; one contracts a debilitating disease. Sometimes suffering simply designates the experience of such objective calamities, *without* referring to the psychological state of the people concerned.

But sometimes suffering has a psychological meaning. It refers to how individuals feel. Roughly speaking, to suffer is to feel bad. This is the sense employed when survivors of those who have died from an accident or violent attack are told, in an attempt to comfort them, that their loved ones "did not suffer." Of course, premature death is normally considered a supreme misfortune, but what is meant here is that the victim lost consciousness before experiencing distress. Suffering, in this sense, is what Jeremy Bentham and Henry Sidgwick had in mind when they spoke of "pain," and what the Epicureans referred to as *lupé*.

This book is concerned with the psychological rather than the objectivist sense of suffering. I focus on suffering in the psychological sense because I want to claim that this particular phenomenon has towering moral significance in its own right, and that we have a powerful duty to stop and prevent it. Epicurus, Bentham, and Sidgwick were right to view it as a paramount evil, albeit they went too far in claiming it is the *only* evil. However, these matters are taken up later. The fact that I have chosen the word *suffering* to refer to this phenomenon tells us nothing about its moral significance and its relation to our duties. Those questions are still on the table.

I shall use the word *happiness* in a parallel way. Happiness is sometimes equated with Aristotle's understanding of *eudaimonia*, which he defined as the expression of human excellence or virtue in action.[1] Sometimes it is equated with success, in the sense of achieving important life goals.[2] But in this book happiness describes a psychological state: roughly, the state of feeling good. It is Epicurus's rather than Aristotle's understanding of eudaimonia. Its closest synonym is "enjoyment," though the latter term with its connotations of mildness and transience fails to capture the full range of positive feelings signified by happiness.[3]

To see the differences between these meanings, consider what we might say about small infants. Aristotle, correctly applying his definition, denied that babies could be happy (attain eudaimonia), since babies lack virtue.[4] Nor can babies be happy in the sense of achieving important life goals. But we frequently observe babies to be "happy" in the psychological sense—when, for example, they are well-fed, gurgling, and smiling. And by "happy" we mean something deeper than that they are feeling pleasure.[5] Indeed a small baby's happiness—during those moments when he or she is happy—often strikes us as purer and more perfect than that which an older person is ever likely to attain.

Some people treat "happiness" as a synonym for "well-being." If we equate these terms, a definition of happiness implies a theory of the human good. Debates among the ancient Greeks about the meaning of eudaimonia assumed this character. However, I will not treat "happiness" and "well-being" as equivalent terms. So by using a hedonistic conception of happiness, I do not mean to suggest that our good consists of happiness hedonistically understood. I am simply naming a dimension of our experience that forms the counterpart to hedonistic suffering and that, in my view, constitutes an important element of well-being. I am not denying that there may be other elements of our well-being, such as moral goodness or the exercise of essential human powers. Even with this disclaimer, some readers may object to a hedonistic conception of happiness as excessively idiosyncratic. But that objection ought not to matter too much, since the main concern of this book is with suffering.

1. Aristotle, *Nicomachean Ethics*, trans. Martin Ostwald (Indianapolis: Bobbs-Merrill, 1962), book I.
2. See John Rawls, *A Theory of Justice* (Cambridge, Mass.: Harvard University Press, 1971), pp. 93, 550.
3. My usage draws closer to, but is still distinct from, L. W. Sumner's understanding of happiness as "a settled sense of satisfaction with the conditions of one's life." Sumner, *Welfare, Happiness, and Ethics* (Oxford: Clarendon Press, 1996), p. 147.
4. *Nicomachean Ethics*, Book I, 1099b–1100a.
5. See section 4.

The limitation of the word *suffering* to psychological distress may seem odd in particular contexts. Victims of violent assault sometimes manage to detach themselves emotionally from what is happening to them; psychologists refer to this reaction as "dissociation."[6] When the detachment is complete, it would not be accurate, according to our definition, to refer to their experience as one involving suffering. I say this even though occurrences of this kind may provoke the greatest outpouring of sympathy from other people, and the sympathy may become more intense as the victims seem to mind less: this might be because we are struck by the contrast between the brutal nature of the injury and the victims' impassivity; or because we are especially frightened by mistreatment that damages or disturbs normal psychology; or because when we see that victims are not protesting the injustice of their situation, we feel instinctively the need to do some of that work for them, even if it is only with our emotions.

We may resist the denial of suffering here, and not just because some of us are drawn to an "objectivist" understanding of suffering. When outrages are committed against the body of a living person and there is strong evidence, perhaps the person's own testimony, to support the view that he feels no distress, then we cannot help being perplexed. We may be told and we may say that he does not feel torment, but we probably do not *believe* it (at least a part of us does not), because it is hard for us to imagine that we could ever be in such a situation and not feel extremely bad. Our ambivalent opinion about the state of his feelings, despite the presence of what normally passes for unarguable evidence that he feels all right, may explain our hesitation to affirm that he is not suffering, even where by suffering we mean bad feeling.

In some people's minds, the word *suffering* necessarily implies that a person has incurred real, and not merely "felt," damage. Though this is partly to be explained by the frequent use of the word in the objectivist sense discussed earlier, it also owes something to the widespread but false belief that distress, whether mental or physical, is invariably the symptom of some determinate injury. This premise appears in the specificity theory of physical pain, according to which pain can always be traced directly to the intense noxious stimulus of specific nerve cells, as typically occurs during injury; and in the psychoanalytic school of psychology, which interprets neurosis, including depression, as the outgrowth of bitter frustrations in the past, the memory of which has been repressed. Both theories have been shown to be inadequate. The link between physical pain and noxious stimuli is a highly variable one; pain often occurs in the absence of injury or long after an injury has healed.[7] And some depressions are best explained, not as the consequence of a past emotional trauma that we have made ourselves forget, but as the result of a simple chemical imbalance in the brain that can be corrected with medication; what is

6. See Judith Lewis Herman, *Trauma and Recovery* (New York: Basic Books, 1992), pp. 42–43.

7. Ronald Melzack and Patrick D. Wall, *The Challenge of Pain* (New York: Basic Books, 1983). See also John D. Loeser and Wilbert E. Fordyce, "Chronic Pain," in J. E. Carr and H. A. Dengerink, eds., *Behavioral Science in the Practice of Medicine* (New York: Elsevier, 1983).

important here is that we would not judge the chemical imbalance to be a problem—we would not even judge it an *imbalance*—if it did not make us feel miserable.[8]

Sometimes, differently from the meaning I intend, "suffering" is used to mean the subjective experience of people who are oppressed or are the victims of injustice. When used this way, the word by its very meaning implies a moral judgment on someone's behavior. To say that some people are suffering is to say that some other people are oppressing them or acting unjustly toward them and that, consequently, these people should change their behavior so as to end the oppression and remove the injustice. To cite someone's suffering is, ipso facto, to make a moral condemnation. Additionally, it presupposes prior knowledge about what constitutes oppression and injustice.

I shall not use the word *suffering* in this way. When someone is suffering, injustice or wickedness may be involved, but it may not. And to the extent that it is, that is a contingent empirical fact, not an implication of the word *suffering*. Suppose, for example, that there is a wicked person inflicting bodily pain and discomfort on you. Now imagine another situation completely identical to this one with respect to what you are thinking and feeling, and which differs from it only in that there is no tormentor—though you are convinced that there is and that he is there hurting you—and that your bodily distress, unbeknownst to you, stems from non-human causes that other people are powerless to prevent. Then we should say that you feel equally bad in both situations, and that consequently your suffering is the same, though the first scenario, unlike the second, includes the element of human wickedness.

2. Suffering as Disagreeable Overall Feeling

> Sometimes we feel good, and sometimes we feel bad, and sometimes we feel neither way at all.[9]

I shall use the terms "happiness" and "suffering" to refer to overall states of feeling at a particular moment. As a first approximation, let us say that happiness refers to a state of feeling good overall, or agreeable overall feeling, while suffering refers to a state of feeling bad overall, or disagreeable overall feeling. I specify overall feeling, because good and bad feelings may be experienced simultaneously, so that the pres-

8. For current theories on depression, see Ronald R. Fieve, *Moodswing*, rev. ed. (New York: Bantam, 1989); George Winokur, *Depression: The Facts* (Oxford: Oxford University Press, 1981); John H. Greist and James W. Jefferson, *Depression and Its Treatment* (New York: Warner, 1984); and Peter D. Kramer, *Listening to Prozac* (New York: Viking, 1993). For a psychoanalytic explanation of depression, see Sigmund Freud, "Mourning and Melancholia," trans. Joan Riviere, in *Sigmund Freud, Collected Papers*, vol. 4 (New York: Basic Books, 1959).

9. Leonard David Katz, "Hedonism as Metaphysics of Mind and Value" (Ph.D. diss., Princeton University, 1986), p. 47.

ence of one or a few bad feelings does not indicate suffering if they are outweighed by positive feelings occurring at the same time, nor does the presence of one or a few good feelings indicate happiness if they are outweighed by simultaneous negative feelings. For example, I may have snapped unjustly at my child and feel guilty as a result. The guilt I experience is itself bad (I may say that "I feel bad" about my conduct), but it is likely to share room with positive feelings (many of which, though present in my consciousness, may not receive direct mental attention). These agreeable feelings are likely to outweigh the cumulative force of my pangs of conscience, and preserve me from a state of suffering. Only if my guilt spreads gloom over my consciousness as a whole—an experience as rare as it is memorably unpleasant—may we confidently infer that I am suffering.

The claim that suffering corresponds to disagreeable overall feeling requires, I think, a small qualification. All suffering is correctly classified as disagreeable overall feeling, but there are certain overall feelings of a mildly disagreeable sort that seem not to deserve the appellation of suffering. If my mood is dominated by a feeling of mild boredom or impatience, it seems odd to say that I am suffering. I am not denying that there is such a thing as mild suffering: I believe there is. The mood that we refer to as "unhappiness" often constitutes mild suffering, for example. But moderate boredom and impatience do not seem to qualify. I conclude that there is a kind of very mildly disagreeable overall feeling that falls short of suffering.

It may be useful to distinguish between the ordinary sense of the word *suffering*, which preserves the previous distinction, and a technical sense of the word that refers to the entire range of disagreeable overall feeling. For the most part I will adopt the ordinary sense, but sometimes (for example, when discussing the measurement of the intensity of suffering) I will have recourse to the technical sense. This is a fairly minor issue, since the disagreeableness of feelings like mild boredom and impatience is indeed very mild. There is not much that separates them from the kind of overall feeling that is neither agreeable nor disagreeable—what Henry Sidgwick called the "hedonistic zero."

Similar remarks about "happiness" do not seem warranted. It does not strike me as odd to refer to the mildest form of agreeable overall feeling as "very mild happiness."

I shall thus distinguish between agreeable overall feeling and disagreeable overall feeling, using "happiness" to refer to the entire range of agreeable overall feeling, and generally using "suffering" as a term that is nearly but not fully coextensive with disagreeable overall feeling.

What makes an overall feeling disagreeable, I believe, is that it is intrinsically worse than unconsciousness.[10] When we ask whether a particular overall feeling is intrinsically worse than unconsciousness, we must consider only the feeling itself, in abstraction from all the goods (or evils) of knowledge, perception, and activity that the person would have to give up if he or she became unconscious. When I

---

10. See the discussion by Stuart Rachels in "Counterexamples to the Transitivity of Better Than," *Australasian Journal of Philosophy* 76 (1998): 71–83, p. 72. Rachels applies this definition to pain.

consider the matter carefully, it seems to me that an overall feeling of mild boredom or impatience may be intrinsically worse than unconsciousness by a slight degree.

It follows from what I have said that all suffering is intrinsically worse than unconsciousness. To say that suffering is intrinsically worse than unconsciousness is not to say that suffering people would be made better off if they became unconscious, for remaining conscious may provide them with certain goods (involving activity, learning, perception, etc.) that make their suffering worthwhile. Sometimes, however, the goods made available by consciousness are clearly not worth their price in suffering. Thus we give patients general anesthesia to spare them the pain and terror of experiencing surgery. (Notice that we would not feel similarly compelled to distribute safe ecstasy-giving drugs if they were available—a clear indication of the moral asymmetry between pain and pleasure.) And when suffering becomes extreme, our desire for unconsciousness may enlarge into a plea for non-existence, as in Job's unforgettable appeal:

> Let the day perish in which I was born,
>   and the night that said,
>   "A man-child is conceived."
> Let that day be darkness!
>   May God above not seek it,
>   or light shine on it.
> Let gloom and deep darkness claim it.
>   Let clouds settle upon it;
>   let the blackness of the day terrify it. (Job 3.3–5)

3. In Search of a Definition of Happiness and Suffering

We can learn by examining Sidgwick's definition of pleasure. Sidgwick followed the philosophical tradition of referring to "pleasure and pain," but his use of those terms corresponds to what I have been calling happiness and suffering. He defined pleasure as

> feeling which the sentient individual at the time of feeling it implicitly or explicitly apprehends to be desirable [or—in cases of comparison—preferable];—desirable, that is, when considered merely as feeling, and not in respect of its objective conditions or consequences, or of any facts that come directly within the cognisance and judgment of others besides the sentient individual.[11]

Sidgwick's definition rightly insists that the assessment of happiness or suffering (in the psychological or hedonistic sense of these terms) depends on the evaluation

11. Henry Sidgwick, *The Methods of Ethics* (London: Macmillan, 1907), p. 131. The interpolated phrase is from p. 127. It should be noted that Sidgwick did not stipulate *overall* feeling. He believed that feelings which differ in their pleasantness may sometimes occur simultaneously, though when they do, they usually "blend into one state of pleasant consciousness the elements of which we cannot estimate separately." Ibid., p. 141. His analysis differs from my own in this regard.

of an individual's feelings in abstraction from all other facts that describe her situation. We easily go astray if we allow considerations external to feeling—Sidgwick's "objective conditions and consequences"—to affect the estimate of happiness and suffering. Only the quality of feeling is relevant.

Feeling should not be confused with "introspectively discernible features of consciousness."[12] Our mental states involve more than feeling. Thus Sidgwick distinguished between feelings, cognitions, and volitions as different elements of consciousness.[13] To have a certain belief or to form a certain will is not to *feel* a certain way. Some of the elements of consciousness not included under the heading of feeling might be deemed independently valuable. The point here is that happiness/suffering tracks the quality of feeling, rather than the quality of mental states per se.

People with painful diseases sometimes turn down strong pain medicine because they fear it will cloud their thinking. Freud, who battled a painful cancer for sixteen years but refused to take anything stronger than aspirin until the very end, reportedly said, "I prefer to think in torment than not to be able to think clearly."[14] Perhaps Freud just meant that his desire for knowledge overrode his desire for comfort. In that case, he wasn't expressing a preference for one set of introspectively discernible features of consciousness over another set, since the actual possession of knowledge, as opposed to the mere belief that one possesses it, is not introspectively discernible. But perhaps Freud was expressing, among other things, a desire for clear thinking, where the kind of lucidity he had in mind *was* an introspectively discernible feature of consciousness.[15] But if he desired clear thinking in this sense, it wasn't as a kind of feeling. What Freud's statement tells us, on the current interpretation, is that his preference for lucidity qua element of conscious experience overrode his aversion to acutely disagreeable feeling qua element of conscious experience.

Agreeable feeling is not the only introspectively discernible feature of consciousness that individuals may find desirable. But the terms "happiness" and "suffering" should be limited to the evaluation of feeling. If Freud indeed preferred tormented lucidity qua conscious experience to comfortable muddle qua conscious experience, it seems most accurate to say that he preferred an experience with greater suffering to one with less. Sidgwick used "desirable consciousness" and "desirable feeling" as interchangeable definitions of pleasure, because he believed that feeling is the

12. I take the term from Derek Parfit.

13. Sidgwick, *Methods of Ethics*, p. 398.

14. This case is discussed by James Griffin, *Well-being: Its Meaning, Measurement and Moral Importance* (Oxford: Clarendon Press, 1986), p. 8. See Ernest Jones, *The Life and Work of Sigmund Freud*, vol. 3 (New York: Basic Books, 1957), p. 245.

15. Some people might deny this possibility, on the grounds that clear thinking is distinguished from unclear thinking precisely on the grounds of its attunement to reality, or of its tendency to connect us to reality; and, to repeat, the correspondence of our thoughts to reality is not introspectively discernible. But let us grant the possibility for the sake of argument: let us suppose that clarity of mind refers to a coherent and orderly structure of thought, with no necessary connection to the truth.

only element of conscious experience that can be regarded as intrinsically desirable or undesirable qua conscious experience.[16] (He thus would have denied that Freud could have a well-informed desire for clear thinking qua element of conscious experience.) I think it is safer to suspend judgment on this question, and therefore to define happiness in terms of feeling rather than consciousness.

Sidgwick's definition usefully focuses our attention on feeling. But it also has defects. Odd though it may sound, I believe that the definition is *too* subjective. It has the pleasurableness of a feeling depend on the individual's judgment of its desirability at the moment of experiencing it. The danger here is that such judgments may be too malleable. Suppose that twenty-four hours from now I could either be having enjoyable sex or listening to some piece of beautifully uplifting music. Each experience may entail a shift in attitude—a change of personality, if you like. While enjoying sex, I may deeply appreciate the goodness of sex and belittle the experience of listening to beautiful music; while transported by music, I may disparage sex. It is not just that the alternative experience will be less vivid in my imagination; the very criteria by which I evaluate and rank different feelings may be altered. But if in one state, I find sex more desirable than music, while in another I find music more desirable than sex, Sidgwick's definition doesn't allow us to compare the intensity of these pleasures. I'm not insisting here on precise comparability. Perhaps neither pleasure is greater or less than, or equal to, the other (see section 6). But Sidgwick's definition doesn't even allow us to postulate a rough comparison.

There is another, related problem with Sidgwick's definition. An adequate definition of pleasure and pain should provide room for interpersonal comparisons. It should allow judgments of the kind that the pain of my torture is more intense than the pain of your headache. But Sidgwick's definition serves us poorly here. If the pleasurableness of a feeling depends on the degree to which the person experiencing it finds it desirable, it is unclear how we can compare pleasures and pains experienced by *different* people. Sidgwick's definition might suggest the following method. To compare my pain with yours, I try to imagine what you are feeling, compare that with what I am feeling, and then determine which feeling I find more undesirable. But even if I could imagine your experience with perfect accuracy, why should *my* ranking have authority? There might not be a problem if everyone would rank accurately imagined feelings in the same way. But people are different from each other, and just as in different moods *I* might rank the same pair of feelings differently, so *different* people with unlike personalities might also rank them differently. If that's the case—and it's not implausible—Sidgwick's definition doesn't allow us to get a handle on interpersonal comparisons.

I believe that Sidgwick's appeal to subjective judgments of desirability introduces an extraneous and distracting element into the definition of happiness and suffering. The assessment of someone's happiness or suffering is not a matter of determining the extent to which the individual finds her feeling intrinsically desirable or unde-

16. Sidgwick, *Methods of Ethics*, pp. 398–99.

sirable; it is a matter, quite simply, of determining what the feeling is like. If we want to determine which of two people is suffering more intensely, we should not ask which person finds the quality of her feeling more undesirable, but rather who feels worse. We should bypass subjective evaluations and head straight for an objective assessment of what it is like to be a particular person feeling a particular way. I shall say more in this chapter and the next about how these objective assessments are formed. I do not deny for a moment that the formation of these assessments is fraught with difficulty, or that we can only hope for partial success.

I have linked happiness with feeling good overall and suffering with feeling bad overall. I've said that one experience involves more intense suffering than another if it feels worse, let's add that one experience involves more intense happiness than another if it feels better. It may be wiser to regard these descriptions as synonyms rather than precise definitions. It may be a mistake, in other words, to attempt analysis of a phrase like "feeling bad" in terms of simpler elements. We know what it means to "feel bad" without breaking it down into simpler elements, and we know that "feeling bad overall" means the same as "suffering." That may be as far as the search for a definition can take us.

The description of happiness and suffering as "feeling good" and "feeling bad" should not be asked to carry more weight than it can support. One way of overloading it is to construe it as a definition stating that the intensity of happiness or suffering corresponds to the intrinsic prudential value or disvalue of one's overall feeling. We should avoid this definition because we sometimes have to distinguish between the degree to which some experience feels good or bad and the degree to which it is worth having or avoiding. As I shall claim in chapter 6, a particular episode of suffering may feel bad to the same degree that a particular episode of happiness feels good, yet the degree to which the suffering is worth avoiding exceeds the degree to which the happiness is worth having. I shall also claim that as suffering increases in intensity, the degree to which it is worth avoiding outpaces the degree to which it feels bad.

4. The Connection of Happiness and Suffering to Desire

There has been a long tradition of drawing a conceptual connection between happiness and the satisfaction of desire, and between suffering and the frustration of desire. It seems natural to suppose some such connection. What sort of connection, if any, might there be?

According to Bentham and J. S. Mill, we desire nothing as an end in itself but happiness and the avoidance of suffering (that is to say, our own happiness and the avoidance of our own suffering). That can't be right as a description of our actual desires, for we care about other things besides the quality of our feelings. We want, among other things, to gain knowledge, to have other people think well of us, to secure the well-being of friends and loved ones. We desire these things for their own sakes, and not just as means to personal happiness. The evidence is that we are sometimes willing to sacrifice happiness in order to obtain these things.

Some may propose a different, though equally strong, connection: happiness is not the sole intrinsic object of our desire, yet we are happy to the extent that our desires (whatever they may be) are satisfied. Right away this needs to be modified, since we can have desires (e.g., for posthumous fame) the satisfaction of which falls outside our experience, and the satisfaction of such desires obviously won't make us happier. So we might revise as follows: happiness is correlated with the satisfaction of desires, the satisfaction of which is experienced by us. But, notice now, it would make no sense to link happiness with the satisfaction of a desire, if we experience its satisfaction after we have ceased having the desire. So we might revise further: happiness is correlated with the satisfaction of desires, the satisfaction of which is experienced by us *while we still possess the desire*. Or more simply: happiness is correlated with the experienced satisfaction of existing desire.[17]

I believe this proposal also fails, by underestimating the seriousness of our non-hedonistic desires. For, as was just noted, sometimes we desire non-hedonistic goods strongly enough that we are willing to sacrifice happiness in order to attain them. It may suffice to recall the example of Freud, who preferred tormented lucidity over confused comfort. For him, greater happiness was *not* tied to the satisfaction of his desires. And many other examples could be added.

Return now to Bentham and Mill. They claimed, falsely, that we desire nothing, as an end in itself, besides happiness and the avoidance of suffering. Perhaps we could assert a more modest claim: that, *other things being equal,* we always prefer an experience involving happiness to one involving suffering, an experience involving more intense happiness to one involving less intense happiness, and an experience involving less intense suffering to one involving more intense suffering. For purposes of discussion, we can refer to this as the claim that, other things being equal, we always prefer to experience greater happiness than less at any given point in time.[18]

If we are drawn to this claim, we must be careful how we interpret it. First, it has to be emphasized that the preference for greater happiness can only be a ceteris paribus preference: our desires for other things besides certain kinds of feelings will

17. R. M. Hare offers a view close to this in *Moral Thinking: Its Levels, Method and Point* (Oxford: Clarendon Press, 1981), pp. 103-4. But Hare may have in mind something other than a hedonistic understanding of happiness.

18. This claim resembles the claim embedded in Sidgwick's definition of pleasure. Sidgwick believed that a more intense pleasure is "implicitly apprehended" by us as being preferable to a less intense pleasure. It is natural to suppose that a pleasure that we "implicitly apprehend" to be preferable is one that we, quite simply, prefer. (Sidgwick himself equates the two descriptions in a number of passages, and nowhere does he distinguish between them.) So it is natural to read Sidgwick as saying that we always prefer more intense happiness to less intense happiness (and less intense suffering to more intense suffering, etc.), other things being equal.

sometimes prevail over our desire for greater happiness. Another way of putting this is that our desire for happiness is a hypothetical preference. Happiness is the kind of overall feeling we *would* generally prefer to experience *if* everything else were equal.

But more than this: the ceteris paribus desire for greater happiness is not always a conscious preference; often it is latent or concealed. There are preferences that lie on the surface of our consciousness: for instance, my preference for ordering asparagus over eggplant at lunch today, or a student's preference for A's rather than B's. But other preferences lie hidden from immediate consciousness and must be elicited by questions. Sometimes, moreover, the questions will not be immediately understood, so an extended effort will be required to make them intelligible; and there is the possibility that on occasion even an extended effort will be incapable of succeeding, so that the preference will remain permanently concealed. The ceteris paribus desire for happiness is very often latent in this way. For example, even when some people's actions are largely driven by the search for agreeable feeling— and even when many of them would acknowledge this if the fact were carefully explained and demonstrated to them—they still may not be conscious of their quest for happiness when making decisions. Instead, people often learn, by a rapid and reliable process that does not register fully in their consciousness, to identify certain objects with their own greater happiness, and then deliberately seek these objects as if for their own sake. Happiness is their underlying but not their conscious motive, and is, without their explicit recognition, promoted by their conscious ends. If some object of desire ceases to be a source of happiness, this will be taken note of, though not at the level of full consciousness, and a new object will be substituted. The shift will appear at the level of consciousness as a basic change of preference, not explainable in terms of a deeper motive; whereas in fact careful introspection would reveal that the shift is only a tactical adjustment made at the behest of the continuous underlying desire for happiness. These people must be *asked* whether they have a ceteris paribus desire for happiness before they are conscious that they do.

We generally think that people plunged into deep misery will always recognize the nature of their condition and struggle mightily to get out. This is indeed usually the case, but there are striking exceptions. People suffering from severe clinical depression often fail to notice that they are depressed, or even sad. They are consumed by thoughts of their own wickedness or uselessness, and do not consider (a) that their beliefs are unfounded, and (b) that they are experiencing great emotional pain. People who are subject to extensive physical and emotional battering, especially children, may lack a clear sense of their suffering. They may sense in a general way that something is wrong with the world, but may interpret that wrongness as an aspect or consequence of some grave personal failing, and so translate their apprehension of wrongness into guilt.[19] It may not occur to them that what is wrong with

19. For a discussion of the "inner sense of badness" frequently experienced by abused children, see Herman, *Trauma and Recovery*, pp. 103–07.

their situation is precisely that they have been placed by the gratuitous actions of human beings in a situation of great wretchedness from which they ought to be rescued. Meanwhile, their guilt may prevent them from thinking how they can escape their present misery and direct their attention instead to the question of how to be less wicked.

Is it correct to say that the victim of clinical depression or emotional and physical battering who fails clearly to discern that she is suffering prefers some happy state to her present condition of suffering? On the one hand, one wants to say yes; in some very deep sense, she does. But on the other hand, it is hard to talk of her having a preference for happiness over her present misery if she does not even grasp that she is suffering. Her preference for happiness (if it can be said that she has one) is a very deeply buried preference, and much therapy may be needed before it will become conscious. She would first have to have a clear image of the quality of her present feelings, together with a clear image of the happiness that is the alternative to her present condition. But because of her present confusion, one is unsure whether *preference* is the most useful concept for analyzing her suffering. My own sense is that it can be misleading.

If we are looking for a conceptual connection between happiness and desire, then, the most that could be claimed is that we have a ceteris paribus preference for greater happiness rather than less at any given point in time, where it is understood that this preference is often latent, not conscious.

Finally, I think it would be a mistake to try to *define* happiness and suffering in terms of the concept of desire. A definition ought to clarify; it ought to bring what it defines into sharper focus. But a definition of happiness and suffering in terms of desire may often have the opposite effect, since the concept of desire can be more elusive than the concept of happiness and suffering. If a newborn infant endures severe burns and exhibits the recognizable signs of acute distress, it is unclear what it would mean to say that she desires to be relieved of her condition, or that she dislikes the state that she is in. This claim seems to presume a degree of self-consciousness and a conceptual apparatus that would be lacking in the child. (The same would hold true for other animals.) But there is no difficulty in understanding and believing the claim that the infant is suffering.

A desire-based definition also serves us poorly for comparing the happiness and suffering of different individuals. As noted before, there are occasions on which it is important to point out that my suffering is more intense than yours. A desire-based definition is ill-suited to such comparisons, for the same reason that a definition based on subjective judgments of desirability is (see the previous section). It might be suggested that subjective desire does indeed provide a basis for interpersonal comparisons: to compare the intensity of happiness or suffering experienced by different individuals, we simply compare the degree to which they *feel* satisfied or frustrated. As I argue later, this would be a mistake.

Economists have used the concept of desire to illuminate many aspects of human experience. But there are limits to what the concept can explain. We need to proceed carefully when postulating a conceptual connection between happiness and desire, and we should avoid the temptation to define happiness and suffering in terms of the satisfaction or frustration of desire.

5. The Relation of Happiness to Pleasure and Suffering to Pain

It is traditional among hedonistic philosophers to refer to the positive and negative dimensions of feeling as pleasure and pain and to treat the concepts of happiness and suffering as derived from them. Pleasure and pain are the building blocks of Bentham's moral, legal, and psychological theory; he sees happiness and suffering as interchangeable with them, though he uses these words more rarely.[20] When Mill states the Greatest Happiness Principle, he explains that "by happiness is intended pleasure, and the absence of pain; by unhappiness, pain, and the privation of pleasure."[21] In Sidgwick's *Methods of Ethics,* happiness has become a computational term: it refers to the surplus of pleasure over pain for a given set of people in a given period of time; and it is this which it is our duty to maximize.[22] Recent hedonistic writers such as Richard Brandt and Leonard Katz have maintained the terminology of pleasure and pain.[23]

But if we are talking about good and bad feeling, I believe that happiness and suffering are better terms. To speak of pain and pleasure for this purpose is to distance ourselves unnecessarily from current ordinary usage. Both words connote the more physical manifestations of happiness and suffering. In everyday talk, pleasure tends to mean gratification of the senses. It is most unmistakably applied to desirable feelings which are primarily physical, notably sex, but also eating and drinking.[24] It seems unsuited to cover all the various states of joy, satisfaction, euphoria, and contentment that come under the heading of good feeling. "Happiness" seems better suited to such a task.

To see the difference between pleasure and happiness, we can note that there is no contradiction in observing of someone that he is addicted to seeking, and adept at finding, pleasure; but that he is nevertheless quite unhappy. Such a person may be burdened by feelings of anxiety, or self-doubt, or pessimism about the future. He engages in those activities designed to gratify the senses that are normally the cause of highly desirable feelings, and are therefore called by us pleasant, but that

20. See Jeremy Bentham, *The Principles of Morals and Legislation* (Buffalo: Prometheus, 1988), p. 2.

21. J. S. Mill, *Utilitarianism,* in *Utilitarianism, On Liberty and Considerations on Representative Government,* ed. H. B. Acton, (London: Dent, 1972), p. 7.

22. "Pain must be reckoned as the negative quantity of pleasure, to be balanced against and subtracted from the positive in estimating happiness on the whole." Sidgwick, *Methods of Ethics,* p. 124.

23. Richard B. Brandt, *A Theory of the Good and the Right* (Oxford: Clarendon Press, 1979); and Katz, *Hedonism.*

24 Compare Sidgwick: "The term Pleasure is not commonly used so as to include clearly *all* kinds of consciousness which we desire to retain or reproduce: in ordinary usage it suggests too prominently the coarser and commoner kinds of such feelings." *Methods of Ethics,* p. 402.

may have lost some of their psychological effectiveness in his case, either through excessive repetition, or because of the pervasive feelings of gloom and despair that they do not quite succeed in dispelling. This person seeks in his pleasure a relief and a distraction from his despondency, but he is never able to banish it entirely. Of course, we do not want to make too much of this story. Many people who devote themselves to the pursuit of pleasure, even those who lead dissolute lives, are also very happy people, despite what our moralizing instincts may tell us.

"Pain," on the other hand, usually means "physical pain." It refers to a specific kind of disagreeable feeling that we locate in our body. Not all kinds of bodily suffering are called pain, however. There is a clear difference between pain on the one hand and physical discomfort and exhaustion on the other hand. A wide variety of physical sensations that cannot be described as painful can nevertheless become intensely unpleasant, even intolerable, as is well known to the victims of certain diseases, abused prisoners, and people made to perform hard and excruciating labor. In the words of one man suffering from chronic itching caused by a malignant skin disorder, "You jump up and scream and holler and you can beat your head against the wall, but when you do all that you're still itching, you're still miserable."[25]

Nor does physical pain cover the many mental kinds of suffering, such as fear, panic, terror, grief, depression, humiliation, loneliness, anxiety, dread. These states are often referred to as species of "mental pain." But physical pain is something sharply distinct, immediately recognizable, and rightly dreaded for its own sake; it deserves the separate attention of "pain specialists" in medicine and other fields. We should not lose sight of it by too readily expanding the sense of pain to cover all forms of distress, both bodily and mental.

Why do moral philosophers—and not only hedonistic ones—refer to suffering as pain? I think they do this because, for a variety of reasons, pain is a particularly useful model for suffering in all its forms. Everyone at one time or another has experienced it (children with particular frequency, since they have not yet learned to avoid hurtful injury). We recognize it instantly, and name it unerringly, when it strikes us. There are certain things known to cause it in virtually all people; and even when it has invisible or unlikely causes, we can recognize its occurrence in other people by characteristic cries, grimaces, and recoiling movements. In our own case we can specify with considerable precision when it comes and goes, when it grows more or less intense, and we are unlikely to confuse it with other bad things that may happen to us. There is also something unmistakably "real" about pain, which, when it is sufficiently intense, can make us forget all our other complaints.[26]

And then, more important, it seems to us that physical pain—at least beyond a certain level of intensity—is always accompanied by genuine distress. In Elaine

25. Quoted in Elisabeth Kübler-Ross, *On Death and Dying* (New York: MacMillan, 1969), p. 151.

26. The philosophical usage may also have its roots in the traditional translation of the Greek *lupé* by utilitarians and others as "pain," whereas in fact its original meaning approximated our everyday sense of "suffering." I am indebted to R. M. Hare for this observation.

Scarry's words, "The first, the most essential, aspect of pain is its sheer aversiveness."[27] Moreover, the intensification of pain commonly entails the intensification of suffering. Pain and suffering begin to appear synonymous.

However, they are not synonymous—not only because there are other sources and varieties of suffering besides physical pain, but also because, as it turns out, a person's degree of suffering does not always correspond directly to the intensity of his or her pain. Many factors that affect the perceived "meaning" of somebody's pain (or the perceived meaning of the situation of someone in pain) can magnify or mitigate that person's distress. These factors include whether or not a person believes that her pain will soon go away; whether the pain is interpreted as the sign of a terminal or life-threatening disease, permanent disability or disfigurement; whether the person is surrounded by friends who seek her well-being, or, on the contrary, by enemies who plan for her destruction; whether the pain is held up as an example of heroism and accomplishment, as it sometimes is in childbirth, or as the deserved punishment of great wickedness. It is speculated that one reason why pain is so peculiarly terrifying to small children is that they see in it a sign of impending annihilation.[28]

During torture all the signs point to destruction, and it is for this reason, among others, that torture appears to me to be the paradigmatic case of suffering. It is a total assault on the psyche. We should not underestimate the extent to which technical advances and deepening expertise have enabled torturers to inflict ever greater amounts of pain on their victims.[29] Nor should we forget that torture extends over long periods of time. As Scarry observes,

> Although a dentist's drill may in fact be the torturer's instrument, it will not land on a nerve for the eternity of a few seconds but for the eternity of the uncountable number of seconds that make up the period of torture, a period that may be seventeen hours on a single day or four hours a day on each of twenty-nine days.[30]

But there are other factors besides the intensity and duration of the pain that make torture uniquely horrible—worse, for instance, than the crippling pain that may result from accidental injury or disease. Torture victims know that their agony is not the result of some haphazard accident or biological breakdown, but the malevolent will of some person or group of people who *could have chosen* to spare their

27. Elaine Scarry, *The Body in Pain: The Making and Unmaking of the World* (Oxford: Oxford University Press, 1985), p. 52.

28. David Bakan, *Disease, Pain, and Sacrifice: Toward a Psychology of Suffering* (Chicago: University of Chicago Press, 1968), pp. 80–81. For an illuminating discussion of the relation of suffering to illness and pain, see Eric J. Cassell, *The Nature of Suffering and the Goals of Medicine* (New York: Oxford University Press, 1991). Cassell reports that the suffering occasioned by pain is greatest when people "feel out of control, when the pain is overwhelming, when the source of the pain is unknown, when the meaning of the pain is dire, or when the pain is apparently without end" (p. 36).

29. Edward Peters, *Torture* (New York: Basil Blackwell, 1985), pp. 161–76.

30. Scarry, *The Body in Pain*, p. 34.

pain but did not, and who *surely will* continue to supply them with fresh amounts of pain in the indefinite future. In torture, the victims are immersed in betrayal—not only from their own bodies, which become the vehicle of their agony, but also from the human presence that would ordinarily be counted on to assist in their rescue, and from the very human artifacts—a table, a bathtub, a telephone—that were originally intended for human comfort and protection but have become in the hands of their captors the instrument of their torment.[31] By the shouts and taunts of their guards, the punitive significance lent to the torture, and the invasive nature of the torture itself, victims are made to feel both humiliated and guilty. They fear the unknown damage being wrought on their bodies. Finally, in many countries they fear, correctly, that their torture will in all likelihood be followed by death—or mutilation leading to death.[32]

Thus intensity of pain is not perfectly correlated with intensity of suffering. This is most obviously true in the case of many minor pains, which adults can psychologically put aside without too much effort and are unattended by any suffering whatsoever. (On the other hand, similar pains might provoke real distress in children.) Some physical pains can even evoke psychological pleasure—as when sore muscles from strenuous exercise remind us that we are on the way to improved health, increased athletic prowess, and greater attractiveness. The most dramatic evidence that pain is distinct from suffering comes from the results of frontal lobotomies designed to alleviate chronic pain. After surgery patients report that they still feel pain but are somehow not bothered by it.[33]

---

31. Scarry describes this effect very well, ibid., pp. 38–45. She shows how torture exaggerates the cognitive alterations and disturbances wrought by pain in general. In severe pain we are deprived of the world. Our pain begins to occupy all our thoughts, and to the extent we remain conscious of any other reality, it seems to us disconnected, unintelligible, false, empty, absurd. The pain victim's disinheritance from the world is more pronounced during torture, when civilized artifacts, elements of a world shared in common, become the source of pain, and torture techniques are given the name of benign collective pastimes.

Other people have remarked on the world-obliterating quality of pain. One cancer patient quoted by Kübler-Ross bitterly complained about the reluctance of the hospital staff to administer pain-killing drugs. The staff feared that drugs would detach patients from reality, she said, but they forgot that severe pain had that effect anyway. *On Death and Dying*, pp. 65–66.

32. The failure to acknowledge the cumulative impact of all these factors on the feelings of the tortured prisoner is reflected in the ludicrous experiment of General Massu in Algeria to submit to the *gégêne*—the torture by field telephone practiced on a massive scale by his subordinates—in order "to see what it was like." Massu ignored "the key factor in torture: that apart from the pain and humiliation involved, its most frightful aspect lies in the uncertainty of its duration. General Massu knew that his sampling of the '*gégêne*' was a mere experiment, sandwiched in between a crowded daily programme, like an appointment with one's dentist. For those Algerians subjected to it in real life, the circumstances were entirely different: '*gégêne*' sessions could go on for hours, be interrupted for hours or days at a time, and be resumed at any moment." Edward Behr, *The Algerian Problem* (London: Hodder and Stoughton, 1961), p. 240.

33. Melzack and Wall, *Challenge of Pain*, p. 168: "When they are questioned more closely, they frequently say that they still have the 'little' pain, but the 'big' pain, the suffering, the anguish are gone."

I do not wish to imply that it is always easy to distinguish pain from attendant suffering. On the contrary, it can be very difficult. The perceived meaning of a pain situation, which can make a person mind his or her pain less, can also decrease the pain itself. Two studies of soldiers wounded in battle—U.S. soldiers on the Anzio beachhead in World War II and Israeli soldiers in the Yom Kippur War—found that the soldiers reported experiencing no pain at all in a much higher proportion than people who suffered similar injuries outside combat. The researchers concluded that the unexpected analgesic reaction of the soldiers was caused by the ironic significance of their wounds: they had emerged from combat alive, and they were going to a safe place far away from the battlefront to receive care.[34] Other psychological variables such as attention, anxiety, the memory of past experiences, and whether or not one feels control over one's pain have also been observed to affect pain intensity.[35] Physiologists of pain now believe that descending control systems from the brain, which can be affected by our cognitive evaluation of the situation we are in, help determine whether a given sensory input will give rise to pain, and of what intensity.[36]

We tend to think that physical pain is more definite, identifiable, and measurable than suffering is. And yet, when we examine the experiences of people in pain we often discover that it is easier to assess their level of aggregate suffering than it is to determine what amount of that suffering consists of pain. We are not sure, for example, whether a certain portion of someone's suffering is made up of pain or pain-related anxiety; yet we are sure that it is suffering, whatever else it might be. And there are some unusual forms of anguish that are subjectively perceived as physical pain, but fall outside our normal conception of it. Though we may hesitate

---

For a probing discussion of these lobotomies and their implications for our understanding of the concept of pain, see Roger Trigg, *Pain and Emotion* (Oxford: Clarendon Press, 1970), chap. 7.

34. Melzack and Wall, *Challenge of Pain*, pp. 35–36. The U.S. soldiers "were not in a state of shock, nor were they totally unable to feel pain, for they complained as vigorously as normal men at an inept vein puncture." (p. 35) The two studies appear in H. K. Beecher, *Measurement of Subjective Responses* (New York: Oxford University Press, 1959); and P. L. Carlen, P. D. Wall, H. Nadvorna, and T. Steinbach, "Phantom Limbs and Related Phenomena in Recent Traumatic Amputations, *Neurology*, 28 (1978): 211–17.

35. Melzack and Wall, *Challenge of Pain*, chap. 2.

36. Ibid., chap. 7. "There is evidence that the sensory input is localized, identified in terms of its physical properties, evaluated in terms of past experience, and modified *before* it activates the discriminative or motivational systems" (p. 167). The observation that psychological processes affect pain perception has been incorporated into Melzack's and Wall's gate-control theory of pain: "The gate-control theory also suggests that psychological processes such as past experience, attention, and emotion may influence pain perception and response by acting on the spinal gating mechanism. Some of these psychological activities may open the gate while others may close it. A woman who one day discovers a lump in her breast, and is worried that it may be cancerous, may suddenly feel pain in the breast. If anxiety is prolonged, the pain may increase in severity and even spread to the shoulder and arm. Later, the mere verbal assurance from her doctor that the lump is of no consequence usually produces sudden, total relief of pain" (p. 247).

whether to call them pain, we have no doubt that they qualify as suffering. Witness the ordeals described by Oliver Sacks in his post-encephalitic Parkinsonian patients:

> Miss R.'s capacity to speak or move, minimal at the best of times, would disappear almost entirely during her severer [oculogyric] crises, although in her greatest extremity she would sometimes call out, in a strange high-pitched voice, perseverative, and palilalic, utterly unlike her husky "normal" whisper: "Doctor, doctor, doctor, doctor . . . help me, help, help, h'lp, h'lp . . . I am in terrible pain, I'm so frightened . . . I'm going to die, I know it, I know it, I know it, I know it . . ." And at other times, if nobody was near, she would whimper softly to herself, like some small animal caught in a trap. The nature of Miss R.'s pain during her crises was only elucidated later, when speech had become easy: some of it was a local pain associated with extreme opisthotonos, but a large component seemed to be central—diffuse, unlocalizable, of a sudden onset and offset, and inseparably coalesced with feelings of dread and threat, in the severest crises a true *angor animi*. During exceptionally severe attacks, Miss R.'s face would become flushed, her eyes reddened and protruding, and she would repeat, "It'll kill me, it'll kill me, it'll kill me . . ." hundreds of times in succession. . . .
>
> In the early years of her illness, Miss H. used to suffer from sudden paroxysms of left-sided pain, associated with anguish and terror, of sudden onset and offset, and lasting some hours; when I asked her about these, many years later, she answered (as she was fond of doing) by a Dickensian example: "You keep asking me," she said, "about the *location* of the pain, and the only answer I can give is that which Mrs. Gradgrind gave: 'I used to feel there was a pain *somewhere in the room*, but I couldn't positively say that I had got it.' "[37]

It should be noticed that there is a latent ambiguity in the word *pain*, such that we are not sure if a "pain sensation" is pain in the true sense of the word if the person experiencing it truly does not mind it or is able to put it out of his mind. Imagine, for example, a hockey player who forgets a painful injury in the excitement of the game. R. M. Hare in an illuminating article has discriminated between two common differing uses of the word *pain:* uses "which refer to the bare sensation, without implying dislike" and uses "which refer to this same sensation, but in addition imply dislike, so that they cannot be had when the sensation is had but not disliked."[38]

We usually say of a pain that *it* feels bad; but we are unsure whether to declare someone to be in pain when his consciousness of *it* is blocked out, partially or in full, by other thoughts, emotions, and sensations strong enough to compete for his attention. But in applying the word *suffering* we have no such hesitation. Suffering just means that *the person* feels bad. And in determining whether someone is suffering, we take a composite reading of all the different sensations, thoughts, emotions

37. Oliver Sacks, *Awakenings* (New York: E. P. Dutton, 1983), pp. 71, 119. See also the discussion of Rachel I., pp. 175–76.

38. R. M. Hare, "Pain and Evil," in Joel Feinberg, ed., *Moral Concepts* (Oxford: Oxford University Press, 1969), p. 32. Trigg reports: "In experiments to measure the threshold of pain, the subjects say that they recognize a sensation as pain and later come to dislike what they say is the same sensation." *Pain and Emotion*, p. 32.

now occupying his mind in order to determine how, on balance, he is feeling. I do not want to exaggerate the independence of suffering vis-à-vis pain. Pain above a certain level of intensity and duration has a way of asserting itself in our consciousness such that it causes even the most stoical among us to suffer. I merely wish to assert that there is some degree of indeterminacy, some "give"—usually small, but occasionally large—in the variation of intensity of suffering with respect to the intensity of pain.

6. Describing Our Lives in Terms of Happiness and Suffering

I propose that all conscious experience can be classified as belonging to happiness, or suffering, or something in between. We may think of a one-dimensional scale with increasing happiness pointing in one direction and increasing suffering pointing in another direction, separated by an intermediate zone that includes feeling neither good nor bad overall and the kind of slightly disagreeable feeling that falls short of suffering. At any moment of a person's conscious life, the quality of his or her overall feeling can be located, in principle, somewhere on the scale.

The location may not be a precise point. As we shall see in our discussion of cardinal intensity, it may be claimed that a person's degree of happiness or suffering may be, even in reality, imprecise. One consequence of this view is that if two people are suffering, and neither suffers more intensely than the other, we cannot assume that the intensity of their suffering is exactly equal. It may be the case that the intensity of the first person's suffering is neither greater than, nor less than, nor equal to, the intensity of the second person's suffering. Yet even in this case a rough cardinal comparison may be possible. We may judge, for example, that in comparison to the second person's suffering, the first person's suffering is somewhere between 30 percent less intense and 50 percent more intense.[39]

The claim that all conscious experience can be located somewhere on the happiness-suffering continuum (which includes a kind of overall feeling intermediate between happiness and suffering) reflects a fairly common way of thinking. Nevertheless, it may encounter several challenges. One is that it utterly fails to capture the content of many important moods and feelings, such as arduous effort, the thrill of danger, nervous anticipation, and rage. This is very true, and importantly so. Happiness-suffering is only one, and often not a very salient, dimension of feeling—especially when, as I think is true in a very large number of cases, people live out the bulk of their lives in a range close to the level of neutral feeling: they may experience stretches of mild, but bearable, unhappiness, and mild contentment, as well as a feeling that is intermediate between happiness and suffering; but they rarely experience intense happiness or acute suffering.

39. I am helped by Thomas Hurka, *Perfectionism* (New York: Oxford University Press, 1993), p. 87.

Certain strong emotions may arise unaccompanied either by happiness or suffering, even though they may carry a great deal of turbulence. When a bad event happens in our lives, for example, we sometimes experience an exaltation of anger or self-pity, an unprecedented pitch of feeling. Our passion seizes possession of us—shakes us with the force of its own intensity, to leave us in the end trembling in exhaustion, drained and disoriented. Yet often in these situations there is no genuine suffering, or only slight suffering, which on a casual survey is easily exaggerated. (Remember that the fact that someone is neither happy nor suffering does not pose a problem for our theory, since we have explicitly allowed for such a category.)

Just as strong emotions can occur in the absence of either suffering or happiness, so extreme suffering may exist unaccompanied by any identifiable emotion, unless suffering itself is called an emotion. Profound apathy and indifference, which we would normally conceive as a lack of emotion, is one of the classic symptoms of depression. Yet as one expert on depression has observed, "Perhaps one of the most important things about the depressed person is that though he appears dull he is clearly in considerable pain. He is not bland or flat, rather he is suffering."[40]

Even when people are very happy or very unhappy, other feelings may be prominent. But I am not denying that different happy experiences (or experiences of suffering) can be very dissimilar. Nor do I wish to imply that happiness–suffering is always the most interesting or most important dimension of feeling. Often it is not: information about it may be comparatively useless to clinical psychologists, for example. I am only claiming that a number of experiences so widely divergent in so many decisive ways may nevertheless have one thing in common: that in addition to all the other crucial things we may note about them we can also observe that they are happy experiences (or experiences of suffering). I distinguish this dimension because I think it has special significance for morality.

There is another challenge to the view that all conscious experience may be described in terms of a single dimension of happiness and suffering: namely, the idea that we can be happy and suffering at the same time. Cheri Register, writing of her own and others' experience with chronic illness, says that despite the unusually cruel burden placed on people like her, they may learn in time how to be "miserable *and* very happy."[41] Register speaks from hard-earned experience, and what she says is undoubtedly true. But it does not mean, I think, that a person in her situation can be happy and suffering, in our sense of the words, at the same time. It means, to speak only of her case, that although she is continually reminded of the terrible unfairness and unrelenting hardship of her condition, she can nevertheless draw satisfaction, when she is not stricken by pain, from all that she has

40. Winokur, *Depression: The Facts*, p. 5. Compare the following observation about a woman with a history of depression: "Before Prozac, she suffered five episodes of major depression, during which she could hardly drag herself off her couch or feel enough to realize she was miserable." "Drug Works, but Questions Remain," *New York Times*, 15 December 1993.

41. Cheri Register, *Living with Chronic Illness: Days of Patience and Passion* (New York: Bantam, 1987), p. 254.

achieved in spite of her illness and from the meaning she has found, with the help of religion, in her life and in her very affliction. She can be simultaneously conscious of the very good things and the very bad things in her life; and the thought of all she has endured, the wisdom she has gained from her illness, and the strong and lasting emotions or "passions" that she among a few has experienced, often leaves her deeply moved, and spares her some of her recurrent depressions and periods of angry frustration. Of course, none of this means that she has cured herself of suffering. When she has an attack of severe pain, she undergoes extreme suffering; and when she is visited by the panic attacks, episodes of melancholic self-pity, and abject depressions that are the emotional spin-offs of her illness, she suffers as well. At these times she is *not* happy. What she means by saying that she can be "miserable *and* very happy" is that she can often think about her illness and still count herself blessed. At such moments of reflection, she may, as I noted, feel deeply moved. The happiness–suffering scale does not record the presence of such strong emotions, which may nevertheless appear to us as being of the very greatest significance. On some of these occasions she may be neither happy nor suffering, literally speaking. On others, she may be mildly happy; and often, in her transport, she may attain a state of joy, which we record somewhere in the range of moderate to extreme happiness.

But may not someone feel happy and unhappy at the very same time? I admit that one can be conscious of good and bad things simultaneously, and even that pleasures and pains, understood in a certain way, may be concurrent. There are any number of experiences that are highly bewildering to us because of the contradictory emotions they contain. I suspect some experiences of childbirth—where intense physical pain is mixed with a feeling of excitement and immense achievement—are like this. Or I may be suffering great physical pain, while savoring the attention of someone I love. Still, introspection tells me that despite the confusion of mixed and contradictory elements, I can nevertheless detect an overall *value* of what I am feeling, a value that takes into account the contrasting impressions that are salient in my consciousness, and that enables me to classify the overall feeling as belonging to happiness, suffering, or something in between. Although certain moments of experience are highly complex, and may join together pleasure and pain, I believe we can still take a reading of the quality of the experience as a whole—where such a reading represents something real about the experience (truly felt), not artificially imposed.

Another challenge to the conception being presented here is the view that happiness–suffering consists not of one dimension, but two. Mill famously asserted that pleasures could be distinguished on the basis of quality as well as quantity. I agree with those commentators who assert that Mill's "quality of pleasure" refers to a dimension outside pleasure itself. According to Mill, one pleasure is of higher quality than another, or "more valuable," if someone who had knowledge of both *would prefer* to experience the former even though the latter exceeded it in the quantity of pleasure felt. But it is clear from Mill's discussion that this preference will be, and ought to be, made on the basis of considerations extrinsic to the quality of the feeling itself: considerations such as what kind of beings we want to be, what kind or traits we want to have, and what kind of faculties we want to develop:

> Few human creatures would consent to be changed into any of the lower animals for a promise of the fullest allowance of a beast's pleasures; no intelligent human being would consent to be a fool, no instructed person would be an ignoramus, no person of feeling and conscience would be selfish and base, even though they should be persuaded that the fool, the dunce, or the rascal is better satisfied with his lot than they are with theirs. They would not resign what they possess more than he for the most complete satisfaction of all the desires which they have in common with him. If they ever fancy they would, it is only in cases of unhappiness so extreme that to escape from it they would exchange their lot for almost any other, however undesirable in their own eyes. A being of higher faculties requires more to make him happy, is capable probably of more acute suffering, and certainly accessible to it at more points, than one of an inferior type; but in spite of these liabilities, he can never really wish to sink into what he feels to be a lower grade of existence.[42]

A good gloss on the meaning of Mill's "higher pleasures" is provided by James Griffin.[43] Griffin has shown that we sometimes step back from the usual interplay of habits and impulses that shape our behavior, and by evaluating our given desires, we form basic preferences about how to live our lives. These preferences are very often determined not by what will give us the greatest amount of pleasure, but simply by what kind of people we want to be and what kind of things we want to do. Recall the example of Freud who preferred to think clearly in torment than to be comfortably confused.[44] Neither Mill nor Griffin is exclusively concerned with the internal state of our feelings; they clearly think other things are important.

As a professed utilitarian with strong Aristotelian sympathies, Mill was under pressure to expand his conception of pleasure. He maintained verbal consistency with utilitarianism by stretching the concept of pleasure implausibly wide. The introduction of a second dimension of pleasure is symptomatic of the strain.[45]

I shall add a few remarks about the way in which happiness and suffering are patterned in our lives. I believe, from introspection, that we often experience happiness and suffering in time segments of more or less unvarying intensity, which give way to each other in rapid, almost instantaneous transitions. I have often noticed this in regard to my affective reaction to bad things that have just happened to me. The onset of a pain or a major physical discomfort can often be one of continuous (even if also rapid) increase, but my affective response may lag behind the increase of pain or discomfort and catch up to it by little jolts that are expressed by thoughts

42. Mill, *Utilitarianism*, p. 9.
43. Griffin, *Well-being*, p. 8.
44. But how clearly can we think when we are in great pain?
45. For a contrary interpretation of Mill, see Rem B. Edwards, *Pleasures and Pains: A Theory of Qualitative Hedonism* (Ithaca, N.Y.: Cornell University Press, 1979).

like "My God!" or "No! I can't bear it!" And there are other examples, some of which have to do with our thought processes in general. Say one feels a pain that, though not strictly unbearable, is of sufficient intensity to make one fairly miserable most of the time; one may attempt to take one's mind off the pain and thereby suppress one's miserable feeling by undertaking an activity requiring great mental concentration. But sometimes the pain reasserts itself in one's mind; the efforts at mental distraction come to naught, and the suppressed misery floods back. Here, too, there is no gentle transition, but a sudden shift in affect.

Encounters with severe physical pain can give rise to quickly succeeding shifts in one's level of happiness or suffering—frequent and dramatic alternations between anguish and relief, or frequent modulations in the intensity of one's suffering. Other events may have similarly spectacular and spasmodic effects on our happiness level. But life is not normally like that. Most people in possession of good health and a decent standard of living and not buffeted by misfortune lead a pretty steady affective life that can be characterized by long periods of mild happiness and mild suffering or neutral feeling.[46] Such a life is, under favorable conditions, the usual reward of adulthood. Children, even when they are well looked after, fall easily into moments of intense suffering and unconsolability. But adults generally learn how to bear and cope with and even ignore the kinds of afflictions—pains, physical discomforts, frustrations, setbacks—that to children can be ominous, terrifying, cruelly insulting, and irremediable.

What about uniform descriptions applied to long periods of times, as when we say, "That summer in the country I was very happy"? Such statements, though useful, tend to be simplifications. It is highly improbable, to say the least, that one's happiness level would not vary at all for such a long stretch of time. Perhaps I was habitually cheerful, felt good about myself, was optimistic about the future, and had plenty to amuse and entertain myself. But one day I was depressed when the bad weather spoiled our plans for an outing I had keenly anticipated, and on another day I burned my finger. "I was very happy that summer" likely means, "I was at least reasonably happy *most* of the time, and I felt *very* happy for longer and more frequent stretches than any time before or since." But to say, "I was happy that summer" by no means carries the implication that on the day in the middle of the happy summer when I felt quite depressed, I was not, in fact, suffering but was happy after all.

We make such simplifications not only to save time and avoid tedium to the people we are speaking to, but also because our memory often plays tricks on us. It tends to cast a haze over long stretches of our past lives and assimilate oscillating

---

46. In Sidgwick's opinion, "So long as health is retained, and pain and irksome toil banished, the mere performance of the ordinary habitual functions of life is, according to my experience, a frequent source of moderate pleasure, alternating rapidly with states nearly or quite indifferent." *Methods of Ethics*, p. 125. Sidgwick may be too optimistic. I suspect that, even in the absence of adverse external conditions or dramatic mental illness, a great many people persist at a level a little ways below the level of neutral feeling.

kinds of feeling into a uniform level of happiness. It is important to recognize the dangers inherent in such simplifications, for we are apt to be all too disloyal to moments in the past when we were very unhappy. Moments of suffering or intense suffering do not cease to be such by virtue of the fact that they are very short, either relatively or absolutely. We sometimes experience physical pains such as slight burns that are intensely unpleasant but are gone in an instant, before we even have time to think about them. Though they last a very short time—sometimes literally a fraction of a second—they are horrible while they last.

Some intense pains take longer to go away: say we get our fingers caught in a closing door. Though it would seem harder, we make a similar effort to consign the experience to oblivion. It hurts; it is unbearable. We devote tremendous psychic energy into forcing, wishing the pain to go away. Then as the pain recedes, and is pushed back by a wave of relief, we begin to feel all right again, and our thoughts make the subtle transition from "Go away, go away" to "It is over, it is over." Now we use our surplus mental energy to carry the process further, and we *do* with a vengeance what we could only desperately *think* before: we put the pain definitively away; we cover it up in oblivion; and we say with triumph, "It is gone!" We avoid the thought, "Well, now I'm a little sore, but—do you know?—just a moment ago it hurt much, much more than it does now; in fact, it hurt so much I couldn't bear it." And so, farther down the road in our distant memory, we are unlikely to recall the pain easily.

There is another way in which we simplify our past record of happiness and suffering. If during a certain period of time our happiness (or suffering) modulated within a certain relatively narrow range, we tend to think that our happiness level remained constant. This kind of simplification poses fewer dangers, I think, because the narrow oscillation that our description leaves out is unlikely to have major moral significance.

7. Happiness and Suffering as Absolute, Not Relative, Terms

Some people might raise the following challenge to the proposal that a person's life can be mapped out in terms of the different levels of happiness and suffering, or absence of either, which a person feels at different times. Happiness and suffering, it will be urged, are not absolute, but relative terms. We use them only in reference to, and in contrast with, each other. And the contrast is always rough and improvised, drawn up from the myopic universe of our ever-receding memory; it does not refer to fixed, determinate, measurable qualities intrinsic to these two things. I wake up, cured of a long, disagreeable illness, and announce, "I'm so happy that I'm better." I say and think I'm happy only because I feel better than when I was in the throes of my fever. But *this* happiness does not measure up to what I knew and felt to be "happiness" in the days before my illness, when I took my good health for granted.

Plato accuses the common run of people of such a sloppy use of the concept of pleasure, or happiness. They mistake the recovery of good health as an occasion of great pleasure, when in fact it only signifies a release from the pain of illness. And they interpret the withdrawal of something pleasant as painful, when in fact it brings nothing more than the cessation of pleasure. In both cases, they have arrived at a feeling of neutrality intermediate between pain and pleasure, but since they define their present state by contrast with the preceding one, they invent for themselves an illusory state of pleasure or pain. They

> have wrong ideas about pleasure and pain and the intermediate state; so that when they are only being drawn towards the painful they feel pain and think the pain which they experience to be real; and in like manner, when drawn away from pain to the neutral or intermediate state, they firmly believe that they have reached the goal of satiety and pleasure; they, not knowing pleasure, err in contrasting pain with the absence of pain, which is like contrasting black with grey instead of white. . . . [Their pleasures] are mere shadows and pictures of the true, and are coloured by contrast which exaggerates both light and shade.[47]

Plato, of course, believes that such sorry confusion can be avoided by a fortunate minority in possession of wisdom and virtue. The pleasures of true knowledge are more intense than any other kind, and they are wholly sufficient in themselves— they do not depend on preceding pains. Thus a wise person, who is familiar with true pleasures as well as illusory ones, intense ones as well as faint ones, has the requisite experience to measure all pains and pleasures correctly. He is not like ignorant people who, "always busy with gluttony and sensuality, go down and up again as far as the mean."[48] Acquainted with the higher pleasures, but also familiar with the "necessary" pleasures (and presumably pains) of common people, he comprehends the whole range of pains and pleasures, and hence can describe human experience accurately in terms of them.

Many readers will refuse to adopt Plato's belief that there is a natural elite that by its vastly superior wisdom and virtue can be neatly distinguished from the bulk of humanity—still less will they believe that a wise few move in a realm of intellectual pleasures the intensity and purity of which are simply unimaginable to the rest of us, and which show our most highly esteemed pleasures to be paltry and insignificant. But such readers may nevertheless be struck by Plato's description of the relativity inherent in ordinary references to pleasure and pain. Rather than suppose that such relativity can be avoided by members of an intellectual elite, they will conclude that it is entirely inescapable.

On this view, our use of the words *happiness* and *suffering*—or pleasure and pain—to describe how we feel at any given time always depends on the contrast with how we felt before, or how we remember having felt, or how we expected to feel. They are fluid concepts that are continually being redefined as we travel be-

---

47. *The Republic*, trans. B. Jowett (New York: Modern Library, 1982), 584e–85a, 586b.
48. Ibid., 586a.

tween fortune and misfortune. "I am happy today" means in effect that I am much improved from how I felt yesterday. But my happiness today is not and cannot be determined by some timeless and universal standard of happiness not rooted in my recollection of my past experiences and my expectations for the future.

I think this view is wrong. Our sense of what it is to be happy and suffering in various degrees of intensity is fairly exact and unvarying. It is not contingent on recent experience. We can tell the difference between a period of suffering that gives way to a neutral state and one that gives way to euphoria. There is a difference between quiet relief and blissful release. Similarly, we know very well when happiness is succeeded by its opposite, depression, and when it is replaced by a return to a feeling of sober normality. And we can distinguish different intensities of our sufferings competently, not by inquiring into their relation to feelings before and after, but simply into *how it felt at the time*. Recollecting our own past illnesses, for instance, we might note that a high fever, though intolerable, was somehow more bearable than a prolonged bout of severe abdominal pain—and we could be confident of this conclusion even though the two experiences were separated by a long period of time, filled with joys and hardships of various kinds.

Of course there is truth in the idea that happiness and suffering are relative to each other. But the truth is not that their very meanings depend on their mutual contrast, but rather that each of these things, or the memory of it, can be the *cause* of its opposite. Plato is clearly wrong if he implies that the mere restoration of health can never signify the occurrence of pleasure (happiness), but only release from pain. The mere consciousness that we have come through a great ordeal such as illness and that it is entirely past us is often the cause of great joy. And then, sometimes it is not: we are of course relieved, but not particularly happy. The fact that we can recognize the difference shows that different intensities of suffering and happiness can be identified on the basis of intrinsic and not merely comparative data.[49]

We can sometimes observe a genuine psychological "pendulum effect," such that the very "force" of extreme suffering seems to intensify the happiness that follows it, and vice versa. Despite what Plato says, there is nothing illusory about these cases. Cheri Register says that in the early days of suffering from a rare affliction of the liver known as Caroli's Disease, before she kept analgesic drugs close at hand, her bouts with extreme pain were followed by a euphoria so intense that she never envied the ecstasies reported by users of hallucinogenic drugs. She could not

> imagine a greater euphoria than that which comes with release from pain. The smile on my face when the pain subsides is not a mask I wear for others, but an expression of supreme joy. Euphoria brings everything around me into sharper focus. I'm back and the world is wonderful.[50]

49. There are more obvious instances of where the mere removal of a painful thing causes genuine happiness, as when we learn that some previous bad news—the diagnosis of terminal illness, or the death of a loved one—is actually false.

50. Register, *Living with Chronic Illness*, p. 231.

On the other hand, it has been observed among manic depressives that periods of manic elation and excitement often swing directly into deep depression. These depressions, even when they last no more than a few minutes, carry the risk of suicide.[51] There is growing evidence that the primary cause of most severe manic depressive cycles is a chemical imbalance in the brain. Nevertheless, we may speculate that the very sequence, mania–depression, makes the depression that follows mania harder to bear. A person who until a moment ago was possessed of absolute confidence and optimism will be singularly unprepared for, and bewildered by, his new feelings of incapacity, worthlessness, and despair. And since we know that mania is typically accompanied by bloated self-esteem, and depression by intense self-depreciation, a depressed person is likely to be overcome with self-disgust when he contemplates his former grandiosity, and his opinion of his own worthlessness is likely to be reinforced by the thought of how wildly he had overestimated himself before.

So we can oscillate between suffering and happiness, and indeed the more extreme versions of these states, where the meaning of these words is not simply relative. But we can also alternate between different degrees of suffering, without it being true that we have reached happiness. Sometimes we are conscious of a diminution in our suffering, and yet perceive very clearly that we are still suffering—that we have not yet arrived at the state intermediate between suffering and happiness, much less happiness itself. A prisoner when her torture is suspended may be left in a state of considerable pain, severe discomfort, and exhaustion. Or she may have fallen unconscious, to awake later in her cell, disoriented, painfully sore, trembling with cold, and feeling despair. She clearly knows that the agony of torture would be worse than what she is experiencing now, but the thought of her relative "good" fortune is not enough to compensate for her continuing wretchedness so as to make her happy.

There are many people who move between more and less extreme levels of suffering without ever, or scarcely ever, rising (or bouncing) to the level of happiness. This is, I think, typically true of prisoners singled out for systematically cruel treatment, such as that found in concentration camps and clandestine jails. I think it is true in general for all people who find themselves in the total power of those who intend them grave harm: victims of sadistic kidnappings, for instance, and severely battered children. I suspect it is true also of people who undergo long and severe episodes of clinical depression, people suffering the ravages of a violent illness, and people perpetually burdened by feelings of humiliation and low self-esteem.

The relativist account has such a hold on our minds that it appears to have given rise to some comforting myths about suffering. Or the causation may be the other way around: because we are so loath to contemplate the existence of severe and lasting suffering, we are inclined to grasp at the relativist account to show that it is not possible. We are often tempted to think that people can get used to their suf-

---

51. Winokur, *Depression: The Facts*, p. 68; and Fieve, *Moodswing*, pp. 56–57.

fering, can learn to bear it. This, I think, is speaking inexactly. What we mean is that people can learn to adapt to hardship, even pain, so that the suffering they feel as a result of it diminishes over time and sometimes fades away entirely. As a matter of observation, this sometimes happens, but sometimes does not. But underneath the claim lies the thought, whether or not it is uttered explicitly, that suffering simply *can't* go on indefinitely, that, by the nature of things, relief *must* come. Now and then we are confronted by an account of someone else's ordeal, and we seek to impress the reality of it on our consciousness. But at some point the suggestion seeps into our minds that the person's suffering surely isn't all that bad, that it surely will not last. After all, we will inevitably go on to something else—to another task, to a meal, and, eventually, to sleep. Surely the person in torment will also take a rest, won't he?

If we enjoy moderately good health and live in a reasonably supportive environment, our energies and strengths are continually being replenished by the restorative processes of our bodies; by the help, praise, encouragement, and courtesy of people we know and meet; and by the innumerable objects of interest and entertainment around us. We may encounter serious blows and setbacks, but even during the worst of these, we know, at some deeper level, that our forgotten sources of support will back us up sooner or later; and if we say the opposite, it is often with the intention and expectation of being contradicted. We are less than fully aware of this steady infusion of support, yet we count on it instinctively, and we slip into the unconscious assumption that it is there for everybody. We see the world through the distorting lens of our good fortune, the reserves of strength that keep us buoyed up; unconscious of the lens, we do not realize that our vision is distorted. It is extremely difficult for us to conceive that someone can be abruptly and decisively let down, that he will be lowered into a state of suffering and left there, without a natural rebound or automatic equilibration.[52]

52. Our unconscious assumption of ever-flowing support explains why the nature of total adversity is always a surprise to us when we experience it ourselves. Jean Améry, seized by the Nazis for his work in the Belgian resistance, describes how all his previous efforts to imagine imprisonment and torture could not prepare him for the first blow delivered by the Gestapo and all that it signified: "The first blow brings home to the prisoner that he is *helpless,* and thus it already contains in the bud everything to come. One may have known about torture and death in the cell, without such knowledge having possessed the hue of life; but upon the first blow they are anticipated as real possibilities, yes, as certainties. They are permitted to punch me in the face, the victim feels in numb surprise and concludes in just as numb certainty: they will do with me what they want. Whoever would rush to the prisoner's aid—a wife, a mother, a brother, a friend—he won't get this far. . . . I don't know if the person who is beaten by the police loses human dignity. Yet I am certain that with the very first blow that descends on him he loses something we will perhaps temporarily call 'trust in the world' . . . the certainty that by reason of written or unwritten social contracts the other person will spare me—more precisely stated, that he will respect my physical, and with it also my metaphysical, being. . . . The expectation of help, the certainty of help, is indeed one of the fundamental experiences of human beings, and probably also of animals. . . . In almost all situations in life where there is bodily injury there is also the expectation of help; the former is compensated by the latter. But with the first blow from a policeman's fist, against which there can be no defense and which no helping hand will ward off, a part of our life ends and it can never again be revived." Jean Améry, *At the Mind's Limits: Contemplations by a Survivor on Auschwitz*

Yet plenty of people *do* remain submerged in suffering that does not gradually diminish. As marathon torture sessions wear on, the victims do not grow accustomed or indifferent to their pain. Even when suffering is recurrent, not continuous, it may retain the same intensity over time. Oliver Sacks describes the countless oculogyric crises of one of his post-encephalitic patients:

> In her oculogyric crises, which tended to come weekly, and to last for twenty-four hours, her face would bear a peculiar look of consternation and horror, she was never able to say what *constituted* or *caused* these feelings, and could only say, "It's pure horror, it's completely past bearing." When I asked her whether she did not get *used* to these feelings, she said, "No, never, not in the least. I have had these attacks for forty-five years now, and *each one is the worst I've had.*"[53]

Similarly, people with chronic illness stress that their recurring attacks of pain do not become more tolerable with time:

> The word "acceptance" is widely used to denote an optimistic attitude toward illness that gets past the initial horror of it and enables you to proceed with life. No matter how philosophical you are, however, pain is never really "acceptable." . . . As I know it, severe pain is isolating and totally absorbing. I can't do anything but hurt. I simply have not learned how to "accept" these awful experiences. They undo me every time.[54]

8. The Variable Intensity of Suffering

I have assumed throughout that suffering may occur at any of several levels of intensity. This is most widely recognized in the case of suffering caused by pain. Patients with chronic pain and their doctors agree that pain itself varies by intensity; they have words to distinguish the intensity of different episodes of pain, and these words also bespeak the level of suffering they feel. These are words such as *mild, annoying, discomforting, troublesome, miserable, distressing, intense, horrible, unbearable,* and *excruciating.* Two pain researchers, R. Melzack and W. S. Torgerson, asked respondents to give number values for the intensity of pain signified by each of the evaluative words listed above. The results enabled them to rank the words in order of increasing severity, as I have done here. Melzack and Torgerson also discovered that five of the words spanning the whole range were so evenly spread apart that they could form the basis of a new pain intensity scale. The five words were *mild, discomforting, distressing, horrible,* and *excruciating.* These words recognizably refer to the intensity of suffering, not just pain.[55]

---

and Its Realities, trans. Sidney Rosenfeld and Stella P. Rosenfeld (Bloomington: Indiana University Press, 1980), pp. 27–29.

53. Sacks, *Awakenings,* p. 300, n. 11.

54. Register, *Living with Chronic Illness,* pp. 180–81.

55. The original study is R. Melzack and W. S. Torgerson, "On the Language of Pain," *Anesthesiology,* 34 (1971): 50–59. It is discussed in Melzack and Wall, *Challenge of Pain,* pp. 56–69.

Melzack and Torgerson also studied the use of words that describe the sensory, not evaluative, qualities of pain. They rated the quantity of pain normally associated with these descriptive words by asking respondents to assign them pain-intensity number values. Words of this kind include *pulsing, throbbing, drilling, stabbing, cutting, cramping,* and *wrenching.* Melzack and Torgerson discovered that within certain categories of descriptive words linked by a common sensory dimension—temporal, spatial, thermal, punctate pressure, incisive pressure, etc.—there was a high degree of uniformity among correspondents regarding the relative intensity of pain associated with different descriptive words. For example, in the category of words that refer to the spatial dimension of pain, most people reported that "shooting" pain was worse than "flashing" pain, which was itself worse than "jumping" pain.

That there are different intensities of pain is well known to the layperson. Many of us have experienced the difference between a cruel debilitating pain and a terrifyingly unbearable one. Cancer pain is known in some cases to become so intolerable that patients, previously known to be happy and stable, are determined to end it by taking their lives.[56] A large increase in pain usually involves a large increase in suffering, though there are exceptions as we saw in section 5.

Suffering varies in intensity not only when it takes the shape of pain, but also when it assumes more purely psychological forms. For some people, this may be difficult to verify by introspection. I have in mind fortunate people who are emotionally stable, have been reasonably successful in their careers, have a solid sense of who they are, and can plan for the future with confidence that their plans will to some extent be realized. Many people in this class persist for the most part within the range between neutral feeling and mild to moderate happiness. Their lives sail along reasonably well. They may encounter frustration, disappointment, and cruel antagonism. But these setbacks, despite the turmoil that may attend them, will not always precipitate them into a state of suffering, and many people in this class who say they do are not reflecting carefully. Sometimes, if their luck has been particularly hard, they may be forced to wade through a period of genuine suffering. Such episodes will be most bitterly resented; they were not what the person had counted on; they seem decidedly unfair. But despite their surprising, insolent character, these episodes are generally, I would insist, of a uniformly mild intensity. One should be careful that one's extreme bitterness does not lead one to interpret these episodes of suffering as being more intense than they are. We are apt to become spoiled and to expect a minimum level of happiness as our due. When made to suffer, we may rail at the injustice of our condition and hence forget that our suffering is actually of a quite mild kind, certainly less severe than the torment and distress that other people must endure.

It is true that the relatively blessed existence of fortunate people can be broken— by disease, by the news of one's imminent death, by the imposition of a particularly

---

56. According to Melzack and Wall, it is rivaled by severe back pain and the pain sometimes present in phantom limb; and all three are exceeded by the average intensity of labor pain: *Challenge of Pain,* pp. 66–67.

harsh burden, by the breakup of a marriage or love affair, or by the death of a loved one.[57] (But, of course, here, too, we must beware of exaggeration. In the last case the internal suffering may be rather less than what is professed. Sometimes, to be sure, it is not.) In such cases, the person may experience a different, more intense kind of psychological suffering than what he or she had known before.

I believe that the experience of these people is to be contrasted sharply with that of people who suffer from chronically low self-esteem and lack hope for the future. Their existence may be one of more or less continuous despondency, during which they remain at a level of mild suffering, punctuated by moments of humiliation and despair, when their suffering becomes more acute.

Some of the best evidence of the variable depth of psychological suffering comes in the testimony of people afflicted with clinical depression, and from the doctors who observe and treat them. Their descriptions of this condition indicate a magnitude of pain wholly different from the typical unhappiness of other people:

If there be a hell upon earth, it is to be found in a melancholy man's heart.[58]

I am now the most miserable man living. If what I feel were equally distributed to the whole human family, there would not be one cheerful face on earth. Whether I shall ever be better, I cannot tell; I awfully forebode I shall not. To remain as I am is impossible. I must die or be better, it appears to me.[59]

I have seen six psychiatrists over the last ten years, and my depression continues chronically without any interruption. Nothing has made it any better—none of the eight drugs I've tried, new and old, none of the psychotherapy, not even shock treatments. This must be what living in hell is like. . . . This illness called depression is not as obvious to an outsider as the sad, disfigured one of an amputated arm or leg, or blindness, or total paralysis from polio. To the person with it, it is a greater torture than solitary confinement for an eternity.[60]

Fifteen percent of the people who suffer depression die by committing suicide, as compared to 1 percent of the general population.[61] It seems likely that relief from pain is one of the motives, though not necessarily a conscious one, that lead depressives to seek death in such high numbers. (Similarly high suicide rates occur among schizophrenics and people with panic disorder.)[62]

57. Mill identified the chief dangers as "indigence, disease, and the unkindness, worthlessness, or premature loss of objects of affection." *Utilitarianism*, p. 15

58. Robert Burton, *Anatomy of Melancholy* (1621), quoted in Greist and Jefferson, *Depression and Its Treatment*, p. 4.

59. Abraham Lincoln, quoted in Greist and Jefferson, *Depression and Its Treatment*, p. 6. It appears that Lincoln as an adult suffered some form of bipolar manic depression: see Fieve, *Moodswing*, pp. 109–16.

60. Woman with depression quoted in Fieve, *Moodswing*, pp. 230, 232.

61. Winokur, *Depression: The Facts*, p. 64.

62. "Panic Disorder Linked to Suicide Risk," *Washington Post*, 2 November 1989.

Intense suffering comes in many different forms: pain, depression, humiliation, ruthless disease, fear of approaching death, imprisonment, torture, military combat, starvation. An important category is terror, such as the terror felt by victims of violent crime. We may sometimes overlook this feeling: the essence of evil in these situations and the place to which we should direct our attention, we may say, is the *object* of a person's terror, not the feeling itself. Perhaps a theory of evil can accommodate both these things. In any event, we must not slight the latter of the two. We are right to hate terror, and we know that it is something real and sufficient in itself, distinguishable from its object. Oliver Sacks reports that many of his patients during their oculogyric crises were struck by overwhelming terror, though they could not say of what.[63] People with panic disorder report frequent and unpredictable episodes of intense irrational fear. I do not know whether their terror is focused on a definite object, real or perceived; but in any case, the intrinsic properties of such an object, if indeed real, would not be sufficient to account for their plight.[64]

I want to stress here what is too often forgotten: namely, that there are kinds of suffering the intensity of which most of us are unable to conceive. This is partly because we tend to forget—largely from fear, I think—the nature of very severe suffering that we have experienced in the past; and partly because there are some forms of suffering the extremity of which is well beyond what we shall ever experience. It is wise to remember Jacobo Timerman's warning:

> In the long months of confinement, I often thought of how to transmit the pain that a tortured person undergoes. And always I concluded that it was impossible.
> It is a pain without points of reference, revelatory symbols, or clues to serve as indicators.[65]

We may compare an inquiry into suffering to the action of peering over the edge of a steep drop in the terrain that falls away indefinitely, or at least as far as the eye can see. Suffering is evil, and it contains within it evil of ever-increasing magnitude. I do not know whether there is a maximum level of suffering that can be experienced. It is sometimes said that the psyche can only take so much suffering; at a certain point we must fall unconscious. This sounds like another comforting myth. Unconsciousness sometimes comes to relieve a person in extreme torment, but sometimes it does not. Though I cannot answer the question whether a maximum level of suffering exists, it seems safe to say that from where we stand, there are forms of suffering the intensity of which will *appear* infinite to us.

---

63. See *Awakenings*, p. 145: "During her oculogyric crisis, Miss A. sat absolutely motionless. Describing it afterwards she said: 'I had no impulse to move, I don't think I could have moved . . . I had to concentrate on the bit of ceiling I was forced to look at—it filled my mind, I could think of nothing else. And I was afraid, deathly afraid, as I always am in these spells, although I knew there was nothing to be afraid of.' "

64. "Panic Disorder Linked to Suicide Risk," *Washington Post*.

65. *Prisoner Without a Name, Cell Without a Number*, trans. Toby Talbot (New York: Knopf, 1981), p. 32.

9. Suffering Distinct from the Frustration of Desire

It is worth repeating and insisting, because error on this issue has become so deeply entrenched, that happiness is distinct from the satisfaction of preferences, and that suffering is distinct from the frustration of preferences. Happiness and suffering refer to how we feel, and our desires range far beyond the quality of our feelings. It is not even wise, I think, to assert that happiness is the only ground on which we intrinsically prefer some feelings to others. Such a claim would be vulnerable to several challenges, not all of them unreasonable. It seems safe to say that we prefer happiness to suffering, all other things being equal; however, this preference is often latent or unconscious.

What explains the habitual identification of happiness with the satisfaction of preferences? I think it has many sources. Part of it can be traced to the doctrine of psychological hedonism vigorously defended by Jeremy Bentham and John Stuart Mill. According to this doctrine, the only things that people desire as ends in themselves are happiness and exemption from suffering. Bentham and Mill hankered after an "external standard" of morality, independent of personal interest and simple prejudice, to replace the customary method of consulting moral intuition, which they conceived to be irrational and skewed toward the status quo. In their view, the tendency to promote pleasure and avert pain was just such a standard. They could lend plausibility to their claim by maintaining that people desired only their greater personal happiness. If happiness is what all people are pursuing—although sometimes not realizing it, or wishing to conceal it—it seems mere spite or perversity to say that they should pursue, or be guided by, something else instead.

Economic theories and methods are another source of the identification of happiness with preference satisfaction. Economists are trained to observe the preferences that people reveal through their choices. Naturally, it enhances the significance and prestige of economic research to identify the satisfaction of revealed preferences with personal happiness. It is therefore tempting to think that the satisfaction of revealed preferences is a sufficient measure of people's relative happiness.

Among people who proceed with greater introspective caution, one common error is expressed as follows: "When we are conscious that a desire or preference of ours has been denied, we experience a feeling of frustration. This feeling of frustration can itself vary in intensity, and one may infer the strength or force of the thwarted desire by estimating the intensity of felt frustration. Intensity of suffering simply matches (or amounts to the same thing as) the intensity of frustration, or the force of the frustrated desire—however you want to put it."

Now I think it is correct to assert that the intensity of suffering *tends* to vary with the intensity of unsatisfied preference. No one likes to suffer (unless she views it as the necessary price to attain something else she dearly desires), and all people have a deep aversion to intense suffering. If you are starving, or are drowning, or even if you get your fingers caught in a slammed door, your desire to be rescued from your predicament will be several magnitudes stronger than almost any preference you will form when you are free of suffering. Nevertheless, the relation between intensity of suffering and the intensity of frustrated desire is not a perfectly direct one. Intense sexual desire seems to be a good example of a case in which the correlation breaks down. Sexual desire can become so overpowering and so obsessive that it may propel those affected by it into foolish, unseemly, unprincipled, and uncharacteristic behavior; yet it would be untrue to claim that the thwarting of such desire leads in most cases to intense suffering, or perhaps even any suffering at all. What it leads to is simply *very intense frustration*, which we are able in our minds to separate quite clearly from the experience of intense suffering.

Suffering is one kind of feeling, and frustration is another. They do not always neatly coincide. Frustration is the resentment, sometimes swelling into rage, which we occasionally feel when some object of desire has been denied to us. At its most powerful, it may seek expression in peevish or petulant behavior, sulking, temper tantrums, or the impulse to strike out at something or somebody. But clearly these signs and the moods they express are not reliable indicators of the incidence and intensity of suffering.

Some people are able to *pump up* the intensity of their desires. They may do this for many different reasons, one being that they believe it increases their chances of eventually attaining the object of their desire. Their desires become more forceful, but the suffering they will encounter if their desires are disappointed does not undergo a proportionate increase. Thus, for example, if a spoiled child throws a temper tantrum because her latest wish has been denied, the frustration she feels may be disproportionate to the suffering she experiences. Similarly, a businessman who enjoys every blessing in life except a promotion that he is obsessively pursuing may feel intense frustration when the promotion does not materialize; in this case his frustration may well be disproportionate to his suffering, because he is psychologically sustained by all sorts of advantages he takes for granted.

Sometimes the reverse may be observed: for certain people in very wretched circumstances, the intensity of frustrated desire may be very low in comparison to the intensity of suffering. They may be so confused or guilt-ridden that they cannot get their thoughts focused on what it is that they want. They may be unaware that a better alternative is possible for them, and they may even lack the sense that they are subjects capable of forming preferences about what kind of life to lead. I believe this is often the case, to varying degrees, in abused children, people suffering severe clinical depression, and people who are made to endure and expect severe deprivation.

Consider the fact that some people suffering from profound clinical depression hardly have any preferences in the first place. If you ask them what they want, they are liable to say that they do not want anything, that nothing matters any more. We say that they have lost their motivation: even the most appealing plan or the most fortunate news you present to them will be viewed with indifference. It is a mistake to think that these people's pain is linked to some object of their hope that continues to be denied to them. They are submerged in a cloud of pain and meaninglessness so profound that it defines their entire outlook and deprives them of the very concept of hope. They are suffering, but it is not the case that they desire anything in particular.

One could say that such people have an underlying, though inarticulate and unconscious, desire to be relieved of their distress. But the point is precisely that this preference is deeply hidden from view, and because it is so effectively concealed or disguised one hesitates to call it a preference in the first place. Much therapy may be needed in order to make it explicit, but by that time the person may be quite changed, and may in fact be suffering less intensely. Certainly it makes no sense to speak of a *feeling* of frustration concerning some desire of which the person has no consciousness.

We can picture to ourselves many situations in which the unsatisfied preferences of one person are stronger than another's, but the second person suffers more. We can try to imagine, for instance, the life of an abused child, who is beaten by her father, has no friends, suffers from guilt as well as very low self-esteem, and does not even have a clear conception that a better life is available for her, much less that she is entitled to one. We can juxtapose her situation against that of a businessman who for several years has been desiring a coveted promotion so strongly that the desire has become an obsession. A large part of his waking hours are devoted to devising strategies for the attainment of his goal and calculating the innumerable ways in which different factors affect his chances for success. The desire is so keen that he not infrequently sinks into moments of bleak dejection and despair, or winds himself up to a state of impotent rage accentuated by acute self-pity; for, after all, he may believe he has been woefully abused and mistreated and that few people have as good a reason to complain of injustice as he does.

In this example it seems plausible to say that the desire of the businessman for a promotion is stronger than the desire of the child for decent care. And yet it is equally probable that the girl suffers more. Because of his obsession, the business-man forgets his relative good fortune. He has food to eat, a safe, comfortable place to live, he enjoys good health (let us say), respect from colleagues and acquaintances, and love from relatives and friends. Moreover, he has the freedom to try various pursuits and entertainments, and to develop untapped faculties. All these blessings, though they are forgotten by him, give him a certain psychological substratum of contentment and security. They keep away uncounted discomforts, fears, and frus-trations. Because he slights his blessings—takes them so utterly for granted—he simply doesn't realize how lucky he is. His blessings make his life much less mis-erable than he is willing to admit or than the obsessive force of his unsatisfied desire would lead us to conclude, if we measured suffering by the strength of unsatisfied preferences.

Meanwhile, the suffering of the abused child, living in fear and confusion, is not adequately measured by the strength of whatever preferences she may have for a stable and secure life. As I noted, she may not be aware that an alternative to her situation is possible. She may not even realize that she is a subject capable of preferences about the kind of life she will have.

(We do not want to stretch the example too far. If the child were much more resilient than we supposed, or if the businessman's obsession led him off the brink to an acute and prolonged mental crisis of a truly wretched kind, then we might have to admit that the businessman's suffering exceeded that of the child—though we would also be perplexed about the moral implications of this.)

Is there no way in which the businessman could discern that his suffering is less intense than the child's? Certainly there is. If he made a careful and intelligent effort to represent to himself the overall quality of the child's feelings, and then contrasted it with a clear-eyed appraisal of the overall quality of his own feelings, he would almost certainly realize that the child suffers more than he. He would undoubtedly be grateful that his experience is unlike that of the child. But whether the businessman from an impartial comparison *would* perceive the child's suffering to be greater than his own, and whether his *actual* level of subjective frustration exceeds that of the child, are two very different questions. The businessman knows that he is in no danger of suffering the child's fate; in fact he is so confident of this that he does not have to think about it. (Most ambitious businessmen and women do not in fact spend much time vividly imagining the experiences of the most wretched people in their midst, and considering how those experiences, by a different turn of fortune's wheel, could have been their own.) The businessman can inflate his desire for a promotion knowing (although he does not say it to himself so plainly) that a comfortable life without a promotion is the worst thing that is likely to happen to him. Not having to fear true calamity, he can afford to invest his current ambition with as much desire and attribute to it as much importance as if its frustration *did* constitute a calamity. This example reminds us that how strongly we desire something is largely a function of what we have come to expect, and what we have come to expect may include a certain prevalent level of happiness or suffering.[66]

It is of the highest importance to be able to distinguish genuine suffering from the pale but deceptive imitation of it. It is of the highest importance to realize that what so often passes for "suffering," for want of a richer vocabulary or clearer powers of discernment, in the experience of people who enjoy a firm material and psychological foundation in their lives, is not genuine suffering and can only be called so by the most distant and strained analogy. I (J.M.) am liable to encounter any number of setbacks and disappointments, mortifications, frustrations, embarrassments even—plans gone awry, hopes dashed, cherished objects torn away—but

66. Buddhists, who are followed in this by Schopenhauer, teach that suffering is caused by the frustration of desire, and consequently that the cure for suffering consists in the renunciation of desire. For the reasons given, I believe that this equation of suffering with frustration is misleading. What is true, and what Buddhism reminds us of, is that a great many people would be a great deal happier if they managed to shed many of their desires, or at least kept them at a certain distance. But it must be remembered that the intensity of frustration can outpace the intensity of suffering, and vice versa. At times the Buddhist teaching seems to be nothing more than the view, urged by the Stoics and others, that our afflictions do not imply suffering if they do not hurt us, and that we have it in our power not to be hurt by them. The extent of such a power, and the usefulness of invoking it, are open to question.

these for the most part are mere squalls played out on the surface of my consciousness. They do not penetrate to the extent of suffering. They will no doubt provoke
loud railing, bitter complaint, and waves of self-pity. But these reactions, out of all
proportion to the objective psychological hurt that has been inflicted on me, are in
themselves nothing more than the proofs and trophies of my good fortune—a good
fortune so firmly established and so utterly taken for granted that minor wounds
take on the appearance of devastating injuries. I exaggerate their import and scale
because I have come to forget the depth of my well-being—all the accumulated
elements of my good fortune, and all the fresh infusions of comfort, ease, and
happiness which flow so punctually and uninterruptedly that I cease to notice them.
I wake up in a comfortable bed under a solid shelter, I clean and refresh myself, I
put on comfortable clothes, I greet cheerful housemates who find enjoyment in my
company as I in theirs, I take a breakfast of my own choosing, I satisfy my curiosity
with a newspaper or radio, I look forward to the day's projects, I see smiling friends
who greet me with affection and respect, the physical world stimulates and livens
my consciousness with a steady stream of rich and variegated and inoffensive sensory
input, and all the while my body toils smoothly and quietly away, performing the
complex rhythms necessary for life, comfort, and basic functioning; swiftly obeying
my commands; and alerting me directly to my surroundings through the unceasing
activity of my senses. I am buoyed by the continuous gratification of innumerable
small unremarked cravings and expectations; the mutual cooperation of a healthy
body and a favorable environment to guarantee basic physical comfort and human
functioning; and the multiple signals, some highly subtle but nonetheless effective,
of my own high worth as an individual. Even if my health falters, I can count on
family, friends, and institutions to help me recover or, if complete recovery is impossible, to help me cope with and adapt to my weakened condition. Add on top
of this, if I am lucky, the blessings of a moderately successful career, the ability to
lead the life I have chosen, the presence of affectionate family and friends . . . These
are the principal elements of a happy life.

   These blessings not only form the foundation of my happiness; to large extent
they *constitute* my happiness. They are present in my thoughts and feelings, though
not fully grasped by them. There is much that goes on in our minds of which we
are not directly aware—much that transpires in our consciousness to which we don't
attend. This is not an unintelligible contradiction; it is a recognizable fact of human
experience. It is a familiar experience, for example, to return to a place where one
had lived earlier in one's life and to notice a sensory fact—a pervasive odor, for
example—which colored or filtered everything else that passed through it, although
at the time one rarely or never had a conscious thought concerning its presence.
The fact, though not consciously noted, was a major element of one's overall conscious state.[67] The same holds true, though to a far greater extent, of the abundant

----

67. A man observed after losing his sense of smell, "I never gave it a thought. You don't normally
give it a thought. But when I lost it—it was like being struck blind. Life lost a good deal of its savour—

blessings in which many of our lives are enveloped. We do not dwell on them, yet they constitute a principal element of our consciousness, and their overflowing goodness spreads happiness over our consciousness as a whole, in a manner not consciously perceived by us.

I do not mean to imply that people who enjoy reasonably good health, the love and respect of others, and secure access to food, shelter, clothing, and medical attention, and are free from grave physical disability or deformity, are utterly immune from genuine suffering—even when they avoid the crushing pain of mental illnesses such as depression, schizophrenia, anxiety disorder, and panic disorder. There can sometimes arise overwhelming disappointments, grief occasioned by the death of loved ones, cruel separations and withdrawals of affection, moments of intense embarrassment or even humiliation, and searing guilt. These events can cause genuine suffering. All I caution is that the intensity of suffering *may* be rather less than what the alleged victim represents to himself, and that claims of having suffered *may* not always be authentic, but may sometimes arise instead from the inflamed imagination of enraged disappointment and an insufficient attention to the whole of one's feelings.

There is a story often repeated in literature in which a person laments her present condition, only to find herself thrust by a cruel fate into a worse one. Then she vows that if only she were restored to her former condition, she would complain less and appreciate the advantages of her situation more. Sometimes this pattern is repeated. Each new affliction brings the belated wisdom that her earlier complaints were excessive. This wisdom is twofold. On the one hand, she learns that she ought to have tempered her bitterness by the recollection that things could be much worse. But on the other hand, she realizes that her former condition was not as intolerable, even in an absolute sense, as she had represented it. Fixated as she was on her grievances, she could spare no attention for the numerous advantages that hoisted the level of her well-being and improved the overall flavor of her existence. She launched her complaints from the pedestal of many blessings and supports, and it is only when they are knocked out from under her that her attention is drawn toward them and she can begin to see the full nature of what she had but now has lost.

There are two issues here, related but different. The first is that we sometimes underestimate our happiness or overestimate our suffering because we take certain blessings so completely for granted that we overlook their beneficial influence on the overall tone of our feeling. Conversely, a truly wretched and disadvantaged person may underestimate her own suffering if she begins to expect a certain level of suffering as a matter of course and does not fully grasp the extent to which her hardship keeps her chained to a level of misery that she otherwise need not feel. The second issue is that we must distinguish between the kind of feeling that

---

one doesn't realise how much savour *is* smell. You *smell* people, you *smell* books, you *smell* the city, you *smell* the spring—maybe not consciously, but as a rich unconscious background to everything else. My whole world was suddenly radically poorer." Oliver Sacks, *The Man Who Mistook His Wife for a Hat and Other Clinical Tales* (New York: Harper and Row, 1985), p. 159.

predominates at the surface of our consciousness and the feelings which suffuse our consciousness as a whole. Sometimes a piece of good news or a personal triumph for which one has been longing a great time is succeeded by a feeling of tense and confused agitation, or even a kind of dejection or despondency, which only belies the profound happiness that is welling up inside oneself. At the end of *Pride and Prejudice,* Jane Austen says of Elizabeth, after Darcy has renewed and she has accepted his offer of marriage, and while she is still struggling with excitement, embarrassment, and the awkwardness of informing her family, that she "rather *knew* that she was happy, than *felt* herself to be so" (chapter 59). The comment is a tribute to the acuity of Elizabeth's self-understanding. Here *happy* means "joyful," not merely "lucky." Austen's novels are steeped in the language of hedonistic psychology; and happiness and misery always carry the meaning of felt joy and wretchedness—essentially the same as, but connoting more permanence and depth than, the minutely measurable concepts of pain and pleasure, words that Austen uses liberally. Darcy has just granted the desire that has dominated Elizabeth's thoughts for the last several weeks, though she has tried hard to deny and repress it for fear of disappointment. Now all her fears are lifted and she can look forward to an indefinite future of burgeoning happiness. Her immediate sensations of tension, nervousness, discomfort, and confusion cover an underlying sense of personal victory and impending happiness, a sense that, as Elizabeth well knows, can only gather strength and confidence over time, and quickly subdue her agitation. This is why the author can rightly say that Elizabeth's mind discerns the true extent of her present happiness, while her immediate sensations tell a different story.

The contrast of surface feelings of one kind with overall feelings of another is a common occurrence. We cry over a sad novel or movie and enjoy ourselves thoroughly. (Admitting this, however, detracts from our enjoyment.) We can indulge in fury without experiencing genuine distress. Father Zossima in *The Brothers Karamazov* says,

> You know it is sometimes very pleasant to take offense, isn't it? A man may know that nobody has insulted him, but that he has invented the insult for himself, has lied and exaggerated to make it picturesque, has caught at a word and made a mountain out of a molehill—he knows that himself, yet he will be the first to take offence, and will revel in his resentment till he feels great pleasure in it, and so pass to genuine vindictiveness. (Book II, Chapter 2)

The attainment of some long-sought-after prize overwhelms us with such awe and excitement that our tension causes us literally to ache; yet we could not honestly deny that we are extremely happy. Melancholy, in one of its senses, means a feeling of subdued or dejected spirits that is actually quite pleasurable on the whole, as Milton observes beautifully in "Il Penseroso." (Why this feeling is pleasurable is hard to explain. We could say, perhaps, that when we are melancholy we gratefully believe that we are restored to a clearer and more sober sense of ourselves and of reality. But this does not capture it all. Sometimes the feeling itself is nice.) Conversely, high and exuberant spirits may coexist with and cover disagreeable feelings of self-doubt, low self-esteem, or general unease. This is what the author of Ecclesiastes has captured so well:

> Sorrow is better than laughter,
>   for by sadness of countenance the heart is made glad.
> The heart of the wise is in the house of mourning;
>   but the heart of fools is in the house of mirth.
> It is better to hear the rebuke of the wise
>   than to hear the song of fools.
> For like the crackling of thorns under a pot,
>   so is the laughter of fools,
>   this also is vanity. (Eccl. 7.3–6)

Pope echoes this thought:

> The broadest mirth unfeeling Folly wears,
> Less pleasing far than Virtue's very tears.[68]

The point is not just that the subdued sage is more fortunate than the giggling fool because of his superior wisdom; it is also that his happiness is deeper, more genuine, more abiding. "By sadness of countenance the heart is made glad . . ." Sorrowful understanding can be the source of a deeper happiness, which cheerful unconcern may not allow us to attain.

10. Suffering Distinct from the Subjective Opinion of Suffering

In adducing arguments against the view that suffering is correlated to the strength of frustrated preferences, we have denied another common assumption: namely, the view that people always know whether or not they are suffering, and know what the degree of their suffering is. In fact, people who are suffering often do not know that they are suffering. They may be stunned out of thought. They may be mute, inarticulate, and confused. Many no doubt sense in a vague and general way that something is wrong—in the world, in themselves, or somewhere else. But their distress takes such a hold of them that they can no longer step outside themselves and acquire the degree of objectivity required to observe that what is wrong (or a large part of what is wrong) is precisely that they are suffering.

Many people do not even think about their lives in terms of happiness and suffering. They think about their plans and desires and commitments and obligations, and the good and bad things that can happen to them, but they do not take repeated measurements of their feelings. Recall Mill's insight: "Ask yourself whether you are happy, and you cease to be so." Before asking the fatal question you were

---

68. Alexander Pope, *An Essay on Man*, IV, 319–20. Of course Pope's poem is not otherwise in agreement with the views of this book.

happy without knowing it; and if you are lucky enough to delay the question, you postpone the knowledge that you had been happy. Our degree of happiness or suffering is a matter of how we feel; knowing our degree of happiness or suffering is a matter of accurately observing how we feel. We ought not to expect that such observation is continuously in operation and that it never deceives us.

Often the cause or object of our suffering takes such complete possession of our minds that it would require an immense and unnatural, perhaps impossible, effort to draw our attention to the suffering itself. Someone fleeing a would-be assassin may feel terror, which can be an extreme form of suffering; but he won't have time to think about how he is feeling, he must think about his pursuer and how to get away. When we are overcome with guilt or shame, we may not dwell on the suffering it causes us, but rather on the reason for our disgrace and the fact that we have been very bad, or ridiculous (whichever is the case).

It is striking that many victims of clinical depression fail to recognize that they are depressed or even sad.[69] Their only thoughts are those of self-reproach—of their own wickedness or failure. Depressed patients commonly express the belief that the world would be a far better place without them: and it is often a conviction of their utter worthlessness, rather than a decision to terminate their pain, which forms the conscious motive of those who attempt or carry out suicide.[70]

It appears that some depressed patients are better able than others to recognize their pain. But we would not conclude from this that the former are more miserable than the latter. The contrary may also be true. A depressed patient might be so dominated by self-contempt that she blocks the bare minimum of introspective concern and curiosity necessary to perceive that she is suffering. When we believe ourselves worthless or hateful we resist the thought that we are suffering. Suffering would entitle us to sympathy and concern, when we know we are entitled to no such thing. Yet self-loathing is in itself one of the worst forms of suffering. We know this in retrospect. We are unaware of it at the time because it is in the nature of self-loathing to blind us to it.

Ironically, when we are able to step outside our state of hurt and point to it, we often succeed in overcoming and transcending it. The failure to perceive this helps account for the dangerous fallacy that anger is a form of suffering. It is not. Anger is what we feel when we transform our mute suffering into an utterable grievance. What before was an undefinable sense of wrongness, now becomes a very definite sense that we are the victims of rank injustice. The badness no longer absorbs us; we have isolated it, located it outside ourselves, and given it the name of injustice or unfairness or wickedness or evil. It consumes our attention, and the fury we vent on it burns up the suffering we felt before.

69. Nathan Billig, *To Be Old and Sad: Understanding Depression in the Elderly* (Lexington, Mass.: Lexington Books, 1987), pp. 19–22; and John White, *The Masks of Melancholy: A Christian Physician Looks at Depression and Suicide* (Downers Grove, Ill.: InterVarsity Press, 1982), pp. 13–14. See also note 40 above.

70. Winokur, *Depression: The Facts*, p. 69.

What I have said needs to be refined. Sometimes we identify the source of our suffering, yet it is so powerful that we cannot conquer it through hatred. This may happen for either of two different reasons. (1) We are unable to *feel* anger, because the suffering is so intense that it absorbs our concentration and leaves us too exhausted for confrontation. Or (2) we can rouse ourselves to anger, but it is not strong enough to cauterize the intense suffering we feel. The latter psychological state is particularly hard on us. Anger, with its accompanying sense of incipient triumph, only magnifies our underlying hopelessness. Our fury expends itself uselessly; it sputters out, leaving us in a deeper despair than before. This is what we call the anger of helpless, or impotent, rage.

What I have in mind is a purer kind of anger: the anger of hatred and indignation. This anger succeeds in displacing suffering; and yet, all too often, it deceitfully calls itself suffering. There are many interrelated reasons for this deceit. The first is cognitive. Since anger often follows on the heels of suffering, and has the person's suffering, or the source of his suffering, as its object, it is natural to confuse the two. The second reason for the deceit is that it may be necessary in order for the anger to operate in the first place. The knowledge that I am suffering fuels my grievance, which stokes my fury, which purges my suffering; this process must be repeated, or else I will fall back into real distress. The third reason is strategic and comes into play when people are pursuing certain goals. Suffering provides greater moral legitimacy for actions carried out in its name than anger does. You will gain greater understanding for your cause or for some desperate or extreme or unusual action carried out in its name if you say it is compelled by a need to relieve your suffering than if you say it is dictated by your anger. So the assertion that you are suffering is valuable rhetoric and you will want to use it for purposes of persuasion and garnering sympathy. But suffering is hard to bear and often intolerable. It is difficult, often impossible, to choose to continue to suffer when you perceive a way out. Anger is one natural way out. It is far easier for people to clamor for action and change from the refuge of their anger than from the impossible resting place of suffering; but their demands will carry greater moral force if they appear to spring from suffering. So there are ample rewards for the deception that our anger is a form of suffering. This is at once a deception of other people and of ourselves: here, as elsewhere, self-deception is a necessary prerequisite, an intrinsic part, of deceiving others.

But sometimes the pretense is dropped. A Palestinian boy in Lebanon gave a surprising but honest report of his feelings at the funeral of thirteen fellow villagers killed by the Israeli army. He "smiled when asked how he felt as a result of the raid. 'Actually, we feel happy. The killing gives us more power to fight them. We actually thank the Israelis, because they woke us up. They taught us how to be strong people,' he said."[71] The boy is happy to be angry. There are any of various

71. "A Village Buries Its Dead: Lebanese Vow Vengeance after Israeli Raid," *Washington Post*, 23 March 1985.

reasons for this. (1) Hatred is preferable to grief. (2) Hatred is an opportunity for the joys of excitement, strife, contention, domination, and moral indignation. (3) Hatred will give the boy's fellow nationals greater force with which to carry out their pre-existing goal of defeating the Israelis. Long ago, Homer understood how anger could be pleasurable, calling it

> bitter gall, sweeter than dripping streams of honey,
> that swarms in people's chests, and blinds like smoke.[72]

There is a whole subclass of rather common emotions that falsely parade as suffering to win increased attention for themselves. I am speaking not only of anger, but also resentment, spite, and bitterness. It is important to recognize that these emotions often include no suffering at all, although the people experiencing them may wish to describe them that way. It is necessary, for instance, to distinguish between an envy that is felt predominantly as a lack in one's own life and hence can be a kind of suffering (albeit not very intense), and a resentment that primarily consists of hatred toward someone whose relative advantage one begrudges and that contains nothing in the way of real pain. These emotions often extort, as their food and fuel, public recognition that they are species of suffering. But this is a misclassification, and it is the source of great mischief.

Real cases of suffering, meanwhile, tend to go unheard. This is not only because people who are genuinely suffering typically lack the resources with which to publicize their condition, but also because, as I have said, many forms of suffering deprive people of the very ability to express, sometimes even think, the fact that they are suffering.

Crying is often viewed as a way to purge or mitigate our misery, and I think this is correct. The irony, of course, is that it is also one of the most unmistakable signals that we are suffering, so that we must often wait till we have found this outlet for our misery before we succeed in provoking the sympathy of other people. Only through our tears does the full force of our suffering "hit" or confront them. It is too bad that sympathy must so often be delayed in this fashion.

When someone is overcome by sobs after a long emotional crisis, he may achieve a degree of detachment from his former suffering self. We feel that he is transported from his situation; we say, for instance, that he is "losing himself" or "letting go." Moreover, his outburst is the irrefutable sign of his suffering. It may be that it is only when a person breaks down that he realizes how much he has been suffering; only then comes the gasp of recognition, "Oh! I am so miserable!" The sobbing permits him to observe his own plight—since he can hear his cries and feel the stinging in his eyes and the wetness on his face—and the effect is often startling. With the realization that he is truly suffering, there may come relief from the

---

72. *The Iliad*, trans. Robert Fagles (Harmondsworth: Penguin, 1990), XVIII, 129–30 (p. 471).

thought that he has now successfully identified the problem and that he is a proper object for sympathy and concern.[73]

But the matter is more complex than this. The recognition of his own suffering may bring relief to a person who is crying, but it may also frighten him by showing him how badly off he is, and thus intensify his distress. The latter effect explains the cycle we often observe in crying. A person bursts into tears, and as he gradually purges himself of his grief, his cries quiet down; then, reviewing his dramatic behavior, he thinks with a shudder how godforsaken he must be to be acting in this way, and he erupts in a fresh outbreak of tears.

When people's sobs become increasingly hysterical, we sense that they have not yet found the relief they thought they could obtain through weeping. Their cries take on a more desperate tone. Their sounds and gestures begin to mimic the signs of physical pain, or fear, or madness. They seem truly lost. They think, it would seem, that by making their behavior more extreme and dramatic, they can attain the measure of solace that continues to elude them.

And then, sobbing is often a sign of hope. People often break down precisely when there is someone to cradle them in their arms. It is as though people will sooner let themselves acknowledge their suffering when they think improvement is on the way. They burst into tears because they want an immediate first installment on the alleviation they think is coming. Now they can afford to open the floodgates of their feelings, as it were, and let themselves be convulsed by the acknowledgment of their misery. And they can do this without fear that they will have to pay dearly for their temporary surrender of control.

73. As Schopenhauer says, though with his customary exaggeration, "We never weep directly over pain that is felt, but always only over its repetition in reflection. . . . Weeping is sympathy with ourselves." Arthur Schopenhauer, *The World as Will and Representation*, vol. 1, trans. E. F. J. Payne (New York: Dover, 1958), pp. 376, 377.

〜〜

THREE

The Measurement of Suffering

1. Other People's Suffering

This chapter addresses problems associated with the measurement of suffering. Specifically, I ask how we can assess whether and with what intensity other people are suffering, and how we should conceive and estimate the cardinal intensity of suffering. I turn first to the issue of interpersonal comparisons.

In order to discover whether and with what intensity someone is suffering, one must determine how that person feels. This seems to present a difficulty: we seem much better placed to observe our own feelings than the feelings of other people. Of course even our assessment of our own feelings can be distorted. An urge to complain, a preoccupation with what we see as our own wickedness, a general incapacity to separate our feelings themselves from their "objective conditions and consequences," a failure to distinguish our feelings as a whole from those that lie at the forefront of our consciousness, or more simply, a lack of practice in introspection into our emotions—these factors and others can lead us to misrepresent the state of our feelings. And when the feelings belong to the past, memory introduces further distortions. Nevertheless, when the feelings are our own, the fact that we feel them (or have felt them) seems to give our assessment of them an anchor in reality. We feel sure that our assessment will approach the truth if only we introspect with sufficient care and guard against conceptual confusions.

But how can we assess another person's feelings? Because they are another person's feelings and not our own, we cannot peer into them directly. And yet we often form judgments about the state of other people's feelings, sometimes with the highest degree of confidence. On what do we base those judgments?

The assessment of other people's feelings in order to determine their degree of happiness or suffering involves the careful sorting of different pieces of evidence. One important kind of evidence is simply what people tell us. If we want to know how another person feels, we can ask her. If the person is introspectively skilled and free from conceptual misunderstanding, if she can communicate effectively and is not attempting to deceive, then we may take her report at face value. If she falls short in any of these areas, we may not want to take her report at face value; however, we may know enough about the nature of her deficiencies as a witness to make the necessary corrections to her account. For example, we may scale down the report of suffering by someone we know to be an inveterate complainer.

Of course this method has serious limits. It leaves out animals, infants, and other people who lack the means of verbal communication. Often there is no time to ask. And sometimes we have reason to doubt another person's testimony without knowing how to correct it.

The other way to assess the feelings of people different from ourselves is to draw on hypotheses about the causes and behavioral symptoms of happiness and suffering. We form many hypotheses about the effects produced on a person's feelings by different mental, physical, and external conditions and events, past and present—what I shall call for short a person's *situation*. (I am obviously using the word in a very comprehensive sense, where it refers not only to external occurrences, but also a person's physical state, her genetic endowment and previous experience, as well as her beliefs, desires, memories, and associations, both conscious and unconscious.) And we form many hypotheses about how different kinds of feeling are reflected in different kinds of behavior. What complicates matters is the vast number of these hypotheses. The more we know about someone's situation and behavior, the more hypotheses come into play, all of which must be accommodated in our final assessment. Contact with hot surfaces normally produces pain, but someone may have a rare neurological condition that reduces sensitivity to heat. Then again, a burn may trigger the memory of a traumatic accident in early childhood, intensifying one's distress. Fear of ongoing pain increases present distress, while expectation of imminent release mitigates it. Howling is a sign of intense pain, but the interpretation of such behavior also needs to take into account the person's cultural background, since different cultures teach different norms regarding the proper response to pain. A practical joker might imitate the sounds of someone in pain in order to fool others. And so on.

Where do these hypotheses come from? Very often they are inferred from other hypotheses: for example, one reason we know that burns are painful is that people cry out when burned, and we know already that crying out is a sign of pain. But, ultimately, our hypotheses about the causes and symptoms of suffering are rooted in two sources: testimony from other people about how they feel in certain situations or while exhibiting certain behaviors, and our own memories of how we have felt in certain situations or while exhibiting certain behaviors. I know in my case that crying out is a response to extreme pain, so I hypothesize that, in general, crying out is a sign of pain. This hypothesis receives support when I observe other people crying out in response to the same events—burns, stubbed toes, crushed fingers—that give me extreme pain, for I have previously hypothesized on the basis of my own experience that these events cause other people pain as well. From the data of many individual experiences—our own and those reported to us by others—we gradually build up a large store of hypotheses regarding the causes and behavioral symptoms of suffering. Armed with this knowledge, we can often determine whether and with what intensity someone is suffering, even if he cannot tell us himself.

I should point out that the identification of certain behaviors as responses to suffering is not simply a matter of correlation. Because we have an intrinsic aversion to suffering, certain responses *make sense*. They are strategies for escaping or reducing suffering. When an infant howls, his parents will try different things to make him stop (either because they think he is suffering, or they can't stand the howling, or both). When he is quiet, they are content to let him stay that way. It is therefore in the infant's interest to howl when he is suffering. (I am not asserting that he employs this strategy consciously. It could be a genetically programmed instinct arising from natural selection.)

A skeptic can object to the methodology described here by pointing out that since we cannot peer into other people's feelings directly, there is no way to verify that they feel just as we do when they find themselves in similar situations or exhibit similar behaviors. We cannot generalize from our own experience to other people's experience. Nor, according to the skeptic, can we turn to other people's verbal descriptions of their own feelings. When someone else reports feeling pain, how can we verify that the word *pain* means the same to him as it does to us? Normally we come to trust other people's testimony because it so often fits the hypotheses we have drawn from our own experience about the causes and behavioral symptoms of suffering. But, as the skeptic has already shown us, this does not count as valid confirmation.[1]

How should we reply to the skeptic? First, we must frankly admit that, because we cannot peer directly into other people's feelings, the verification requested by the skeptic is impossible. The skeptic claims that because such verification is impossible, any assessment of another person's feelings is unwarranted. At this point we should simply stick by our intuitions and say that this claim is absurd and frightening in its implications. If someone screams in response to a severe physical injury, it would be crazy to suspend judgment about the state of her feelings. Indeed, the reasoning employed by the skeptic calls into doubt the existence of other minds altogether.[2]

John Harsanyi has provided some helpful remarks about the reasoning we employ when we estimate other people's level of psychological well-being.[3] (He speaks of

1. See J. L. Cowan, *Pleasure and Pain: A Study in Philosophical Psychology* (London: MacMillan, 1968), pp. 36–43.

2. Many people have made this point. See, for example, John Rawls, *A Theory of Justice* (Cambridge, Massachusetts: Harvard University Press, 1971), p. 91.

3. John Harsanyi, "Cardinal Welfare, Individualistic Ethics, and Interpersonal Comparisons of Utility," *Journal of Political Economy* 63 (1955): 309–21, section 5. See also Allan Gibbard's extremely helpful discussion in "Interpersonal Comparisons: Preference, Good, and the Intrinsic Reward of a Life," in

the mental state of "satisfaction," but his comments apply equally well to happiness and suffering.) First, Harsanyi says, imagine another person whose situation (in the comprehensive sense) and behavior are identical to my own in every observable respect. In such a case, we should assume that both of us feel alike, for it would be completely gratuitous to assume a difference in feeling if there were no observable difference in our respective situations and behaviors.[4]

Of course, this scenario will never arise. There will always be some difference between my situation and behavior—my state, for short—and another person's. However, I can search my previous experience to see if I ever differed from my present state in the past in the same way that the other person differs from my present state. If my search is successful, memory may tell me that those differences corresponded to certain differences in feeling, and I should assume, for reasons given in the previous paragraph, that the other person's feelings differ in the same way.

But in reading another person's feelings out of my own feelings in a similar state, I need not limit myself to states I have actually experienced. Some of the hypotheses I derive from past experience about the correlation of states and feelings extend beyond my actual experience. For example, I found in the past that the painfulness of a burn varies with the length of exposure to the source of heat. Extrapolating, I determine that a longer exposure to the heat source than I have ever experienced will produce a more painful burn than I have ever experienced. The general question is: "How would I be feeling if I were in this other person's state (placed in her situation, and behaving as she does)?" My past experience often gives me an idea of how I would feel even though I never occupied the same exact state.

But sometimes another person's state may contain a feature where my past experience seems to give me no idea of what difference in feeling, if any, is associated with that feature. How do I proceed then?

First, I should go back and search more carefully. I may find that I can redescribe the feature in a way that exposes links to my own experience or, alternatively, that more thorough rummaging of my memory will uncover buried clues.

But in addition I can *ask* the other person what change in feeling is associated with the feature. And I can ask the same question of other people whose experience includes the feature or at least gives them enough information for a prediction of the change in feeling associated with it. We rely on this method a great deal. We continually ask other people how they feel and listen when they tell us unbidden. Now, very often we check their reports to see if they mesh with the hypotheses we have formed from personal experience (and from the reliable reports of other people). We want to make sure that their reports are not skewed by sloppy introspection, faulty conceptualization, ineffective communication, or deception. And often we

John Elster and Aanund Hylland, eds., *Foundations of Social Choice Theory* (Cambridge: Cambridge University Press, 1986), pp. 183–90.

4. Harsanyi, "Cardinal Welfare, Individualistic Ethics, and Interpersonal Comparisons of Utility," p. 317. Harsanyi adds: "In the last analysis, it is on the basis of this principle that we ascribe mental states to other human beings at all: the denial of this principle would at once lead us to solipsism."

reject other people's reports (sometimes too hastily perhaps) if we think they contradict our pre-existing hypotheses. But we do place *some* independent trust in other people's reports. We come to trust the reports of other people—people we know and people in general—because we see them using the words *pain* and *suffering* to characterize
states where those feelings are predicted by the hypotheses we draw from our own experiences and where there is little reason to expect failures in introspection, conceptualization, communication, and honesty to distort their testimony. We conclude that
those words mean the same to them as to us. We then study other people carefully—
individuals and categories of people—for signs telling us whose testimony we can
trust more and whose we can trust less. (When we cannot take other people's testimony at face value, we may still know enough about the distortions at work to trust it
after making the necessary corrections.) Sometimes we trust other people's testimony
to the extent that it serves as an independent confirmation of hypotheses we have
drawn from our own experience, or even a spur to critical re-examination of those hypotheses in case of contradiction. And sometimes we trust other people's testimony to
the further extent that it forms the basis of hypotheses about certain features of personal states where our own experience offers no guide.

Now suppose that I can form no idea of the change in feeling associated with a
particular feature of another person's state, even after the most careful study of my
own experience and other people's testimony (including the testimony of the other
person in question, supposing it is available). I think that in such a case we should
assume that no change in feeling is associated with the feature. Here, as Harsanyi
points out, we should appeal to "the a priori principle that, when one variable is
alleged to have a certain influence on another, the burden of proof lies on those
who claim the existence of such an influence."[5] And to cover features that consist
of different behavioral responses, we should appeal to the further a priori principle
that when one variable is alleged to reflect another, the burden of proof lies on those
who claim the existence of such a relationship.

I have tried to describe in a very general way the method we use to assess other
people's feelings for purposes of determining whether and with what intensity they
are suffering. It is this general method that lies behind the most sophisticated techniques of physiologists, psychologists, and sociologists to take an accurate reading
of other people's feelings. And it is the same method used to understand the feelings
of animals.[6]

5. Ibid., p. 319. Harsanyi uses this principle to claim that we should not associate differences in
psychological well-being with "variables that, for any particular individual, are not capable of change,"
Ibid. I think it is clearer to say that we shouldn't associate differences in psychological well-being with
any variables where personal experience and other people's testimony give us no idea of the impact of
those variables on people's well-being.

6. In the case of animals, attention needs to be paid to the organization of the nervous system. For
a careful and illuminating discussion, see David DeGrazia, *Taking Animals Seriously* (Cambridge: Cambridge University Press, 1996), chaps. 4 and 5. See also Marian Stamp Dawkins, "The Scientific Basis
for Assessing Suffering in Animals," in Peter Singer, ed., *In Defense of Animals* (Oxford: Basil Blackwell,
1985).

It is sometimes alleged that we cannot hope to comprehend the experience of people whose culture or life circumstances are radically different from our own. I think this view should be resisted. We can learn what it is like to live or grow up in a radically different setting by breaking that experience down into its simplest elements—for often we can find parallels to those elements in our experience, though obviously combined very differently and mixed with foreign elements—and then imagining the cumulative effect on ourselves of those elements in the particular way they are combined. We can learn from the testimony of the other people themselves, and if they speak to us in a strange language with strange concepts, we can ask a skilled anthropologist to help explain, or turn to someone who has lived his or her life in both settings and can serve simultaneously as informant and interpreter. Of course, our efforts to understand are fraught with difficulty. We are prone to many kinds of mistakes. (I have examined some of the principal mistakes in chapter 2.) But these mistakes can be anticipated and corrected. There is a crucial difference between saying it is *difficult* to understand the experience of people from radically different backgrounds, and saying it is *impossible*. For that matter, I do not think it is impossible to form some idea of the experience of other animals—ask most pet owners—though of course the difficulties are much greater than in the case of other humans.[7]

2. The Question of Cardinal Intensity

In this book I shall assume that we can measure the intensity of happiness and suffering not only in ordinal terms, but also in cardinal terms. An ordinal measure ranks experiences of happiness or suffering in order of intensity. A cardinal measurement records the size of the difference between those intensities. I shall assume, furthermore, that cardinal measurements of happiness and suffering can be rendered in terms of a ratio scale. A ratio scale permits us to say that the intensity of one person's suffering exceeds that of another person's suffering by a certain proportion. Ratio scales presume the existence of a non-arbitrary zero.[8] On the happiness-suffering scale, I shall locate this zero in the space between agreeable overall feeling and disagreeable overall feeling (Sidgwick's "hedonistic zero").

Even if we agree that the intensity of happiness and suffering can be measured in terms of a cardinal ratio scale, we may have different conceptions of what the scale refers to. In the rest of the chapter, I explore four different conceptions of

7. See DeGrazia, *Taking Animals Seriously*, and Dawkins, "The Scientific Basis for Assessing Suffering in Animals."

8. An example of a ratio scale is the scale used for measuring height: a six-foot person is twice as tall as a three-foot person. An example of a cardinal measure that does not use ratios is the geographic concept of longitude. Milan is west of Venice, and the distance in longitude between Milan and Venice exceeds that between Padua and Venice by a certain ratio, but it's not the case that Milan is *more west* than Venice by any ratio. We record longitude with reference to the zero of the Greenwich Meridian, but the location of zero at that particular meridian is arbitrary.

cardinal intensity: the intuitive measure, the preferential measure, the global evaluative measure, and the local evaluative measure. (There may be others.) On the intuitive measure, the intensity of suffering is linked to "how much someone hurts," while the intensity of happiness is linked to "how good a person feels." These estimates are directly produced by intuition, hence their name. The other three measures look for some basis other than intuition to estimate intensity. The preferential measure links cardinal intensity to individual preference rankings regarding alternative distributions of happiness and suffering of varying degrees of intensity over time (or alternative probability sets of happiness and suffering of varying degrees of intensity). The two evaluative measures link cardinal intensity, not to individual preferences, but to an *objective* value-ranking of alternative distributions of happiness and suffering of varying degrees of intensity over time. However, the local evaluative measure, unlike the global evaluative measure, derives its estimates only from short-term trade-offs involving relatively brief, unvarying, and uninterrupted episodes of happiness and suffering.[9]

The four measures of cardinal intensity need to be distinguished because each has the potential to diverge from the rest. Discussion of important prudential and moral issues can be muddied if people slide unconsciously from one measure to another. In the following discussion I will be concerned to point out the differences between the four measures and to compare the merits of each. For reasons I hope to make clear, I generally favor the intuitive measure, and this is the measure usually employed in the book. But the intuitive measure is not without defects, nor are the other measures lacking in virtues. The distinction between the four different measures will be relevant in subsequent chapters, most particularly chapter 6, where we examine the relative moral importance of happiness and suffering.

I want to emphasize that the rest of this chapter addresses one very specific concept: the intensity of someone's happiness or suffering at a particular time. Intensity is only one morally important dimension of suffering: another is duration, and there may be others as well. Parts of the following discussion may be misunderstood if this specific focus is not borne in mind.

3. The Intuitive Measure

I believe we can make direct intuitive judgments of the proportional intensity of happiness and suffering. What do these proportional judgments mean? It helps to consider some techniques used in the field of pain therapy and research. In order to assess the effectiveness of various treatments, clinicians sometimes ask their patients for cardinal estimates of the intensity of their pain. For example, patients are

9. The rest of this chapter emerged from a long and extensive conversation with Derek Parfit about the meaning and measurement of intensity. Parfit urged me to be clearer about this issue, and it was he who brought to my attention the three measures other than the intuitive measure. The following discussion owes an enormous amount to his challenges and suggestions.

asked to rate the intensity of their pain on a scale from zero to one hundred, or to mark a point on a ten-centimeter line with "no pain" on one end and "pain as bad as it could be" on the other. In other studies patients are asked to say by how great a fraction (one-third, one-half, two-thirds) their pain is reduced by the injection of an analgesic drug. Most patients are able to respond to these kinds of questions with little hesitation.[10] These estimates of pain intensity are best interpreted, I believe, as a statement of how much the pain *hurts*. If one pain is twice as intense as another, it hurts twice as much, and so forth.[11] We can also say that a pain that is doubly intense "feels twice as bad."

I believe the concept of pain intensity gives us a model for thinking about the intensity of suffering. Whereas pain is a particular disagreeable feeling, suffering is disagreeable feeling *on the whole*. Pain may be one feeling among many, and sometimes it is outweighed by feelings of a positive kind, so that a person can experience pain without suffering. Suffering is the state in which the negative feeling exemplified in pain characterizes our feelings on the whole. To assess the cardinal intensity of suffering, we can ask the same sorts of questions used by clinicians to assess the cardinal intensity of pain, with the following difference. Whereas for the purpose of measuring pain intensity we ask how much *it* hurts (that is, the pain), for the purpose of measuring the intensity of suffering we should ask how much *the person* hurts, overall.[12]

When we ask how intensely someone is suffering, then we are asking how much she hurts. One kind of suffering is twice as intense as another if the person experiencing it hurts twice as much, or if she feels "twice as bad." Intensity of suffering, we might say, corresponds to the "immediately felt badness" of the suffering. Similarly, intensity of happiness corresponds to the "immediately felt goodness" of happiness. One kind of happiness is twice as intense as another if it feels "twice as good," and so forth. There is thus an evaluative component to what I am here calling the intuitive measure of intensity. Nevertheless, the intuitive measure needs to be clearly distinguished from the evaluative measure, which I discuss in a later section. On the evaluative measure, to say that one kind of suffering is twice as intense or "feels twice as bad" as another just means that it would be equally bad to undergo two hours of the less intense suffering as one

10. Mark P. Jensen and Paul Karoly, "Self-Report Scales and Procedures for Assessing Pain in Adults," in Denis C. Turk and Ronald Melzack, eds., *Handbook of Pain Assessment* (New York: Guildford, 1992); and Ronald Melzack and Patrick Wall, *The Challenge of Pain* (New York: Basic Books, 1982), pp. 57, 60. Jensen and Karoly report: "Patients are usually able to provide pain intensity estimates relatively quickly," "Self-Report Scales," p. 136.

11. Jensen and Karoly write, "Pain intensity may be defined as *how much* a person hurts" ("Self-Report Scales," p. 136). I prefer a slightly different formulation, for reasons that appear that in the next paragraph. But it's clear that Jensen and Karoly mean the same thing as I do.

12. Pain researchers sometimes distinguish between pain intensity and pain affect. Pain affect has been defined as "the emotional arousal and disruption engendered by the pain experience" (Jensen and Karoly, "Self-Report Scales," p. 143). It might be thought that pain affect corresponds to suffering, but this would be inaccurate. Pain affect refers to the *effect* of pain on a person's overall feeling. But this is different from a direct assessment of the overall feeling itself, which is what suffering refers to. Notice, for example, that suffering can have sources other than physical pain. Pain affect at most refers to the *contribution* of physical pain to suffering.

hour of the more intense suffering. But the intuitive measure keeps the measurement of intensity analytically separate from judgments concerning the optimal balance of suffering of various degrees of intensity over time. On the intuitive measure, saying that it is equally bad to endure two hours of suffering of intensity x as one hour of suffering of intensity $2x$ is a *substantive* claim, which may either be true or false. As I discuss in chapter 6, I lean toward the view that this claim is in fact false, at least where significant intensities are involved. That is, I am inclined to agree with someone who would say that "suffering A feels twice as bad (is twice as intense) as suffering B; however, two hours of B are definitely preferable to one hour of A. Even three or four hours of B may be preferable to one hour of A." Later in this chapter I explain how such a view is possible.

The intuitive measure is different from the evaluative measure, as I define those terms. Nevertheless, as I have said, there is an evaluative component to the intuitive measure, since it records *how bad* a person feels at a particular time. One could be forgiven for wanting to call it the "evaluative measure" (though I reserve that term for something else). I do not intend to have the last word on terminology, and it is possible that further refinements of what I here call the "intuitive" and "evaluative" measures will bring them closer together.

Some people may express skepticism about the existence of a ratio scale that records intuitive judgments of the intensity of happiness and suffering. However, I believe most of us take the existence of such a scale for granted. Compare the suffering typically caused by the application of torture with the suffering of ordinary stomach cramps. Most of us would want to say that the former suffering is not only *more* intense than the latter, but *several times* more intense.

Though we may feel unable to measure cardinal differences in intensity with precision, we are often capable of providing rough estimates. We often feel sure that a cardinal measurement can be correctly described as falling within a certain range. These are what I call *vague* cardinal measurements.

For example, we know that when a major academic failure brings sharp disappointment and a sense of personal inadequacy to an ambitious student, such disappointment may sometimes involve real suffering, but we know that the effective application of torture would in almost every case multiply the intensity of the student's suffering several times over. Even with more information than I have given here, we may be unable to say whether the intensity would differ by a factor of three, or five, or ten, or more. Still, we could assert confidently that the increase in intensity would be no less than, say, 100 percent, or 150 percent.

There are, on the other hand, certain experiences of suffering that we know to be roughly equal in intensity. This is especially the case when the experiences being compared are our own. We may be unable to tell which episode of suffering, if any, is more intense than another, or we may be able to perceive that one is slightly more intense than the other. But in either case, we can state that the intensity of suffering does not vary by more than a certain amount, say 30 percent or 40 percent.

We can also make vague cardinal measurements of the intensity of happiness. (Once more, I remind my readers that I have in mind the hedonistic or Epicurean sense of happiness: happiness as feeling good.) It is hard to produce powerful examples here, because the sources of happiness vary more than those of suffering. Nevertheless, some experiences of happiness stand out for their intensity: the joy that can be awakened, for example, by a personal reconciliation, or the recovery of a loved one from a dangerous illness; the joy that a composer may feel upon creating a beautiful piece of music; the joy that can overwhelm people in the presence of great natural beauty. Here the novelist A. S. Byatt describes the happiest moment in her life: "I found myself alone in this house, and there was total silence, and the sun was absolutely blazing, and I walked up and down the stairs absolutely boiling with the sense that I belonged to myself and could finish any thought."[13] If we compare these sorts of experiences with milder pleasures such as resting in one's chair after a hard day's work, we may decide that the former are several times more intense than the latter. In addition, we can identify episodes of happiness that seem roughly equal in intensity.

There are two ways to interpret vague cardinal measurements. On the first interpretation, a vague cardinal measurement always implies that a precise measurement is possible in theory. Our use of a vague measurement only signifies our uncertainty of what the precise value is. On another interpretation, however, a vague cardinal measurement does not necessarily imply the existence of a precise value. It could be that Smith's suffering is between two and five times more intense than Jones's, without it being the case that Smith's intensity of suffering exceeds that of Jones's by a *precise* factor somewhere between 2 and 5. I shall not try to determine which of these two interpretations is the correct one.

Some people may object that the experience of suffering is too heterogeneous to be conceived as a single magnitude the intensity of which can be measured in cardinal terms. I agree that suffering is highly heterogeneous—experiences of suffering differ along many dimensions besides that of intensity of suffering—but I deny the inference that cardinal measurements of its intensity are meaningless. Once again, it helps to consider physical pain. As medical researchers have stressed, pain, too, is a highly heterogeneous experience. In an article devoted to this topic, R. Melzack and W. S. Torgerson write:

> To describe pain solely in terms of intensity . . . is like specifying the visual world in terms of light flux only, without regard to pattern, color, texture, and the many other dimensions of visual experience. . . . The word 'pain' . . . refers not to a specific sensation which can vary only in intensity, but to an endless variety of qualities that are categorized under a single linguistic label. There are the pains of a scalded hand, a stomach ulcer, a sprained ankle; there are headaches and toothaches. Each has unique qualities. The pain of a toothache is obviously different from that of a pin prick, just as the pain of a coronary occlusion is uniquely different from the pain of a broken leg.[14]

13. "What Possessed A. S. Byatt?," *New York Times Magazine*, 26 May 1991.
14. R. Melzack and W. S. Torgerson, "On the Language of Pain," *Anesthesiology* 34 (January 1971): 50–59.

But although pain varies greatly in quality, it is still plausible to claim that its intensity can be measured in cardinal terms: we can compare experiences of pain differing greatly in kind along a common dimension of overall intensity. (In their article, Melzack and Torgerson assume the existence of this dimension.) This claim gains support from the readiness of most patients to give cardinal estimates of the intensity of their pain. I believe a similar claim is plausible in the case of suffering: experiences of suffering differ along many dimensions, but one of these is the intensity of suffering itself, which can be conceived in cardinal terms. Once again, if we can give cardinal estimates of the intensity of pain, it is plausible that we can do the same for suffering. The only difference is that in the former case we assess a specific feeling, whereas in the latter case we assess feeling overall.

The heterogeneity of suffering is not a good reason for rejecting a common measure of cardinal intensity. But it may lend support to the view that the proportional difference between the intensity of some or perhaps all episodes of suffering is, even in reality, imprecise. Compare the suffering of someone prostrate with grief over the death of her child, and the suffering of another person dying from cancer in great pain. Suppose we know enough to assert that neither person suffers more intensely than the other. Some people would infer from this that the intensity of these people's suffering is exactly equal, but other people may refuse to draw this inference. They may claim that the intensity of the cancer patient's suffering is neither greater than, nor less than, nor exactly equal to the bereaved parent's suffering. These people would claim that if the cancer patient experiences a marginal reduction in the intensity of her pain and the attendant suffering, it would be wrong to conclude that her suffering now becomes less intense than that of the grief-stricken parent. Those who reject precise cardinality, however, can still use a notion of rough or imprecise cardinality. They might judge, for example, that in comparison to the grief-stricken parent's suffering, the cancer patient's suffering is somewhere, say, between 30 percent less intense and 50 percent more intense. As I have said before, rough cardinal comparisons are hard to avoid. That is so either because precise cardinal differences always exist in reality but are hard to locate, or because precise cardinal differences do not (always) exist even in reality. I shall not try to determine which of these explanations is correct, but people who are impressed by the heterogeneity of suffering may incline toward the latter one.

I believe the same remarks apply to happiness. Happiness, like suffering, is highly heterogeneous, but as in the case of suffering, I believe there is a common dimension of intensity that applies to highly dissimilar kinds. The heterogeneity of happiness, like that of suffering, may imply that only rough proportional estimates of intensity are possible, even in principle.

Our use of vague proportional measurements permits us to construct a numbered scale to describe the approximate intensity of different episodes of happiness and suffering. This scale has two parts, separated by a zero point. Distances above zero are proportional to the intensity of happiness. Distances below zero are proportional to the intensity of suffering. I have in mind something like the integer scale of positive and negative numbers, where happiness corresponds to the domain of positive numbers and suffering corresponds to the domain of negative numbers.

One question is whether our proportional judgments of the intensity of suffering presuppose something closer to the ordinary sense of the word, in which we distinguish between suffering proper and a kind of slightly disagreeable feeling (like mild boredom or impatience) that falls short of suffering; or whether they presuppose something closer to the technical sense of the word, which corresponds to the entire range of disagreeable overall feeling. I am unsure of the answer. In this book, the happiness-suffering scale will refer to suffering in the extended, technical sense. Thus the negative numbers begin in the range of slightly disagreeable overall feeling that is ordinarily distinguished from suffering proper. The decision to include slightly disagreeable overall feeling in the negative portion of the scale will make little difference to the measure of the intensity of suffering, except where very mild suffering (in the ordinary, not technical, sense) is involved. This is because in comparison to moderate and intense suffering, the slightly disagreeable overall feeling that falls short of suffering in the ordinary sense is very close to the hedonistic zero.

Now let us see how the happiness-suffering scale can be drawn up. Start with the portion that measures suffering. All we do is take a particular episode of suffering of unvarying intensity and assign its intensity an arbitrary number value. Other intensities of suffering are then assigned number values (which may either be precise or rough) that record the proportional difference between them and the baseline intensity. For example, we might take an episode of mild suffering and give it a value of one. Suffering twice as intense would be given a value of two. Suffering only half as intense would be given a value of one-half. And so forth.

The construction of the happiness intensity scale is analogous to that of the suffering intensity scale. We can assign an arbitrary value to some specific episode of happiness, and then measure the intensity of other episodes of happiness according to the proportional differences between them and the base level.

The difficulty lies in calibrating the suffering scale with the happiness scale. We want the same unit of incremental intensity to apply to the entire scale, so that we can say, for example, that an increase in the intensity of one person's happiness equals or exceeds a decrease in the intensity of another person's suffering. In order to arrive at a common unit of incremental intensity, we need to determine when some episode of happiness equals some episode of suffering in intensity. For if we can do that, we can assign those intensities the same (though opposite) magnitude and calibrate the rest of the scale accordingly.

Though it is impossible to be precise about this, I believe we can form a rough idea of when an episode of happiness and an episode of suffering share an equivalent intensity. To start with, notice that we sometimes judge certain episodes of suffering to be more intense than certain episodes of happiness, and vice versa. The suffering of torture is more intense than the ordinary happiness of spending an evening with one's friends. Byatt's happiness during the happiest moment of her life is more intense than the suffering involved in a mild bout of depression. Now imagine an episode of extreme happiness and an episode of mild suffering. Then imagine that the happiness gradually decreases in intensity until it becomes mild, while the suffering gradually increases in intensity until it becomes extreme. At some point, or over some range, the intensities will cross, whereupon we should say that they are equivalent, or roughly so. It is hard to give a clear example of such a crossing. Suffice it say that if we are unsure whether some episode of happiness is more intense than some episode of suffering or vice versa, this may be evidence of rough equivalency. This could be the case, for example, in a comparison of Byatt's happiness during the happiest moment of her life and the suffering involved in some fairly debilitating bout of depression.[15]

4   The Preferential Measure

In the last section I argued that we can form intuitive estimates of proportional differences in the intensity of happiness and suffering. These estimates reflect nothing more than intuitive judgments of "how good one feels" or "how much one hurts." However, it may be suggested that there are other ways of measuring cardinal intensity that do not rely so directly on intuition, but that tie our estimates of cardinal intensity to people's well-informed, self-regarding preferences, or to our judgments of what makes a person's life go better or worse. Because these alternative measures define cardinal intensity in terms of other concepts, they supply us with a method or algorithm for measuring cardinal intensity. In this section I discuss one of these measures—the preferential measure. In the following two sections I take up the evaluative measure.

The preferential measure is best introduced by some examples. Suppose I could either experience one hour of suffering at a certain intensity x or two hours of suffering at a lower intensity y. If I prefer two hours of the less intense suffering to one hour of the more intense suffering, this shows, according to the preferential measure, that the more intense suffering is over twice as intense as the less intense suffering. Here is another example. Suppose I could either experience five hours at the hedonistic zero, or four hours of happiness at intensity x together with one hour of suffering at intensity y. If I prefer five hours at the hedonistic zero—that is, if I prefer to give up the four hours of happiness in order to avoid the one hour of suffering—this shows, according to the preferential measure, that the intensity of suffering is over four times greater than the intensity of the happiness.

15. One complication that should be mentioned is the sense shared by many people that the intensity of happiness can expand very little in comparison with the intensity of suffering. Adam Smith writes: "What can be added to the happiness of the man who is in health, who is out of debt, and has a clear conscience? . . . Though little can be added to this state, much may be taken from it. Though between this condition and the highest pitch of human prosperity, the interval is but a trifle; between it and the lowest depth of misery the distance is immense and prodigious." *The Theory of Moral Sentiments* (Oxford: Oxford University Press, 1976), I.iii.I.7–8. This view gives support to the theory of diminishing marginal returns that I discuss in chapter 6.

In these examples, we should assume that my preferences are *well informed* and *non-discounting*. Well-informed preferences are those based on an accurate understanding of the alternatives being compared. Non-discounting preferences (or preferences made in the absence of a discount rate) are those that do not assign greater weight to our interests in the near future than to those in our distant future, but instead assign equal weight to our interests throughout the future.

There is an alternative version of the preferential measure that does not refer to alternative distributions of happiness and suffering over time, but rather to probabilities. Suppose that I can choose between a 100 percent chance of less intense suffering, on the one hand, and a 50 percent chance of more intense suffering together with a 50 percent chance of being at the hedonistic zero, on the other hand, where all the durations are the same. If I prefer the first option, this shows, according to the preferential measure, that the more intense suffering is over twice as intense as the less intense suffering. Or suppose that in place of a guaranteed period at the hedonistic zero, I am offered an 80 percent chance of happiness at intensity x together with a 20 percent chance of suffering at intensity y during the same period. If I decline the gamble, this means, according to the preferential measure, that the intensity of the suffering is over four times greater than the intensity of the happiness. In these examples, as in the previous ones, we should assume that my preferences are well-informed and non-discounting.

We can now state the definition of the preferential measure in each of its two versions. The first, non-probabilistic version calculates the cardinal intensity of happiness and suffering in such a way that it is always the case that people's well-informed, non-discounting preferences favor the maximum surplus of happiness over suffering in their own lives, when everything but the pattern of happiness and suffering in their own lives is held equal. The second, probabilistic version calculates cardinal intensity in such a way that it is always the case that people's well-informed, non-discounting preferences favor the greatest *expected* surplus of happiness over suffering in their own lives, other things being equal. In both versions, the relevant quantities of happiness and suffering refer to the product of intensity and duration. The non-probabilistic and probabilistic versions of the preferential measure are mutually compatible. Most of my comments will be addressed to the former, since it is more plausible and easier to discuss than the latter.

Both versions of the preferential measure conflict with observations we are often prepared to make about people's preferences regarding the intensity of happiness and suffering. These observations presuppose intuitive estimates of cardinal intensity. This shows that the preferential measure diverges from the intuitive measure. In fact, as I will argue, the preferential measure and the intuitive measure are concerned with two entirely different things.

I'll begin with the second, probabilistic version of the preferential measure. It calculates cardinal intensity on the assumption that people always seek the maximum expected surplus of happiness over suffering in their own lives, other things being equal. This conflicts with our observation that people can have diverse attitudes toward risks involving happiness and suffering. Recall one of the earlier examples.

If I turn down an 80 percent chance of happiness of intensity x conjoined with a 20 percent chance of suffering of intensity y, the probabilistic preferential measure reports that y is more than four times greater than x. However, we can imagine someone who would decline the gamble even if the happiness and suffering under consideration were *equal* in intensity. One possible reason is that the person has a strong aversion to risks that involve the danger of suffering. To retain the probabilistic measure, either we would have to claim, implausibly, that everyone has a neutral attitude toward risks, or we would have to acknowledge that we are using the concept of cardinal intensity differently from the sense ordinarily employed. In the latter case, our concept of intensity incorporates, or partly reflects, people's dissimilar attitudes toward risks. But then intensity of happiness and suffering seems a misleading term. It would be clearer to use a more flexible term like "cardinal utility."[16] However, there are reasons for doubting that even cardinal utility, flexibly understood, is reliably measured by the probabilistic preferential measure.[17]

Now turn to the first version of the preferential measure. It assumes that people seek the maximum surplus of happiness over suffering in their own lives, other things being equal. But this conflicts with the observation that different people with well-informed preferences may favor *different* distributions of happiness and suffering over time, other things being equal. In order to experience a given amount of happiness, for example, different people will be willing to put up with different amounts of suffering. Some people will be willing to put up with more suffering and others with less.

At least some people will report well-informed preferences on the intuitive measure that are unintelligible on the preferential measure. Recall one of the earlier examples. If I prefer five hours at the hedonistic zero to four hours of happiness of intensity x with one hour of suffering of intensity y, the preferential measure declares that the suffering is over four times as intense as the happiness. However, when I employ intuitive judgments of cardinal intensity as described in the last section, I may genuinely prefer to avoid the four hours of happiness joined with one hour of suffering even if I judged them *equal* in intensity. If such a preference is possible, it shows that the preferential measure diverges from the intuitive measure.

Here it helps to draw a comparison with physical pain. As I have suggested, the cardinal measurement of the intensity of suffering is analogous to the cardinal measurement of the intensity of pain, which has been made the subject of numerous experiments. In none of the studies I have consulted is it suggested that either the experimenters or their respondents linked the cardinal measurement of pain inten-

16. John Harsanyi uses the probabilistic preferential measure to calculate "cardinal utility" in "Morality and the Theory of Rational Behaviour," in Amartya Sen and Bernard Williams, eds., *Utilitarianism and Beyond* (Cambridge: Cambridge University Press, 1982).

17. See the editors' Introduction and articles by Edward F. McClennen and by Daniel Kahneman and Amos Tversky in Peter Gärdenfors and Nils-Eric Sahlin, eds., *Decision, Probability, and Utility* (Cambridge: Cambridge University Press, 1989).

sity to the assumption that people seek to minimize the total duration of their pain multiplied by its intensity. And I would in fact be surprised if many of the respondents made explicit or implicit use of this formula. Thus I would be surprised, for example, if the majority of a group of respondents who were asked to compare the proportional intensity of a more intense pain with that of a less intense pain reasoned to themselves: "I would prefer x hours of the less intense pain to one hour of the more intense pain. Therefore, the more intense pain is over x times more intense than the less intense pain." Indeed one could imagine the respondents forming preferences that flatly contradict the preference-based view. For example, someone might prefer three hours of a moderate pain to one hour of another pain that he judges doubly intense.

I believe that the same remarks apply to happiness and suffering. We could imagine someone who prefers three hours of moderate suffering to one hour of suffering that he judges doubly intense. He may even prefer *ten* hours of the moderate suffering to one hour of the suffering that he judges doubly intense.

Some people may claim that these preferences don't make any sense. To discuss this objection, I shall introduce the following example. On the claims I have been making, we can imagine two dissimilar characters, Bold and Timorous, of whom the following is true when we use the intuitive measure of hedonic intensity. Bold would accept one hour of suffering of intensity x in order to experience four hours of happiness of the same intensity x. Timorous, however, would not. He would rather give up four hours of happiness of intensity x than endure just one hour of suffering of intensity x. The preference attributed to Timorous is not intelligible on the preferential measure, but it is intelligible—so I claim—on the intuitive measure.

Someone may object: if we assume for the sake of argument that the happiness in question really does have the same intensity for Bold and Timorous, the fact that Bold is willing to endure one hour of suffering in order to experience four hours of that happiness, whereas Timorous is not, shows that the suffering in question *cannot* have the same intensity for these two people, on *any* plausible understanding of intensity. The suffering as experienced by Timorous must be *more* intense than the suffering as experienced by Bold. That is what is revealed by Timorous's unwillingness to endure one hour of that suffering even for the sake of four hours of the happiness.

I believe this assertion rests on a fundamental mistake. It is true that Timorous's aversion to a package combining four hours of happiness (of a particular intensity) with one hour of suffering (of a particular intensity) reveals a strong aversion to the one hour of suffering. The assertion in the previous paragraph assumes that Timorous's strong aversion to the one hour of suffering must reflect nothing more than the phenomenological features of the suffering: it is the phenomenological features of that suffering and those features only that are reflected in Timorous's aversion to the one hour of suffering (even when it purchases four hours of happiness). What this assumption misses is that Timorous may have what might be called a *higher-order* aversion to suffering—which is to say, an aversion not fully predicted by the phenomenological features of his suffering alone. We could imagine Timorous saying something of the following sort: "I'm sure that Bold would suffer just as much as I would—even when we take into account variable factors such as hardiness of constitution and emotional fortitude that differently determine the quality of our respective feelings. However, to a greater extent than Bold, I have made it a priority to minimize the amount of suffering I will experience, even if this costs me a substantial amount of happiness." What I am trying to bring out here is the independent and flexible nature of our preferences—something that is not understood by the view I discussed in the previous paragraph.

Recognizing the independence of our preferences with regard to the distribution of happiness and suffering over time allows us to record several familiar contrasts in attitude. We have already met Bold and Timorous, who disagree about trade-offs between the enjoyment of happiness and the avoidance of suffering. Other characters may disagree about trade-offs concerning the duration and intensity of happiness, or the duration and intensity of suffering. Whereas Provident would prefer four hours of moderate happiness to one hour twice as intense, Restless would prefer the reverse. Whereas Tough would choose one hour of fairly intense suffering over four hours half as intense, Fragile would choose the opposite. Restless's preference might be explained by saying that he has a higher-order preference for intense happiness, and Fragile's preference by saying that he has a higher-order aversion to intense suffering.

The same reasons why some people don't want to maximize their *actual* surplus of happiness over suffering can also explain why some people don't want to maximize their *expected* surplus of happiness over suffering. If someone prefers not to maximize her expected surplus of happiness over suffering when this increases the probability of suffering, one reason for her preference may be that she has a higher-order aversion to suffering. Even if in a particular trade-off the suffering feels no more bad than the happiness feels good, she may want to go to greater lengths to avoid the suffering than to experience the happiness. So she will choose to reduce the likelihood of experiencing the suffering even if this reduces her expected total surplus of happiness over suffering.

If we recognize that the intuitive and preferential measures diverge from each other, this leaves us to choose between them. I personally favor the intuitive measure. I shall suggest a number of reasons to favor this measure, but the most fundamental of these is the belief (which I cannot prove, though I have tried to make it plausible) that what the intuitive measure reports really is the intensity of happiness and suffering, whereas what the preferential measure reports really is not. What the preferential measure reports is—our preferences. The following arguments return us, in one way or another, to this guiding idea.

One advantage of the intuitive measure is that it allows us to refer to more aspects of our experience. The preferential measure defines the intensity of happiness and suffering in terms of our preferences. The intuitive measure does not define the intensity of happiness and suffering in terms of our preferences, but treats it as a distinct and independent dimension. I believe this dimension is real. (I have tried to make its reality plausible in this section and the previous one.) If we use the intuitive measure, we can refer to this distinct dimension, and also say everything that would have been reported by the preferential measure, just by reporting the content of the relevant preferences. But if we use the preferential measure, we have no way of referring to the dimension that corresponds to the intuitive measure. Use of the preferential measure obscures an important dimension of our experience. Thus, for example, it conceals what is really involved in the differences between Bold and Timorous, Provident and Restless, Tough and Fragile.

It may be suggested that the preferential measure is better suited to discussions about prudence and morality, since it derives the intensity of happiness and suffering from our preferences, which are morally and prudentially significant. But this suggestion is mistaken in two ways. First, nothing about the intuitive measure prevents us from attributing moral and prudential significance to individual preferences. The fact that the intuitive measure of hedonic intensity isn't *defined* in terms of preferences doesn't hinder us from giving preferences their due weight. Second, the preferential measure, far from improving our discussion of morality, actually lands us in moral trouble. The reason why is that the dimension described by the intuitive measure, which the preferential measure conceals, possesses independent moral significance. Because the preferential measure conceals this dimension, it yields perverse moral implications in certain kinds of interpersonal trade-offs.

Recall Bold and Timorous. On the intuitive measure of intensity, Bold is willing to endure one hour of suffering of intensity x in order to experience four hours of happiness of the same intensity x, while Timorous is not. If we use the preferential measure of intensity, however, this description of Timorous's preference is disallowed. It must be revised. Three kinds of revisions are possible. Speaking of Timorous, we must either say (1) that the intensity of suffering we initially pegged at x is in fact greater than $4(x)$; or (2) that the intensity of happiness we initially pegged at x is in fact less than $1/4(x)$; or (3) that the intensity of suffering is greater than x, and the intensity of happiness is less than x, such that the intensity of suffering is more than four times greater than the intensity of happiness.

Any one of these revisions would have perverse implications in particular trade-offs affecting Bold and Timorous. Consider the first revision: the intensity of Timorous's suffering is in fact greater than $4(x)$. Suppose now that we have to choose between two hours of suffering for Bold or one hour of suffering for Timorous. If we follow the intuitive conception of hedonic intensity (relying on the pre-revision measurements), we should choose one hour of Timorous's suffering. If we follow the preferential conception, however, we should choose *two* hours of suffering for Bold (because this suffering, though twice as long, is less than four times as "intense"). This is perverse. On the intuitive, non-preferential understanding of intensity, this is the *same* intensity of suffering. But we choose to have Bold suffer for two hours rather than Timorous suffer for one. What are we doing? In effect, we are penalizing Bold for his particular preference regarding trade-offs between happiness and suffering.

Now consider the second revision: Timorous's happiness is less than one-fourth as intense as Bold's. Suppose we can either give two hours of happiness to Timorous or one hour of happiness to Bold. If we follow the non-preferential understanding of hedonic intensity (again relying on pre-revision measurements), we should give two hours of happiness to Timorous. But if we follow the preferential view, we should give one hour of happiness to Bold (because his happiness, though, twice as short, is more than four times as "intense"). Again, because on the intuitive conception we are dealing with the same intensity of happiness, this seems perverse.[18] Only this time, it is Timorous who is penalized for his particular preferences regarding trade-offs between happiness and suffering.

Finally consider the third revision: Timorous's intensity of suffering is greater than x (Bold's intensity of happiness/suffering), and his intensity of happiness is less than x, such that his suffering is more than four times as intense as his happiness. Now because Timorous's suffering is more than four times as intense as his happiness, either his suffering is more than twice as intense as x, or his happiness is less than one-half as intense as x, or both of the above. In either case, we encounter perverse moral implications in certain interpersonal trade-offs affecting Bold and Timorous, for the same kind of reasons described in the two previous paragraphs.

These kinds of interpersonal trade-offs show us the irreducible moral significance of the intuitively estimated, non-preferential dimension of hedonic intensity. If we want to discuss individual preferences, we need to refer to them as a separate dimension. This is precisely what the preferential measure prevents us from doing, by collapsing both dimensions into one.

Before closing this section, I shall address one final argument for the superiority of the preferential measure. The intuitive measure, it may be pointed out, makes it appear that people sometimes prefer to suffer *more* rather than *less*, and sometimes prefer *less* happiness to *more*. Recall our characters Fragile and Restless. The intuitive measure allows us to say of Fragile that he prefers four hours of moderate suffering to one hour doubly intense, while it allows us to say of Restless that he prefers one hour of intense happiness to four hours half as intense. If we calculate the quantity of happiness and suffering by multiplying intensity by duration, the intuitive measure implies that Fragile prefers more suffering to less, while Restless prefers less happiness to more. This, however, is an odd implication that we can avoid by adopting the preferential measure.

This argument is not as decisive as it sounds. (For simplicity, I shall limit my response to the case of suffering; the parallel response regarding happiness is easily imagined.) It is true that in ordinary speech we tend to assume that, other things being equal, people desire to reduce their suffering, and never to increase it. However, we need to identify the usual context and meaning of this assumption. For

---

18. Or rather I should say: perverse, if we believe that under these circumstances it is right to maximize overall happiness. A strict egalitarian might prefer to minimize the difference in happiness between Bold and Timorous. However, a strict egalitarian would also find the application of the preferential view perverse, though for different reasons. On a non-preferential conception of hedonic intensity, a strict egalitarian, applying pre-revision measurements, would award one hour of happiness to Bold. The preferential view, however, would dictate giving two hours of happiness to Timorous. From the strict egalitarian perspective, *this* is perverse.

one thing, when we talk about reducing or increasing suffering, we typically imagine a simple kind of change. If we talk about a reduction in someone's suffering, for example, we usually imagine a reduction of intensity without an increase in duration, or a reduction of duration without an increase in intensity, or a reduction of both duration and intensity. In these simple comparisons, it is just as true on the intuitive measure as it is on the preferential measure that people always prefer to suffer less rather than more, other things being equal. (The only exception is comparisons that involve variations in timing: e.g., changes in sequence, or temporal concentration versus dispersal of suffering. But these comparisons are rarely imagined either.) To the extent we are imagining the simpler kind of comparison, the assumption that people always prefer to suffer less rather than more does not favor the preferential measure over the intuitive measure.

There may be occasions when we are aware of a complicated contrast in which dimensions such as intensity and duration vary in opposite directions and yet we still assume that, other things being equal, people will prefer whichever option "reduces" or "minimizes" their suffering. But when we make this assumption, seemingly quantitative words like *reduce* and *minimize* may not be referring to the mathematical product of intensity and duration. In our ordinary speech, we often give these words an evaluative meaning. If we say, for example, that one alternative brings a person "less" suffering than another, we may just be expressing a global evaluative judgment that the suffering it contains is less bad to undergo. If we assume that people's well-informed preferences regarding happiness and suffering always indicate what is best for them, we can safely assume that, other things being equal, people always prefer to suffer less rather than more, provided we use the words *less* and *more* in the evaluative sense just described. On this interpretation, the assumption conflicts neither with the preferential nor the intuitive measure of hedonic intensity.

The assumption that people always prefer less suffering to more, other things being equal, becomes untrue on the intuitive measure only when it refers to the product of intensity and duration, and is applied to all imaginable cases. However, I do not think that the assumption understood in *this* way is deeply ingrained in our thought, and thus I do not think there is any great cost to giving it up. Whatever cost there may be is outweighed by the enhanced clarity of the intuitive measure of hedonic intensity.

5. The Global Evaluative Measure

As an alternative to both the intuitive and preferential measures, some people may propose an evaluative measure. As I mentioned before, this measure comes in two versions. In this section I shall discuss the global version, which is the most direct counterpart of the preferential measure. In the next section, I discuss the local version, which seeks to repair some of the difficulties of the global version.

The global evaluative measure is structurally similar to the preferential measure, though different in content. Recall that the preferential measure calculates the cardinal intensity of happiness and suffering in such a way that it is always the case that people's well-informed, non-discounting preferences favor the maximum total surplus of happiness over suffering in their own lives, other things being equal. The global evaluative measure calculates the cardinal intensity of happiness and suffering in such a way that it is always *better* for individuals to experience the maximum total surplus of happiness over suffering, other things being equal. Whereas the preferential measure refers to individual preferences regarding the distribution of happiness and suffering, the global evaluative measure refers to an *objective* judgment about what makes people's lives go better and worse.

Suppose that I could either experience two hours of less intense suffering or one hour or more intense suffering. If it is better for me to experience two hours of the less intense suffering, then, according to the global evaluative measure, the more intense suffering is over twice as intense as the less intense suffering. Or suppose that in place of five hours at the hedonistic zero, I could experience four hours of happiness at intensity x with one hour of suffering at intensity y. If it is better for me to experience five hours at the hedonistic zero, this shows, according to the global evaluative measure, that the suffering is over four times as intense as the happiness.

In the last section I argued that the preferential measure of intensity diverges from the intuitive measure of intensity. Does the global evaluative measure also diverge from the intuitive measure? How we answer this question depends on whether we think that, on the *intuitive* measure of hedonic intensity, it is always better for an individual, other things being equal, to experience the greatest possible surplus of happiness over suffering. This is a substantive moral question, which lies beyond the purview of this chapter. In chapter 6 I shall claim that the answer to this question is no. For now let us just note that *some* people (such as me) think that the answer to this question is no, and that when *these* people measure the intensity of happiness and suffering, their global evaluative estimates will diverge from their intuitive estimates. Suppose Fragile thinks that four hours of moderate suffering are better than one hour of suffering that is only twice as intense on the intuitive scale. If Fragile uses the global evaluative scale, he must say that the more intense suffering is, not twice as intense, but over four times as intense. In Fragile's opinion, therefore, the global evaluative measure diverges from the intuitive measure.

Here some people may object: How can Fragile claim on the intuitive measure that four hours of moderate suffering are better than one hour of suffering that is only twice as intense or that "feels only twice as bad"? Doesn't Fragile's evaluative ranking show that, in his judgment, the more intense suffering feels over four times worse—is over four times as intense? This objection echoes one from the previous section in casting doubt on the independence of the intuitive measure; my reply shall resemble the one I gave before. What the objection misses is the possibility that people may form *higher-order* judgments about the advisability of pursuing happiness and avoiding suffering. Fragile may believe that one kind of suffering "feels only twice as bad" as another, but that the necessity of avoiding it is over twice as great. If judgments like Fragile's are correct, then judgments about the advisability of pursuing happiness and avoiding suffering cannot be automatically equated with the intrinsic quality of the relevant feelings. There is some independence of the former from the latter.

The same kind of higher-order judgments that apply to trade-offs involving more intense and less intense suffering may also apply to trade-offs involving happiness and suffering. Some people's higher-order judgments may tell them that it can be more important to avoid suffering than to attain happiness of equal intensity. Thus Timorous may believe that it is better to avoid one hour of suffering at a certain intensity than to gain four hours of happiness at the *same* intensity.[19]

This discussion shows that different senses can be given to the word *bad*. (Similarly for the word *good* applied to happiness.) In discussing a particular kind of suffering, we can refer either to its "immediately felt badness" or to its "overall prudential badness." In claiming that the global evaluative measure may diverge from the intuitive measure, I am claiming that these two senses of "bad" may also diverge.

The distinction between these two senses of the word *bad* is clearest when we consider the views of those who claim that suffering is not intrinsically evil. These people claim that we have no reason to avoid suffering itself, but they can hardly deny that suffering feels bad, for that is what it means to suffer! They simply make a distinction between immediately felt badness and overall prudential badness. That suffering feels bad, they claim, is no reason why we should avoid it. We can certainly understand this view, even if we think it is seriously mistaken.[20]

On the view that Fragile holds and that I shall later endorse, a distinction is once again made between immediately felt badness and overall prudential badness. However, Fragile and I put the distinction to an opposite use from that of the ascetics described in the previous paragraph. Whereas the ascetics claim that suffering lacks intrinsic prudential badness notwithstanding its immediately felt badness, Fragile and I claim that the prudential badness of suffering is *disproportionate* to its immediately felt badness. Judgments of overall prudential badness can diverge from

---

19. It is in this vein that Schopenhauer quotes Petrarch's line, "A thousand pleasures are not worth one pain" (*The World as Will and Representation*, vol. 2, E. F. J. Payne, trans. [New York: Dover, 1958], p. 576). Schopenhauer alters the poet's meaning, since Petrarch intended the romantic claim that one pain (in loving Laura) is worth *more* than a thousand pleasures. (See Sonnet 231.)

20. On what Thomas Hurka calls pure perfectionism, there is no intrinsic value to pleasure and pain: "From a perfectionist standpoint, pleasure and pain can appear to be mere biological signals of good and poor functioning—indicators of what has moral importance, but not significant in themselves" (*Perfectionism* [New York: Oxford University Press, 1993], p. 190). Some Christian theologians are led to deny the intrinsic evil of suffering in their effort to solve the problem of evil. Bentham discusses an extreme version of asceticism, according to which pleasure is actually bad and pain good (*The Principles of Morals and Legislation* [Buffalo: Prometheus, 1988], chap. 2, pp. 9–13).

judgments of immediately felt badness, and they can diverge in either of two directions.

As I have argued, some people's normative views will lead them to record different estimates of intensity on the global evaluative measure than on the intuitive measure. In chapter 6, I will claim that the correct normative view does indeed entail this divergence. Consequently, it makes a difference which measure we choose. Is one of them preferable to the other?

My own preference lies with the intuitive measure. Perhaps the main reason (the importance of which becomes more salient in chapters 6 and 7) is that the intuitive measure appears to me to do a better job of showing what is really involved in higher-order judgments about the undesirability of suffering, and intense suffering in particular. I believe that the global evaluative measure obscures what is involved in these higher-order judgments, because it folds them into the measurement of intensity itself.

This may not strike some people as a decisive criticism. However, the global evaluative measure faces other difficulties. One of these stems from the fact that the global evaluative measure, if it is to avoid perverse moral implications, must be non-preferential. That is to say, it cannot make the truth of what is better or worse for a person depend, even partially, on the person's own preferences. Recall Bold and Timorous. On the intuitive measure of intensity, Bold's well-informed preferences favor one hour of suffering of intensity x with four hours of happiness of the same intensity x over five hours at the hedonistic zero. Timorous's well-informed preferences run the other way. Some people may be inclined to say that here Bold's well-informed preferences determine what is best for Bold, while Timorous's well-informed preferences determine what is best for Timorous. But if we believe this, the global evaluative measure requires us to adjust the intensity estimates for Timorous so that his suffering is more than four times as intense as his happiness. And if we do this, we open the way to the perverse moral implications described in the last section.

An adherent of the global evaluative measure is therefore obliged to hold the view that the goodness or badness of alternative patterns of happiness and suffering cannot vary with individual self-regarding preferences. I happen to favor this view, but I lack a conclusive argument for it. The view is controversial, and it therefore seems to me an awkward feature of the global evaluative measure that it obliges one to hold it. It is bizarre to have the *concept* of intensity roped together with the view that individual preferences cannot alter the value of individual patterns of happiness and suffering. It is odd that someone who denies this view is disqualified even from *discussing* the intensity of happiness and suffering. The view should not be enforced by definitional fiat; it should be defended on substantive grounds.

I believe this constitutes a serious objection to the global evaluative measure. However, there are even more serious difficulties. The global evaluative measure makes it impossible to ask certain important moral questions. One such question is whether the order in which happiness and suffering (or more and less intense suffering) succeed each other can affect the value of the overall pattern. For example:

given an episode of happiness of a particular intensity and duration, and an episode of suffering of a particular intensity and duration, is it worse for the suffering to follow the happiness rather than vice versa? If we use the global evaluative measure of intensity, this question is unintelligible: there is no way of *conceiving* that the sequence, in itself, makes a difference, since the product of intensity and duration, by definition, contains the whole truth about value. However, this is a genuine moral question, about which people have intelligibly disagreed. (My own view is that sequence, in itself, does not affect value.)

It is important to avoid confusion here. If a painful experience follows a joyful experience rather than vice versa, and the person is aware throughout the sequence of what lies in store, his happiness may be diminished by the anticipation of suffering, and his suffering aggravated by his not being able to look forward to happiness.[21] Awareness of the future (and perhaps the past) can affect the quality of our experiences. But this fact is different from the claim that sequence *in itself*—that is, apart from its psychological effects—alters value. It is the latter idea that the global evaluative measure can't successfully accommodate.

Compare the two sequences, happiness-then-suffering and suffering-then-happiness, where the quality and duration of the suffering, similarly of the happiness, are the same in either sequence. (Imagine that we somehow prevent or cancel any differences caused by anticipation of the future or recollection of the past.) The global evaluative measure can't successfully accommodate the idea that the first sequence is worse than the second, unless we try saying that the *mere fact* that suffering follows happiness renders the suffering more intense or the happiness less intense. But that's an odd thing to say. Surely the intensity of happiness or suffering depends on what it is like at the time, and is not affected by the *mere fact* of what occurs at other times.

Another important moral question concerns the chronological concentration of suffering. Imagine suffering of a particular unvarying intensity and a fixed total duration. Does combining the suffering into one uninterrupted period make it worse than it would be if it were scattered over time and interspersed with islands of relief? Some people may believe that the answer to this question is yes. Consider childbirth, where a mother experiences intense pain during contractions and relief in between; one may think that her pain is significantly less bad than a somewhat briefer cumulative duration of equally intense suffering gathered into one uninterrupted period. (I say "equally intense suffering" advisedly; we must factor in the possibility that the pain of labor contractions is mitigated by the consciousness of imminent though temporary relief.) Some people may think, in other words, that the temporal concentration of suffering sometimes makes that suffering worse. This is a view which merits serious consideration, whether or not we decide to accept it. (In a later chapter, I examine the view at length and remain undecided whether or not to accept it.)

21. As Milton says of Satan, cast out of heaven into hell: "his doom / Reserved him to more wrath, for now the thought / Both of lost happiness and lasting pain / torments him."

On the global evaluative measure of intensity, however, the view is simply incoherent. If the badness of suffering equals the product of intensity and duration, then the temporal concentration of suffering cannot in itself alter its disvalue. It may help to look at an example. Compare (on the one hand) two hours of continuous suffering at intensity x, with (on the other hand) one hour of continuous suffering at intensity x, followed by one hour of continuous relief at the hedonistic zero, followed by one hour of continuous suffering at intensity x. Assume that the second alternative is just twice as bad as one hour of continuous suffering. If, as some are inclined to think, the first alternative is worse than the second alternative, this means that two hours of uninterrupted suffering are more than twice as bad as one hour of uninterrupted suffering. That idea can't be accommodated on the global evaluative measure of intensity. We might try saying that when the uninterrupted suffering lasts two hours the intensity during the first hour is higher than it would be if the suffering lasted only one hour. But that can't be right. Surely the intensity of the suffering at any point during the first hour must be a function of what it is like at the time and can't be affected by what does or does not happen in the future.

As the preceding discussion has shown, the global evaluative measure of intensity rules out a number of important moral questions. This inflexibility is a good reason, I think, for rejecting the global evaluative measure.

The underlying problem, in my view, is that the global evaluative measure proceeds from the wrong direction. It begins by asking us to judge the overall value of an individual's pattern of happiness and suffering; from that judgment it then derives an estimate of the intensity of the person's happiness or suffering at a particular time. It adopts what we might we call a bird's eye view of intensity. For discussing the intensity of happiness and suffering, I believe that a worm's eye view is more appropriate. We should calculate intensity by looking directly at the relevant experience, without any preconceptions about how its intensity contributes to the value of the larger pattern. The worm's eye view (which I associate with the intuitive measure) permits us to consider a variety of views regarding the ways in which intensity, duration, and timing affect the value of different patterns of happiness and suffering.

One argument for the global evaluative measure is that it preserves the result that it is always better, other things being equal, for a person to experience more happiness rather than less, and less suffering rather than more. On a different measure of intensity—say, the intuitive measure—we might have to give up this claim. I shall later maintain that on the intuitive measure we *should* give up this claim, if quantity refers to the product of intensity and duration. But (it may be argued) that would be strange. It would be strange to think that it can be better, other things being equal, to experience less happiness rather than more, or to suffer more rather than less.

For reasons offered in the last section, I do not find this a decisive argument. Though in our ordinary speech we often assume that it is better to suffer less rather than more (or to experience more happiness rather than less), we often have in mind simple comparisons in which the claim remains true on several different measures of intensity, including the intuitive measure. Moreover, phrases like "more suffering" and "less suffering" are often intended in an evaluative, non-quantitative sense; "more suffering" may just mean "suffering that it is worse to undergo." The idea that the badness of suffering (or goodness of happiness) corresponds directly to the product of intensity and duration is not, I think, implicit in our ordinary speech.

6. The Local Evaluative Measure

The global evaluative measure, I have argued, prevents us from asking certain important questions. To overcome this defect, some people may propose a variant of the global evaluative measure, which I shall call the local evaluative measure.

Both the global evaluative measure and the local evaluative measure make use of the idea that it is better, other things being equal, to experience the greatest possible surplus of happiness over suffering. I shall call this the maximization thesis. (The preferential measure, which holds that we always *prefer* the greatest total surplus of happiness over suffering, makes a maximization assumption of a different kind.) The global evaluative measure stipulates that the maximization thesis is *always* true. The local evaluative measure stipulates, more modestly, that the maximization thesis is true where relatively short, unvarying, and uninterrupted episodes of happiness and suffering are involved.

Suppose we want to compare two kinds of suffering, one more intense than the other. If five uninterrupted minutes of the more intense suffering are worse than twenty uninterrupted minutes of the less intense suffering, this means, according to the local evaluative measure, that the more intense suffering is over four times as intense as the less intense suffering. Or suppose that we want to compare happiness of a certain degree of intensity with suffering of a certain degree of intensity. If twenty minutes of the happiness together with five minutes of the suffering are worse than twenty-five minutes at the hedonistic zero, then according to the local evaluative measure the suffering is over four times as intense as the happiness.

I have some of the same misgivings about the local evaluative measure as I do about the global evaluative measure. Like the global evaluative measure, the local evaluative measure obscures what is involved in higher-order judgments about the undesirability of suffering and of intense suffering, by collapsing them into the measurement of intensity itself. And like the global evaluative measure, it preemptively rules out the view that the value of alternative patterns of happiness and suffering can be altered by people's self-regarding preferences.

In the last section, I criticized the global evaluative measure on the grounds that it prevents us from asking certain important questions: namely, whether changes in sequence and temporal concentration can affect the value of alternative patterns of happiness and suffering. The local evaluative measure appears designed in such a way that we can ask these questions. But the local evaluative measure is not as much of an improvement in this regard as it initially appears. It is less inflexible than the global evaluative measure, but it is still too inflexible.

To begin with, it is hard to see how the local evaluative measure can be neutral on the question of whether the sequence of happiness and suffering affects the value of the overall pattern. To compare the intensity of happiness with that of suffering, we need to ask how much suffering it is worth experiencing for the sake of a given amount of happiness, and we can only imagine the suffering preceding the happiness or vice versa. Some people may think that the sequence can affect the value of the overall package. But this thought is ruled out by the maximization thesis.

This problem arises for the local evaluative measure when we compare happiness to suffering, though not when we compare happiness to happiness or suffering to suffering. That's because in order to compare the intensity of two different kinds of suffering, or happiness, we don't need to imagine one following the other. We just ask at what point the prolongation of the less intense suffering would make it worse than the more intense suffering, or at what point the prolongation of the less intense happiness would make it better than the more intense happiness.

The global evaluative measure prevented the thought that the temporal concentration of suffering sometimes makes that suffering worse. The local evaluative measure doesn't exactly prevent this thought, because it applies the maximization thesis only to uninterrupted suffering. But the local evaluative measure admits the view about concentration only at a cost. One would think that on any evaluative measure of intensity, the overall prudential badness of suffering is directly proportional to the intensity of suffering, when other factors are held constant. One would think, for example, that if suffering x is four times as intense as suffering y, then five minutes of suffering x are four times as bad, prudentially, as five minutes of suffering y. The association of intensity with badness presumably forms part of the rationale of the evaluative measure. However, if we want to be neutral on the question of temporal concentration, we must be prepared to abandon this association. We must be prepared to say, for example, that where suffering x is only four times as intense as suffering y, it may be over four times as *bad*.

Why is this? If the temporal concentration of suffering sometimes makes that suffering worse, then (as we saw in the last section) the badness of uninterrupted suffering can be disproportionate to its duration. Thus twenty uninterrupted minutes of suffering y may be *more* than four times as bad as five uninterrupted minutes of suffering y. The local evaluative measure tells us that if five uninterrupted minutes of suffering x are equal in badness to twenty uninterrupted minutes of suffering y, then x is four times as intense as y. But if twenty uninterrupted minutes of y are over four times as bad as five uninterrupted minutes of y, then five uninterrupted minutes of x will also be over four times as bad as five uninterrupted minutes of y.

The reason for this odd result is that the local evaluative measure uses variations in duration to calculate intensity. This would be less problematical if we could assume that badness is directly proportional to duration. But if the relation is not directly proportional, then the local evaluative measure of intensity partly reflects the *independent* impact of variations in duration. This suggests that the local evaluative measure is not as narrowly focused as it ought to be. It, too, admits the distortions of the bird's eye view. It seems better, for purposes of measuring intensity, to focus exclusively on the quality of the experience at a particular time, without referring to other dimensions such as duration or timing.

There are other, related problems. The local evaluative measure tells us that a certain kind of suffering is equal in intensity to a certain kind of happiness, if five minutes of the happiness are worth exactly five minutes of the suffering. (By this I mean that there would be no difference in value between experiencing five minutes of the happiness with five minutes of the suffering, on the one hand, and experiencing ten minutes at the hedonistic zero, on the other.) Now suppose we think that twenty uninterrupted minutes of the suffering are over four times worse than five minutes of this suffering. We might also think twenty uninterrupted minutes of the happiness are *not* over four times *better* than this happiness. The local evaluative measure, however, disallows this combination of views. For on this set of views, twenty minutes of happiness at intensity x are not worth twenty minutes of suffering at the same intensity x—a claim which is unintelligible on the local evaluative measure.[22] The local evaluative measure permits the view that the badness of uninterrupted suffering can be disproportionate to its duration, only under a rather stringent condition. The condition is acceptance of the view that at all levels of intensity the badness of suffering is disproportionate to its duration by the same ratio, and that the goodness of happiness, at all levels of intensity, is disproportionate to its duration by this ratio also. I believe this makes the local evaluative measure too inflexible.

In the last section I argued that the global evaluative measure is too inflexible because it prevents the thought that the badness of suffering is disproportionate to its duration. The local evaluative measure allows this thought, though only with the proviso that the goodness of happiness must be disproportionate to its duration by the same ratio as the badness of suffering is disproportionate to its duration. Even then, the thought is allowed only under the strain of decoupling the intensity of suffering from its badness. This seems to me to be an intolerable strain. If one thinks that the badness of suffering can be disproportionate to its duration, there doesn't seem to be much point in using the local evaluative measure.

I have presented several criticisms of the evaluative measure of intensity, in both its global and local versions. One can imagine that, under certain circumstances, the weight of some of these criticisms would be reduced. Use of the evaluative measure would be less problematic if one thought there was good reason to believe that the

---

22. Someone might reply that this claim is not unintelligible on the local evaluative measure. On the local evaluative measure, it may be claimed, the maximization thesis does not apply to twenty-minute units, but only to shorter periods of time. But the story I have told about extending five minutes to twenty minutes could also be told about extending one minute to five. To get around the problem I have identified, the local evaluative measure would have to specify a particular unit of time to which the maximization thesis uniquely applies. It would no longer be the "local evaluative measure," but the "one-minute evaluative measure," say, or the "thirty-second evaluative measure." I assume that no one would be drawn to such a measure.

value of individual patterns of happiness and suffering *cannot* be altered by variations in individual preference, sequence, or temporal concentration. But notice that in order to defend this belief one would need to use the language of the intuitive measure, because only that measure permits the alternative possibility to be comfortably expressed. One would have to start out with the intuitive measure before switching over to the evaluative measure. Any advantages we associate with consistent usage would weigh in favor of using the intuitive measure throughout. Notice, too, that if we believe that value is unaffected by sequence or temporal concentration, there is no longer a significant difference between the global evaluative measure and the local evaluative measure, and consequently no reason for preferring the latter to the former. Finally, the circumstances I have mentioned as possibly mitigating certain criticisms of the evaluative measure do not touch my central objection: namely, that the evaluative measure obscures what is involved in the higher-order undesirability of suffering.

7. Conclusion

In the bulk of this chapter I have examined four different ways of conceiving the cardinal intensity of happiness and suffering: the intuitive measure, the preferential measure, the global evaluative measure, and the local evaluative measure. I have dwelled on the difficulties inherent in the last three.

The intuitive measure is not without difficulties. The comparative estimates it allows us to make are vague; perhaps they are never better than extremely vague. But I believe this limitation is unavoidable. It doesn't reflect a defect in the measure used, but rather the inherent difficulty of measuring suffering. It is worth pointing out that the preferential and evaluative measures will also be vague to the extent that our preferences and evaluations are vague or uncertain, or both.

It may be thought that the intuitive measure faces difficulties not shared by the other three. There may be outright skepticism about the existence of the dimension that it presupposes. At least, there may be skepticism that any such common dimension exists for feelings of happiness and suffering that differ sharply in content. I have tried to allay such skepticism in section 3, but some may remain unconvinced.

The skepticism may run strongest with regard to comparisons between happiness and suffering. It may be thought that there is no way of comparing the intensity of happiness with that of suffering except on the terms laid out by the preferential and evaluative measures. I do not share this skepticism. It seems to me that one can have a sense, however vague and imperfect, of the extent to which the "immediate felt goodness" of an experience of happiness compares in intensity or degree to the "immediately felt badness" of an experience of suffering—a sense that is prior to and independent of judgments about what duration of the suffering is worth putting up with for the sake of a fixed duration of the happiness. Like Schopenhauer (mis)quoting Petrarch ("one thousand pleasures are not worth one pain"), I believe that one can distinguish an assessment of the inherent magnitude of different episodes of happiness and suffering from a higher-order judgment that the avoidance of suffering is more important than the pursuit of happiness.

In most of the subsequent discussion, unless otherwise noted, I shall have in mind the intuitive measure when discussing the cardinal intensity of happiness and suffering. This is partly because of my belief that the other measures are burdened by difficulties that outweigh any difficulties associated with the intuitive measure. It is partly because of the related belief that the intuitive measure allows us to focus more clearly on a number of important issues. And partly it is for the simple reason that I am most used to thinking in terms of the intuitive measure—it is in terms of this measure that I have pondered these questions for many years.

I will sometimes refer to the other three measures. We need to be aware that the same substantive views may be expressed very differently depending on which measure is used. We should also keep in mind that certain influential discussions of happiness and suffering may have presupposed one or more of the three alternative measures; ignoring this possibility could lead us to serious misinterpretations of those discussions. But there is also a virtue in sticking primarily to one measure. Doing so allows a clearer story to be told. The story that lies ahead will be told primarily in terms of the intuitive measure of cardinal intensity.

FOUR

The Moral Significance of Suffering

1. The Personal and Impersonal Badness of Suffering

The underlying claim of this book is that the badness of suffering, in the particular way that it is bad, gives rise to a prima facie duty to prevent suffering. I develop this claim in chapter 5. In this chapter, I prepare the way by examining certain questions relating to the badness of suffering.

The claim that we have a prima facie duty to relieve suffering can be seen as resting on three assertions. First, suffering is bad for the individual who experiences it. Second, suffering is bad from an impersonal perspective. Third, the impersonal badness of suffering implies a prima facie duty on our part to prevent suffering. This chapter is concerned with the first two claims.

The first claim is that suffering is bad for the individual who experiences it. To be more precise: suffering is an *intrinsic* bad for the individual who experiences it. This claim needs to be carefully distinguished from two other claims, both of which are true, and neither of which is incompatible with it. These are the claims that suffering can be instrumentally good and that it can be instrumentally bad. Suffering is instrumentally good when it enables the sufferer to attain a genuine good such as virtue or wisdom. It is instrumentally bad when it deprives the sufferer of a good or exposes him or her to a different sort of evil: for example, when it disables the person from achieving some valuable goal.

What I claim is that suffering is intrinsically evil for the individual who experiences it—evil in itself. I'm afraid I have no argument for this claim. This doesn't strike me as a great embarrassment, since few moral claims appear to me more certain. Rather than argue for this claim, I shall simply assert it, and hope that enough of my readers agree.

If there is resistance to this claim, it may be tied to the view that suffering has an improving effect on us. It makes us wiser or more virtuous or cleanses us morally.[1] I have two things to say in reply. First, not all suffering makes us better. How is an abused child or a tormented animal improved by her suffering? Much suffering makes us worse. It makes us bitter or vengeful or manipulative or crazy, or renders impossible the activities and experiences that *would* improve us.

Second, if suffering sometimes makes us better, that doesn't disprove the claim that suffering is bad for us in itself. It is important, as I have mentioned, to distinguish the intrinsic evil of suffering from whatever instrumental value it may possess.

We can distinguish between two kinds of reformative suffering. *Educative suffering* is that which makes us wiser or more virtuous. An example of educative suffering is a painful emotional crisis that causes us to reflect on our previous life, amend past faults, and alter our priorities. *Redemptive suffering* is that which, when we have committed a grave moral crime, functions (it is claimed) as an indispensable element of our moral regeneration. The theory is that, without this kind of suffering, the criminal cannot become good again.

Literature is filled with examples of educative suffering. Both tragedy and comedy narrate the painful learning of valuable lessons. And we can think of many real-life people who attribute important wisdom to painful crises in their past. Redemptive suffering, memorably discussed in the novels of Dostoevsky, is more mysterious. Why do we think that a criminal must suffer in order to become good again? One reason may be that such suffering is indispensable to the criminal's understanding of the nature of what he has done. He must understand the great wrong he has committed, and such understanding cannot be genuine unless it is accompanied by suffering—by a certain self-loathing; by a certain anxiety, which feels it can never be allayed, to be restored to the condition of goodness; and by an overwhelming regret of what has occurred. The criminal who can preserve equanimity in spite of what he has done is lacking in a kind of knowledge that he, above all people, ought to possess: the knowledge that he has done wrong. This explanation makes redemptive suffering closely related to educative suffering. But there may be deeper, more metaphysical reasons for the redemptive power of suffering.

There is value connected to both kinds of reformative suffering, but the value does not reside in the suffering itself. In the case of educative suffering, it derives from the close causal connection between suffering and the important goods of knowledge and virtue. Suffering can be the necessary means to valuable knowledge and enhanced virtue—or an unavoidable consequence of whatever else produces those goods. Perhaps the overall package is worth having; perhaps the knowledge and virtue are worth their cost in suffering. But the suffering *is* a cost. In itself, it seems to me, it cannot be seen as anything other than evil.

1. The latter idea is a theme in several spiritual traditions, notably Christianity. In St. Paul's words, "We also boast in our sufferings, knowing that suffering produces endurance, and endurance produces character, and character produces hope" (Rom. 5.3–4).

The case is more easily made with respect to redemptive suffering. For our belief in the potentially redemptive character of suffering depends precisely on the view that suffering is an evil to the person who experiences it. The criminal must pass through evil in order to become good again. So again, although suffering may lead to consequences that are desirable on the whole, suffering in itself must be viewed as evil.

Though intrinsically evil, educative and redemptive suffering may sometimes be worth having, all things considered. But in deciding whether reformative suffering is worthwhile, we must guard against the temptation to falsify. In too many discussions of reformative suffering, the suffering itself is minimized or even forgotten. We hear about its *meaning* and *point*—aspects that are often discovered only retrospectively. The consciousness of subsequent benefits is somehow imposed on our recollection of the experience itself. We become like veterans who bask in wartime memories while managing to forget their bewilderment, discomfort, pain, and terror. The actual experience leaches out and is replaced by a precipitate of a different composition, disguised in the form of the original, but wholly unlike it in substance.

I have asserted that suffering is bad for the individual who experiences it. To this assertion, I add another: that suffering is bad from an impersonal perspective. Suffering isn't bad only for the sufferer. It is bad, period. The prevention of suffering is an improvement, not just from the perspective of the individual whose suffering it is, but an improvement in the state of the world.

Once again, I find myself without an argument. I don't know what I could say in support of a claim that seems so self-evidently true. This matter is eloquently discussed by Thomas Nagel, and I would not be able to improve on what he says.[2] I take comfort in Nagel's admission that he, too, finds the impersonal badness of suffering self-evident.

Those most likely to deny the impersonal badness of suffering are those who deny the very possibility of impersonal values. But attention to suffering makes it hard to preserve skepticism about impersonal values. That is why Nagel begins his defense of impersonal values with the example of pain.

When I assert that suffering is bad from an impersonal perspective, I mean (as before) that it is intrinsically bad. From an impersonal perspective, suffering, though intrinsically bad, may be instrumentally good. It may make good things possible. Indeed, from the impersonal perspective, it may be a price worth paying for the good things that it makes possible.

There may be doubts, however, that suffering is on *all* occasions an intrinsic evil, impersonally viewed. These doubts need to be taken seriously. The strongest of these doubts are connected to common attitudes toward punishment. Most people think that it is right to punish criminals for the crimes they have committed, and

2. *The View from Nowhere* (New York: Oxford University Press, 1986), pp. 159–62.

punishment is normally thought to entail suffering. Belief in the appropriateness of punishment might seem to presuppose the view that the suffering of the criminal, in consequence of his crime, is a good thing from the impersonal point of view.

That needn't be the case, however. There are, I believe, three main arguments for punishment. The first defends punishment as a means of deterring crime. Punishment frightens the criminal from committing future crimes, and it deters others from following his example.[3] Those who justify punishment as a means of deterrence usually add that criminal guilt is a necessary condition of legitimate punishment: one should never "punish" an innocent person, even as a means of deterring crime. A deterrent justification of punishment is compatible with the view that suffering is always evil in itself. It is bad for the wrongdoer to suffer, but we should nevertheless punish him in order to avert greater evils in the future. Some of those who subscribe to the deterrent justification of punishment may still distinguish between the suffering of the guilty and the suffering of the innocent. Though suffering visited on the guilty as punishment is to be regretted in itself, it is less bad than suffering, of equivalent intensity and duration, endured by the innocent. Perhaps this thought helps shore up the prohibition on "punishing" the innocent. But to judge the suffering of the guilty as less bad than the suffering of the innocent, other things being equal, is not (or not necessarily) to judge it a positive good.

A second argument for punishment is to say that it *benefits* the criminal. Plato takes this position in the *Gorgias*.[4] Punishment repairs the damaged soul of the criminal; it is a medicine that restores him to moral health. The most sense I can make of this view is that it attributes educative and redemptive powers to punishment. But then, as we saw above, the criminal's suffering is not good for its own sake; it is good as a means of moral regeneration.

The third argument for punishment cites the need for retribution: whether or not deterrence is achieved, criminals should be punished because that is what they deserve. The moral appropriateness of retribution can be understood in two different ways. Some retributivists, like Kant, see punishment simply as a matter of duty; others, like G. E. Moore, regard it as a *good thing*.[5] Kant's view doesn't necessarily contradict the claim that suffering is always evil (though it does contradict the notion that we always have a duty to relieve suffering), whereas Moore's view seems to contradict it directly. Notice that Moore's view, in contrast to Plato's, retains and indeed emphasizes the thought that punishment harms the criminal. For Moore, the value of punishment *depends on its being an evil to the criminal*. It is *good* that he

---

3. Punishment can have the added function of incapacitating the criminal. Strictly speaking, this function is distinct from deterrence, since one can imagine forms of incapacitation that are not unpleasant. (Think of being confined to a luxury resort.)

4. See also Jean Hampton, "The Moral Education Theory of Punishment," *Philosophy and Public Affairs* 13 (1984): 208–38. Reprinted in A. John Simmons, Marshall Cohen, Joshua Cohen, and Charles R. Beitz, eds., *Punishment* (Princeton, N.J.: Princeton University Press, 1995).

5. Immanuel Kant, *The Metaphysics of Morals*, trans. Mary Gregor (Cambridge: Cambridge University Press, 1991), pp. 140–45; G. E. Moore, *Principia Ethica* (Cambridge: Cambridge University Press, 1903), p. 214.

endure evil in payment for his crime. There is here a sharp distinction between personal value and impersonal value. The criminal's suffering, though bad for him, is good from the impersonal perspective.

Of the various justifications for punishment, only a view of Moore's kind obliges us to say that the suffering of the guilty is impersonally good. If we adopt this view, then we must say that suffering is not *always* evil from an impersonal perspective: the suffering of the guilty provides us with at least one exception. Some readers may be drawn to such a view. For my part, I confess to finding something perverse and inhumane in a view that, acknowledging someone's suffering to be an evil to that person, nevertheless converts it into a good thing. I also suspect that the view is nourished by certain feelings, like the desire for revenge, that should not be accorded moral authority, though they often appear in moral dress.[6]

Suppose we agree that suffering is both a personal and an impersonal evil. (Some people will want to make an exception in the case of retributive suffering.) What factors determine the *degree* of suffering's badness? I shall assume that the badness (both personal and impersonal) of an individual's suffering varies with intensity and duration. The question is whether other factors also affect the badness of individual suffering. (I postpone the question of aggregation: that is, how to evaluate the suffering of more than one person.)

It is sometimes suggested that suffering resulting from human cruelty is intrinsically worse than suffering that arises naturally, or accidentally, or as a side-effect of people's actions. It is true that deliberately inflicted suffering generally seizes our attention and horrifies us more than other kinds. However, there are a number of ways to explain this reaction without positing an intrinsic moral difference between suffering that is and is not caused by human cruelty.

For one thing, we are appalled by the wickedness of the perpetrator. There may be several reasons why this should be so; at least one of them is the duty to relieve suffering itself. If someone by an act of cruelty causes another person's suffering, he presumably had the power not to. Moreover, his behavior is presumably susceptible in some degree to the influence of other people's reaction to it—their condemnation, approbation, or indifference, not to mention material forms of punishment or reward. To deter him in the future, and those who may be inclined to imitate

6. One source of retributivism, I have often thought, is the unacknowledged hope of canceling past crimes—of making it the case that they never happened. When we punish a criminal with imprisonment, physical violence, or death, we unequivocally trample and suppress the will that had lately asserted itself with such grievous consequences. If now we have such utter control over the criminal that we can hurt him *at will*, and he is powerless to resist or retaliate, then surely it *cannot* have been true that just a short while ago he had *us* at *his* mercy, and that through stealth and violence he was able to plot and carry out our damage. Punishment effects such an utter reversal of the previous relation of the criminal to his victim—or to society at large inasmuch as it identifies with the victim—that the former situation now seems implausible and unreal, the idea of it laughable and absurd. Perhaps, then, the crime and the suffering or damage it caused never happened. Or so we think, in our unconscious.

him, we may make him feel the heat of our displeasure. Beyond that, we can declare that there is an intrinsic evil residing not only in the suffering he causes, but also in the very *act*, the *intention* leading to it. We can announce that he is *wicked* to have acted as he did, and we can try to bring him to a state where that wickedness is something he fears. Needless to say, this deterrent strategy works much less well against human actions that lead to suffering unintentionally, and it does not work at all against natural causes of suffering such as earthquakes, storms, viruses, and falling trees.

Because cruelty is a source of suffering against which social punishment and condemnation is especially effective, our heightened fear of it is well-invested. Fear increases our vigilance, and vigilance insures that we will punish it more swiftly and more consistently. If we directed the same kind of fear and vigilance toward other kinds of suffering, we would be using our emotional energy and our attention inefficiently.

There is another, less commendable factor behind our vigorous repudiation of cruelty. Cruelty is only one of several human attitudes causally linked to suffering. Another harmful attitude is indifference, which causes us to overlook our indirect contributions to suffering and weakens our determination to prevent it. But cruelty, unlike indifference, is a disposition from which most of us fancy ourselves immune. And because it seems foreign, it is easier to condemn. We prefer to condemn those dispositions that seem furthest from our character, whereas if the harmful disposition is one that we recognize in ourselves, we are likely to soften our criticism or suspend it entirely.[7]

In one respect, deliberately inflicted suffering *is* worse than other kinds, but the reason is not the distinction itself. It is that, when other factors are more or less equal, deliberately inflicted suffering is so much more *intense* than other kinds. We are social creatures. We come to expect and depend on the help of other people. When under normal conditions we are struck down by suffering, we are sustained by the hope that other people will come to our aid and remove our pain. The influence of this hope in mitigating our suffering, and sometimes dispelling it entirely, can scarcely be exaggerated. But when other beings do not act to relieve our suffering, but are themselves the source of it, our hope is turned directly on its head. It is not just withdrawn, it is metamorphosed into its opposite. Every unconscious expectation of being helped stands revealed to us for the first time in the moment of its being directly contravened. It is brought forth, exposed, and mocked.[8] The helping human presence on which we had counted has become a tormenting presence. And our fear is redoubled by the knowledge that the agent of our suffering is not some blind and haphazard force of nature, but a determined, consistent, and

---

7. "Most people have a considerable amount of indulgence towards all acts of which they feel a possible source in themselves, reserving their rigour for those which, though perhaps really less bad, they cannot in any way understand how it is possible to commit." John Stuart Mill, "Nature," in *Collected Works of John Stuart Mill*, vol. 10 (Toronto: University of Toronto Press, 1969), p. 401.

8. See the passage from Améry's *At the Mind's Limits*, quoted in chapter 2, n. 52.

self-knowing human will. It is this—the suspension of hope and the hammered concentration of fear—that makes deliberately inflicted suffering such a deserving object of our terror.

I am skeptical that there is an intrinsic moral difference between deliberately inflicted suffering and other kinds.[9] However, some people may argue that suffering arising from the cruelty of other people belongs in a larger category that does possess intrinsic moral significance. Usually when we are the victims of other people's cruelty, our suffering is in no sense self-inflicted. And some people will claim that there is a moral distinction between suffering that victims bring on themselves and suffering that they cannot reasonably be expected to avoid. Thus suffering caused by inflated ambitions, profligate habits, or risky behavior should be viewed differently from suffering caused by inherited poverty, bad luck, or unjust treatment. Suffering where the victim need not and ought not to have adopted the attitude or taken the action that led to his suffering is just not as bad as other kinds are.

We do react differently to these two categories of suffering. The question is how we ought to make sense of this response. On one view, there is no intrinsic moral difference here. The suffering is equally awful in either case, at both the personal and the impersonal level. Even if we adopt this view, however, there are good reasons—drawn once more from the duty to relieve suffering generally—why we should extend greater sympathy and help to those who could not reasonably be expected to have avoided their predicament. Suffering is an evil, and we must do what we can to prevent it. People must be discouraged from incurring suffering through their own folly and vice. They must be especially discouraged from perpetuating it when the means of ending it lie within their own power. If we give them the expectation that we will rush to their aid whenever they land themselves in trouble, or extend their own misery, we will continue to promote their wasteful and irresponsible behavior; and we will, moreover, be forced to neglect many of those whose suffering cannot be avoided by their own efforts. It is best to give people an incentive to prevent their own suffering and to give priority of assistance to those unable to do so.

On another view, there is an intrinsic moral difference: suffering is morally less bad when responsibility for it can be traced back to the victim. This view finds a natural home in a moral outlook that stresses our role as agents and not merely subjects of positive and negative experiences.[10] Such an outlook values our ability to shape our own lives. It values a state of affairs in which, as Will Kymlicka puts it, our fates are determined by our own choices rather than circumstances external to us.[11] While this outlook need not go so far as to call self-induced suffering a

9. This is not to deny that evil is involved in the *infliction* of suffering.

10. See Christine M. Korsgaard, "Personal Identity and the Unity of Agency: A Kantian Reply to Parfit," *Philosophy and Public Affairs* 18 (1989): 101–32, p. 101. Reprinted in Korsgaard, *Creating the Kingdom of Ends* (Cambridge: Cambridge University Press, 1996), p. 363.

11. *Contemporary Political Philosophy* (Oxford: Clarendon Press, 1990), p. 56. For an excellent discussion of the overall issue, see George Sher, *Desert* (Princeton, N.J.: Princeton University Press, 1987).

positive good, it may hold that suffering that arises through the victim's own imprudence or carelessness, and is therefore in some sense chosen, is *less bad* than suffering that is imposed by forces beyond the victim's control, and is therefore in no sense chosen. The extent to which we discount the evil of self-induced suffering largely depends, I think, on the degree to which we emphasize the moral importance of agency.[12]

There is another factor that may affect the badness of an individual's suffering—not at the personal but at the impersonal level. This is the factor of distributive justice. Other things being equal, suffering may be worse—worse from the impersonal perspective—when it befalls someone whose life has gone worse overall. An episode of suffering of a certain intensity and duration may appear worse if it is added to a life already characterized by misery and deprivation, than if it is added to a life otherwise characterized by happiness and accomplishment. This idea lies behind the intuition that it is worse to pile up a fixed sum of suffering in one person's life than to spread it out among several. I pick up this theme in chapters 6 and 7.

I have discussed a number of factors that have been thought to affect the badness of suffering. Other factors might be examined, for people seem to find many grounds for deeming some forms of suffering morally less serious than others. In general, I think we need to be careful not to let a certain stinginess creep into our judgments. When people deem certain kinds of suffering "less significant," often the real reason is an inner conviction that *they* would not suffer with anything like equal intensity in the same situation. But this reason incorporates an inexcusable bias toward the speaker's own psychology. We must not care only about afflictions to which our own personalities render us susceptible.

Some people may say that the *background* of a person's suffering has a role in determining how bad it is. Suffering in the context of deprivation is worse than suffering in the context of plenty. So, for example, we should not view the passing boredom, frustration, disappointment, or embarrassment of a prosperous businessman who enjoys every material comfort in the same way as we view the harrowing plight of a street person. The plight of the street person, we are urged, is worse.

Here it is important to distinguish between different issues. First, we might see the street person's suffering as worse because he has experienced more suffering in his life as a whole. This raises the issue of distributive justice, to which I alluded earlier.

Second, a plausible reason for thinking that the street person's suffering is worse is just that it is more intense. Remember that we are interested not just in surface feelings, but the overall state of feelings. We should expect that the businessman

---

12. Of course there is the question of *how much* of the victim's suffering is ultimately his fault. Here there is the broadest possible spectrum of views—everything from the position that denies the existence of free will, to views like the Christian teaching that our suffering is punishment for Adam's disobedience, in which we all participated, or the Hindu doctrine that our suffering is recompense for misdeeds in previous lives.

enjoys a solid psychological substratum of security, comfort, and self-esteem. Even in the worst crises, he has deep reserves of hope and self-esteem on which he can draw. The street person, however, must wage a constant struggle for survival and comfort. His self-esteem sinks from his continual awareness of the contempt, fear, and revulsion he inspires in other people. He is exposed to dangers, hardships, and humiliations that are hard for us even to imagine.

Someone might say, however, that what makes the street person's suffering worse is not just the greater intensity of his suffering. What also makes it worse is that it takes place in the context of extreme material deprivation. I think that there is an important claim here, but it needs to be expressed more clearly. The claim is not that the street person's deprivation is a feature internal to his suffering that makes it worse qua suffering, regardless of intensity. The claim is that material deprivation is a feature external to suffering that is morally significant in its own right. This is no longer a question of the moral distinction between different *kinds* of suffering, but rather a question of whether the badness of suffering adequately accounts for the badness of deprivation. I take up this issue in the final section of this chapter, after considering some general issues concerning well-being and ill-being and taking another look at the badness of suffering.

2. The Desire Theory of Well-being

Suppose we think that suffering harms those who experience it. Are there other evils that can befall a person? If so, what are they, and how should we balance them against suffering? What are the positive goods of life, and how do we balance them against life's evils? How in general do we determine what makes a person's life go better or worse?

I believe that an adequate answer to these questions must take a pluralist form. There are different kinds of harms and benefits, which cannot all be reduced to one ultimate value. The most fruitful work in value theory in recent years has come from philosophers working to develop and refine pluralistic accounts of the good.[13]

13. Among the most important treatments are Elizabeth Anderson, *Value in Ethics and Economics* (Cambridge, Mass.: Harvard University Press, 1993); John Finnis, *Natural Law and Natural Rights* (Oxford: Clarendon Press, 1980); James Griffin, *Well-being: Its Meaning, Measurement, and Moral Importance* (Oxford: Clarendon Press, 1986); Thomas Nagel, "The Fragmentation of Value," in *Mortal Questions* (Cambridge: Cambridge University Press, 1979); Nagel, *The View from Nowhere*; Martha Nussbaum, "Human Functioning and Social Justice: In Defense of Aristotelian Essentialism," *Political Theory* 20 (1992): 202–46; Thomas M. Scanlon, "The Moral Basis of Interpersonal Comparisons," in Jon Elster and John E. Roemer, eds., *Interpersonal Comparisons of Well-being* (Cambridge: Cambridge University Press, 1991), and "Value, Desire, and Quality of Life," in Martha Nussbaum and Amartya Sen, eds., *The Quality of Life* (Oxford: Oxford University Press, 1993); Amartya Sen, *Commodities and Capabilities* (Amsterdam: North-Holland, 1985); and Sen, *Inequality Reexamined* (New York: Russell Sage, 1992). Another important account is Thomas Hurka, *Perfectionism* (New York: Oxford University Press, 1993). Hurka limits his discussion to the examination of one overarching good—human perfection—but his account of perfection embraces diverse elements, and he allows the possibility that human perfection may need to be combined with other values in the most adequate theory of the human good.

If these philosophers have erred, it is, I believe, in not attaching sufficient importance to the badness of suffering. (Nagel, who gives it prominence in some of his writings, is a partial exception.)

The obvious difficulty with pluralistic theories is vagueness. There is not only the difficulty of specifying a complete and accurate list of goods, but also of knowing how to balance different values against each other. This is a problem that even the best pluralistic theories have not avoided. The vagueness of pluralistic theories may make monistic theories seem attractive by comparison. Monistic theories seem to leave no loose ends; they always allow us, in principle, to measure someone's level of well-being by determining how well he or she scores on the one ultimate value. However, the most eligible monistic theories of well-being are not, in the end, very plausible. And as Amartya Sen remarks, "It is better to be vaguely right than precisely wrong."

In this section and the next, I examine two monistic theories—the desire theory and the theory of value hedonism—that might seem congenial to a view that gives prominence to the badness of suffering. I draw on the work of a number of contemporary philosophers to argue that neither theory is very satisfactory. I then argue that although suffering is not the sole evil that can befall us, we tend nevertheless to underestimate its moral importance.

Many people are drawn to the view that how well-off someone is depends on the extent to which his or her desires are satisfied. For example, the harmfulness of a person's suffering depends on the strength of her desire to get rid of it; whether it is worse for someone to experience suffering or evil of another kind depends on which she would rather avoid; and so forth. On closer examination, however, this view needs to be qualified. And once we have made the necessary qualifications, we emerge with an account of well-being in which desire plays a much reduced role.[14]

Economists and those influenced by them sometimes identify well-being with the satisfaction of desires that people are conscious of having. This is implausible, since people's conscious desires can be mistaken in obvious ways. They can be based on false beliefs, as when I want to cross a bridge not knowing that it will fall under my weight. They can also be based on introspective failure, as when I pursue a career in medicine, not grasping until the end that what I really wanted all along

---

14. There are many criticisms of the desire account in the recent literature. See, for example, Anderson, *Value in Ethics and Economics*, pp. 229–40; Jon Elster, "Sour Grapes—Utilitarianism and the Genesis of Wants," in Amartya Sen and Bernard Williams, eds., *Utilitarianism and Beyond* (Cambridge: Cambridge University Press, 1982); James Griffin, "Against the Taste Model," in Elster and Roemer, eds., *Interpersonal Comparisons of Well-being*; Warren Quinn, "Putting Rationality in Its Place," in *Morality and Action* (Cambridge: Cambridge University Press, 1993); Scanlon, "The Moral Basis of Interpersonal Comparisons" and "Value, Desire, and Quality of Life"; Amartya Sen, "Rational Fools: A Critique of the Behavioral Foundations of Economic Theory," *Philosophy and Public Affairs* 6 (1977): 317–44; Sen, *Commodities and Capabilities*; and Cass R. Sunstein, "Preferences and Politics," *Philosophy and Public Affairs* 20 (1991): 3–34. The frequency of these criticisms is testimony to the allure of the targeted view.

was to win the approval of my parents, and that there were cheaper and more effective ways of doing this.

To avoid the problem of mistaken desires, many value theorists propose that well-being should be identified not with the satisfaction of desires that people consciously have, but rather with the satisfaction of desires they *would* consciously have if they formed their desires on the basis of full and accurate information, sound logic, and clear self-understanding. The move from actual to well-informed desires can be justified in one of two ways: either as a move to people's *true* desires (what they really want, whether or not they are conscious of wanting it), or on the grounds that only well-informed desires count for purposes of moral evaluation.

The move to well-informed desires does not get rid of our problems, however. Here is a problem noted by Allan Gibbard.[15] We can imagine that I might have a well-informed desire for a situation in which many people are rescued from extreme suffering even though I suffer a modest diminution of my overall well-being. But we cannot make room for this idea unless we grant that the fulfillment of certain well-informed desires does *not* redound to the good of the desirer.

It is not plausible to claim, in response to this example, that I must be mistaken in claiming that I become worse off when the other people are rescued from extreme suffering. As Gibbard writes, "Even if I am made miserable by the misery of others, that may not be my sole reason for wanting them to be happy. . . . A person may really want others to be less miserable, and not simply be made less miserable by their misery. In that case, he may prefer a policy that he knows will leave him less well off than some alternative, simply because it will be much better for others."[16]

If we are defending a desire-based theory of well-being, we might try to get around this problem in a number of ways. To rule out my desire for other people's well-being, we could decide to exclude morally motivated desires. But it is possible that I might prefer the greater well-being of others not because of a moral motivation—not, for example, because I think the resulting outcome is more just, or because I think it is my duty to seek such an outcome. I might be moved by sympathy alone—by the mere desire to spare other people from extreme suffering.

Alternatively, we could exclude desires that refer exclusively to other people's interests and include only those that pertain to our own. But what, then, *are* our interests? This question is dangerously close to the one we started out with. It does not seem much of an advance to explain well-being in terms of interest. To avoid this kind of circle, we could identify well-being with the satisfaction of desires that, in Nagel's phrase, lie "closest to home": desires that concern the longevity, health, happiness, liberty, power, and self-respect of the desirer, and the success of his or her core projects. But by now, it seems to me, we are already distancing ourselves

---

15. Gibbard, "Interpersonal Comparisons: Preference, Good, and the Intrinsic Reward of a Life," in John Elster and Aanund Hylland, eds., *Foundations of Social Choice Theory* (Cambridge: Cambridge University Press, 1986), p. 173. See also L. W. Sumner, *Welfare, Happiness, and Ethics* (Oxford: Clarendon Press, 1996), pp. 133–35.

16. Gibbard, "Interpersonal Comparisons," p. 173.

from the desire account. We have begun to characterize well-being in terms of a list of particular goods. We might claim that desire is still a *necessary condition* of well-being: unless I desire my own health, for example, it is not good for me. But many people will find this implausible. And even if we make such a claim, it is important to note that desire is no longer doing all the work. In order for something to benefit me, I must desire it *and* it must be the right kind of object. We leave our account of well-being incomplete if we do not specify what kinds of things are potential bearers of value.

One of the main deficiencies of a desire account is that it offers a poor basis for interpersonal comparisons.[17] On the desire account, an individual is better-off than she otherwise would be if her desires are realized more fully. But how do we determine whether one person is better off than another? How can *individual* desires furnish comparisons of well-being across persons?[18]

It might be suggested that we can derive interpersonal comparisons from a desire account if we equate relative well-being with one's relative feeling of satisfaction: someone is worse off than another if he is more strongly dissatisfied with his situation, if he has a stronger desire to exchange his present situation for something else. But this approach leads us badly astray. Recall the example in chapter 2 of the ambitious businessman on the one hand and the abused child and the depressed person on the other. As I argued there, it is not hard to imagine circumstances in which the businessman, though suffering far less than the abused child or the depressed person, has a much stronger preference for his promotion than the abused child and the depressed person have to be removed from their respective conditions. The businessman, in his raging ambition, may have let his desire for the promotion swell into an obsession. Yet we can imagine that he does not suffer very much, perhaps not at all, because he forms his desire against a background of health, material comfort, underlying self-esteem, and love and respect by others, blessings that sustain his overall state of psychological well-being, though he takes them so completely for granted that he pays them little notice. Meanwhile, the battered child, though suffering intensely from the treatment she receives, may fail, for any number of reasons, to form a strong preference for the termination of her abuse. She may not be aware that a better situation is possible for her. She may be hindered from imagining better situations, let alone forming preferences for them, simply because her mind is so fully occupied by thoughts of her own wickedness or naughtiness. And as we noted in chapter 2, severe clinical depression is often characterized

17. See Torbjörn Tännsjö, "Classical Hedonistic Utilitarianism," *Philosophical Studies* 81 (1996): 97–115, p. 113, n. 2. Here I revisit a theme discussed in chapter 2, sections 3-4.

18. This problem helps explain why economists, who often construe well-being in terms of desire, sometimes use Pareto criteria to compare the value of alternative outcomes involving several people. Pareto criteria allow us to rank alternative outcomes without interpersonal comparisons of well-being. Outcome A is Pareto superior to outcome B if there is at least one individual who fares better in A than in B, and no one who fares worse in A than in B. The obvious problem with Pareto criteria is that they leave so many alternatives unranked—all the alternatives in which at least one person fares better and at least one person fares worse.

by the inability of its victims to form strong preferences about anything. Some depressed people do not even realize that they are suffering from depression or sadness. Instead they are consumed by thoughts of their own worthlessness.

If we measured people's ill-being by the strength of their desire to be rescued from their predicaments, we would get the ludicrous result that the battered child and the depressed person are better off than the frustrated businessman. Many other contrasts like the one above could be described. One factor often at play is that people who have come to expect continued suffering by dint of long experience may tame their desire for happiness in order to avert too much disappointment, whereas those who have come to expect a certain fairly high level of happiness may be furious when temporarily deprived of it. Thus when we guide our judgments of ill-being by the strength of people's desires for improvement, we favor the pampered at the expense of the deprived.

A better test of relative ill-being is to ask the people whose experiences are being compared which they would rather avoid, provided they have an accurate and vivid understanding of each of the alternatives. This saves us from reaching a wrong judgment in the example discussed above. Presumably, the businessman, the child, and the depressed person, if they were offered the choice, would all prefer to be the businessman. (Notice, though, how hypothetical this is, since in real life the depressive quite possibly and the abused child almost certainly would not be competent to make the comparison.)

This method, though an improvement over measuring ill-being according to subjective dissatisfaction, still faces problems. Because people's preferences can conflict, the method will sometimes yield indeterminate results. Suppose we are trying to decide who is worse off: Smith experiencing some form of safe inactivity (let's call it X) or Jones experiencing some form of dangerous activity (which we'll call Y). If we ask them which they would prefer to avoid, Smith might prefer to avoid X while Jones prefers to avoid Y. Even if we asked them to put themselves in each other's shoes, so that they ask whether they would rather avoid being *Smith* experiencing X or *Jones* experiencing Y, their preferences might still conflict, because of contrasting higher-order preferences. Smith might have a special loathing for enforced inactivity, and Jones might have a strong aversion to dangerous activity. Smith might compare enforced inactivity as experienced by herself to danger as experienced by Jones and still, because of her higher-order preference for activity, prefer Jones's experience to her own. Whereas Jones making the same comparison might, because of a higher-order preference for safety, prefer *Smith's* experience to her own.[19]

James Griffin's informed desire account in *Well-being* gets around this problem by emphasizing that the relevant preferences must be based on an adequate understanding of the alternatives. If Smith and Jones saw matters clearly enough they would recognize the intrinsic desirability of both security and activity. And if they clearly beheld the particular alternatives in question—a particular experience X involving safe inactivity and a particular experience Y involving dangerous activity—

---

19. See Gibbard, "Interpersonal Comparisons," pp. 175–78; and Griffin, *Well-being*, pp. 108ff.

they might both decide that in this case, the benefits of activity outweigh those of security so Y is preferable to X. (Or they might both decide the reverse.) On the other hand, individual differences between Smith and Jones may rule out such a simple judgment. Though Y is normally better than X, Jones may be so prone to terror that Y is not a good bargain for her. But then the reason doesn't lie in the simple fact that she prefers X to Y. The reason is that, because of her psychological makeup, the normal benefits of Y are not available to her, or such benefits are paired, to an abnormal degree, with the evils of anxiety. Now we can return to the original question: If Smith prefers Y to X, and Jones prefers X to Y, who is worse off, Smith experiencing X, or Jones experiencing Y? According to Griffin, the answer is reached by assessing the goods and evils potential in either experience, and the degree to which Smith and Jones, given their individual characteristics, have access to the goods and are vulnerable to the evils. We compare the intrinsic desirability and undesirability of the features of X-as-experienced-by-Smith with the intrinsic desirability and undesirability of the features of Y-as-experienced-by-Jones. We may then be in a position to conclude that, all things considered, one of these experiences is less bad than the other.

Griffin solves the indeterminacy problem, but only because he moves far away from the ordinary conception of a desire-based theory of well-being. He explains well-being less in terms of individual preferences than in terms of the intrinsic value of certain outcomes. In fact, though he professes to be an informed desire theorist of well-being, he winds up developing a pluralistic theory of the good. He offers a list of prudential values that he thinks constitute the essential interests of all people: accomplishment, autonomy, basic physical capacity, liberty, understanding, enjoyment, and deep personal relations.[20] Griffin is reluctant to privilege intrinsic value over desire at the deepest level of justification.[21] So one might say that his theory of well-being is rooted in what we *ultimately* desire, whether or not we realize it. But notice that Griffin would not have told us very much if he had ended his account there. He needed to spell out the substance of his theory of the good in order to make his meaning clear. The most helpful theory of the human good equates our well-being with a list of particular goods, rather than the content of our desires, whatever they may be.

3. Value Hedonism

But perhaps we shouldn't be too ecumenical in drawing up our list of goods. According to the school of value hedonism—which includes Epicurus, Bentham, and Sidgwick—there is only one intrinsic good and only one intrinsic evil. They are, respectively, happiness and suffering. Other things are good only insofar as they

---

20. Griffin, *Well-being*, p. 67.
21. See Ibid., pp. 26–31.

lead to happiness or reduce suffering, and evil only insofar as they lead to suffering or diminish happiness.

We can distinguish between two kinds of value hedonism. *Classical value hedonism* holds that happiness and suffering are equally important from a moral point of view. What I call *negative value hedonism* holds that suffering carries greater moral significance than happiness, so that the alleviation of suffering takes precedence over the promotion of happiness. In a later chapter I defend the priority of suffering over happiness. But for the time being I put this question aside.[22] Classical and negative value hedonists agree that only happiness is intrinsically good and only suffering is intrinsically bad. Value hedonism has attracted many critics, and they can claim a solid ally in common sense. The critics assert that there are other intrinsic goods besides happiness,[23] including knowledge, liberty, virtue, friendship, and life itself. The value of these goods cannot be reduced to their tendency to promote happiness or prevent suffering. The proof is that these goods often appear worth having, even if we must sacrifice some happiness in order to attain them. We think that a life in pursuit of the truth can be worthwhile, even if it increases our suffering. We think that turbulent liberty can be better than comfortable slavery. Nozick's famous experience machine is intended to show that happiness can't be the *sole* intrinsic value.[24] Imagine that by connecting your brain cells to a special machine you could detach yourself from reality and lead an imaginary existence characterized by much greater happiness than what you would experience in real life. Most people recoil at the idea of plugging themselves in. This shows, in Nozick's words, that "we want to *do* certain things" and "to *be* a certain way" and, not least, to preserve contact with reality.

When value hedonists are told that we value other things besides happiness, they typically respond that such views result from intellectual confusion. The confusion is of two kinds. First, the alleged non-hedonic intrinsic goods are *generally* correlated with happiness. They tend to produce happiness. For example, we desire knowledge, and so are happy to get it; it also increases our power to obtain other ends we have. Liberty is generally a prerequisite of happiness, since it enables us to pursue our chosen goals and protects us from harm by other people. And so on. We thus tend to form a close association in our minds between happiness and these other things. But often the association falls beneath the level of consciousness. This leads us to ascribe an independent value to these other things, whereas if we reflected with sufficient care, we would see that their value stemmed entirely from the happiness they make possible. Of course, these other things do not *always* cause happiness; sometimes indeed they produce suffering. But this only shows that mental associ-

22. The question is quite complex, as I show in chapter 6. One problem is determining to what extent classical value hedonists and negative value hedonists are divided by substantive and not merely verbal disagreement.

23. To simplify discussion, I shall sometimes use the term "happiness" in its expanded sense, to refer not only to the achievement of positive happiness, but also the alleviation of suffering.

24. Robert Nozick, *Anarchy, State, and Utopia* (New York: Basic Books, 1974), pp. 42–45.

ations can be very crude, and fail to leave room for exceptions. Consciously or unconsciously, we associate these other things with happiness, even if they do not always bring happiness. This causes unreflective minds to assert that they are valuable even when they do not bring happiness.

Second, we may confuse *moral* requirements to seek knowledge, protect liberty, respect life, and the like with the claim that these things are good in themselves. But the moral requirement to safeguard these things need not derive from their being intrinsically good. We can have a duty to seek knowledge, because, armed with knowledge, we are better able to help other people. We can have a duty not to invade someone's liberty, simply because of the respect we owe her as an autonomous being, or, to use an indirect consequentialist justification of the kind often favored by value hedonists, because the protection of liberty leads to the greater happiness of both the individual and society over the long term. But it is hard to distinguish the moral injunction to protect or secure something from the thought that it is intrinsically good. So because we acknowledge duties to protect life, liberty, knowledge, and other essential goods, even when they do not lead directly to happiness, we easily slip into the thought that these things are good independent of their tendency to promote happiness.

Value hedonists can develop arguments of considerable sophistication. But the more I reflect on things such as knowledge, liberty, and accomplishment, the more implausible value hedonism appears. Griffin states the case very well. Of knowledge, he writes, "Simply knowing about oneself and one's world is part of a good life. We value, not as an instrument but for itself, being in touch with reality, being free from muddle, ignorance, and mistake." Of liberty, "Choosing one's own course through life, making something out of it according to one's lights, is at the heart of what it is to lead a human existence. And we value what makes life human, over and above what makes it happy. . . . Even if I constantly made a mess of my life, even if you could do better if you took charge, I would not let you do it." Of accomplishment, "We all want to do something with our lives, to act in a way that gives them some point and substance."[25]

Virtue, too, seems an intrinsic good—or at least a good whose value cannot be explained in hedonistic terms. When someone commits a terrible crime, it is hard to avoid the thought that something has gone dreadfully wrong with his life. We wonder whether it can be put back together. This has nothing to do with whatever guilt or punishment the criminal may subsequently suffer. (Indeed some may believe that the absence of guilt compounds the evil, and that guilt prepares the way for moral regeneration.)

Then, too, there is the value of life. Classical value hedonism implies that the prolongation of life is a benefit only if what is added contains a positive surplus of happiness over suffering. (Negative value hedonism implies that even with such a surplus, additional life is a harm, unless the ratio of happiness to suffering is sufficiently great.) Yet this seems to understate the value of life. It seems odd to say

25. Griffin, *Well-being*, pp. 67, 64.

(as classical value hedonism implies) that longevity becomes a harm the moment that the surplus of happiness over suffering dips below zero. (In the case of negative value hedonism, the implausibility is only heightened.) Something seems to have been left out. At least one reason for valuing life is that it makes possible the *non-hedonistic* goods of experiencing the world and of acting in it.[26] Reflection on the value of life doubly undermines value hedonism: value hedonism sometimes under-represents the value of life, and it does so because life includes other goods besides happiness. (I return to the question of life and death in chapter 6.)[27]

4. Underestimating the Evil of Suffering

Suffering is not the only intrinsic evil. (Nor is happiness the sole intrinsic good.) Nevertheless, I believe that most of us tend to underrate the evilness of suffering. The reason is that it is difficult for us, when not actually suffering, to recollect what suffering really is. We employ numerous psychological mechanisms to conceal from our consciousness the true nature or meaning of suffering, to falsify and deny it. We do this without renouncing the word, however. The word comes to designate, in our minds, only a faint copy or superficial image of the real thing; but having forgotten what the original is, we mistake it in the copy. We ascribe to "suffering" a certain gravity of evil; but it is slight compared to what we would ascribe to suffering itself, if we could only recall its true meaning.

A little reflection will disclose the great efforts we go to—some conscious, some not so conscious—to shield ourselves from the perception of other people's suffering. People of a generally kind and benevolent disposition are sometimes heard to say, "The terrible tragedies described on television and in the newspapers—child abuse, starvation, plagues, torture, massacres—are too horrible for me to think about. I simply have to tune out. I look for absorbing projects or forms of entertainment to cheer me up and help me forget." Yet this sentiment reveals much more awareness than other prevalent attitudes do. Very often, not content to skirt around the consciousness of great tragedies, we seek them out, to denature and falsify them in our minds, so that our terror of them can be less. Think of how many movies represent scenes of great suffering that are sweetened with stirring music and clever direction so as to coax moving tears from the audience's eyes. We feel the effects of such scenes in heated indignation (if injustice is the culprit), quivering sympathy, and a small kind of hurt, a kind of painful tenderness for the

26. See Nagel, "Death," in *Mortal Questions*. For probing discussions of the value of life and longevity, see F.M. Kamm, *Morality, Mortality*, vol. 1 (New York: Oxford University Press, 1993), part 1; and Jeff McMahan, *Killing at the Margins of Life* (New York: Oxford University Press, forthcoming).

27. Another difficulty with value hedonism stems from the fact that it is usually advertised as a comprehensive theory of value, and not just a theory of well-being. It therefore assumes that the only values in existence are harms and benefits to individuals. Yet we may think that there is value inherent in distributive justice, or the preservation of natural variety, or great works of art, that is not reducible to benefits obtained by specific individuals.

victim. Yet a dispassionate analysis will reveal that the complex of our ostensibly empathetic emotions is very different, in kind as well as degree, from the more banal horror being experienced by the character on screen. The irony is that a more literal representation might not impress us at all. In order for us to be impressed by the "reality" of what we see, it must be represented in false terms. *True* suffering is simply too horrible for us to acknowledge; but a false and pleasing simulacrum of it will be gladly admitted into our consciousness.

The falsification of suffering is everywhere—in movies, in poetry, in novels, on the nightly news. Accounts of disaster routinely veer from a discussion of the agony and plight of the victims (which quickly becomes tiresome) to the description of some moving act of kindness or bravery. Often it is these descriptions that affect us the most and that provoke the greatest outburst of emotion. These are the images we often take away and that become our image of "suffering." Suffering comes to be closely associated with stirring images of hope in adversity, acts of moral heroism and touching kindness, gestures of human dignity, sentiments of noble sympathy and tremulous concern, the comfort and consolation of tears. It turns into something beautiful. It becomes poetry. People begin to refer to "sublime suffering."[28] Suffering, in other words, becomes just exactly what it is not.

But there are other mechanisms that we use to block out the consciousness of suffering. Besides the technique of transformation, there is the technique of denial. A very common form of this is, when faced with evidence of other people's suffering, to think that their suffering is their own fault. It must be a result of their own laziness, or vice, or selfishness, or some other defect of character. "Who that was innocent ever perished?" is the cruel and cutting remark which Job hears from his companions (Job 4.7). If the present victims made a point of improving themselves and ridding themselves of their flaws (or if they had done so in the past), they need not be suffering. The insidious suggestion behind these thoughts is that it is within the power of these people not to suffer, and that they only continue to do so because they are unwilling to give up their wicked and benighted ways. But if it is within their power to remove the cause of their suffering, if it is a matter of *choice* that they continue in their present path, how much can they really be said to be suffering, how unbearable is their situation after all?

The impulse to blame the victim for his own plight (and the imputation may not *always* be unreasonable, but the instinct behind it is generally stronger than the warrant of evidence) is also part of a general tendency to put distance between the victim and ourselves. We want to know that the victim is very different from ourselves, so that the faculty of sympathetic identification need not be awakened. Upon learning of some frightening accident, how often we quickly check to confirm that the circumstances that rendered the victim vulnerable do not apply to our own case.

---

28. This is Carlyle's absurd characterization of Job's experience. Anyone paying attention to what Job has to say about his ordeal knows that there is nothing sublime about it. The book's author is partly to blame, however, by giving Job such beautiful poetry in which to express himself. But would we read the story and be as affected by it otherwise?

If the misfortune sprang from the victim's own folly or wickedness, so much the better! Because the victim is so different from us, and we cannot easily imagine encountering the same misfortune in the same way, we can forget his story straight away and promptly banish the perception of his suffering from our minds. Job understands the reason for his companions' insistence that he is to blame for his own misfortune: "You see my calamity, and are afraid" (Job 6.21).

Think how difficult it is for us to preserve the awareness of another person's suffering, even when we seem to have every motive for doing so. Even when we are in the immediate company of a loved one who is suffering—say, from sickness—and whom we are determined to help, our awareness of his or her suffering may only be a flickering one. Often it serves as the initial impetus to beneficent action and is then forgotten as we become mentally absorbed in the performance of those tasks necessary to alleviate his or her suffering; the perception may recur thereafter only through forcible external reminders, such as the renewal of the victim's complaint. Sometimes our attempt to relieve the other person's suffering is unsuccessful, or only partly successful. In this case, since we have nothing left to do, it might be expected that we are brought back—by default, as it were—to a perception of the person's suffering. Yet we often find that such perception is displaced by a feeling of bored irritation or distractedness—that is, absorption in thoughts unrelated to the victim's present plight. The same pattern of psychological reaction can be observed when the effort of alleviation takes a long time.

It is true that there are generous souls who, either by vocational choice or the force of circumstance, devote long hours to the assistance of others who are suffering. I would hazard that most of these people, in order to carry out their work without succumbing to exhaustion, must acquire the capacity to distance themselves psychologically from the suffering that they strive continuously to relieve. Or rather, they must develop a double psychology: the ability to be simultaneously aware of and oblivious to the other person's suffering.

Every day I think about torture, marveling that its persistence is tolerated, and wondering how it can be stopped. But it would be more accurate to say that I think about "torture," not the real thing. The word *torture* passes before my brain, together, sometimes, with words that describe certain of its methods. Sometimes there are vague, filtered momentary visual images of its methods being carried out. But there is no real perception or consciousness of torture. I know this, because very rarely, not more than about four times a year, the consciousness returns—sometimes by reading the testimony of a survivor, sometimes without any apparent cause. There is no special insight, simply a reminder of what torture is, and that it occurs. Then a feeling of desperate uneasiness and unbearable anxiety seizes hold of me to be freed from the awareness of torture. Slowly, mercifully, the awareness subsides. If I am lucky, the determination to try to combat torture remains, but the consciousness of what it is is gone. What is remarkable is that often upon returning to the personal descriptions that trapped my awareness when I first read them, I no longer experience the same reaction. It is as though one encounter were sufficient to deaden my sensibilities and shield my consciousness from future reminders. The words bounce on my brain and bounce right off again; they are incapable of conveying their meaning to my understanding.

The introspection of my own case, the behavior of other people, and the observation of general cultural practices convince me that we have a deeply rooted psychological need not to be aware of suffering. (Except when we are suffering ourselves—then, too, we have a strong need to imagine the non-existence of our suffering, but we also have a powerful reason to acknowledge it, inasmuch as doing so may be a necessary element of making it go away.) Sometimes, as in the case of sentimental falsification or blaming the victim, the psychological mechanisms we employ to satisfy this need are transparent. At other times, no such mechanisms are visible, but our obliviousness in the face of such clear and plentiful evidence of other people's suffering cries out for an explanation and suggests that our need or desire not to be aware of it is the underlying cause. I suggest that this need may be linked in turn, though at a deeply unconscious level, to a fear of our own suffering. Deep in our unconscious, we think that the existence of suffering *anywhere* means that we, too, are going to suffer. (In other words, there is a part of us that is unable to distinguish between the existence of suffering anywhere and our own suffering.) And so the best way to assure ourselves of our safety is to deny that there is or has been any suffering going on at all.

If this suggestion is correct, the thought process that leads to the suppression of awareness of other people's suffering is not only unconscious; it is deeply irrational. Some people might think that there are good reasons for the suppression. For example, our tendency to look for differences between the victim's situation and our own, in order to confirm that we are not vulnerable in the same way that he is, might be explained as the natural consequence of our desire to avoid suffering, and hence to reassure ourselves of our greatest possible immunity to it. The influence of this motive, rational in its way, cannot be denied; but it is only part of the story. Why, for instance, is the successful location of a significant difference between the victim and ourselves often followed so quickly by oblivion of his plight, or at least an end to genuine awareness? Moreover, this motive fails to explain all the other mechanisms and manifestations of the impulse to block out consciousness of other people's suffering.

It may be suggested that we flee awareness of other people's suffering simply because we find such awareness unpleasant or distressing. That may be part of the explanation. One has to emphasize, however, that although the awareness of other people's suffering sometimes causes us distress, that distress rarely constitutes more than a kind of discomfort or unease, and rarely rises to the level of suffering. Even when it qualifies as suffering, it rarely acquires any more than a very minor degree of intensity. It must be stressed that if the suffering of the victim is extremely intense, then the intensity of suffering of the perceptive onlooker (if her perceptiveness is the only source of her suffering) can only be *very small* next to that of the victim.

Sympathy is sometimes defined as the suffering we experience as a result of contemplating the suffering of other people and animals. If this were what sympathy meant, there would be even less of it—much less of it—than the small amount actually found! But suffering in the onlooker is by no means a necessary condition of sympathy. In fact, sympathy usually exists without it. Sympathy just means the sincere desire to see another person's or animal's suffering removed. It does not even require the genuine awareness of another person's (or animal's) suffering. One can have the superficial verbalized knowledge that another person is suffering; one can trust, on the basis of previous perception, that such suffering is a horrible evil; and one can therefore have a sincere abiding desire for the removal of that suffering. It is thus possible to feel sympathy while skirting genuine awareness. Yet some people's unconscious fears may prevent even this; they would rather flee all references to suffering than let themselves feel a proper concern. It is a great error to suppose that sympathy is psychologically costly. Yet there are powerful hidden psychological forces that are forever causing it to be suppressed.

In reality, the vivid perception of other people's suffering poses little danger to ourselves. Nevertheless, if my earlier suggestion is correct, our unconscious believes that it poses a very grave danger. With impressive regularity and rapidity it raises barriers to divert such knowledge away from us. It encourages the use of stratagems to forget, to deny, and when that doesn't work, to falsify the reality of other people's suffering. This is why the effort of grasping the reality of suffering is not so much uncomfortable as it is difficult. I believe an understanding of this fact lies behind the assertion of certain Christian theologians and other thinkers that a willingness to suffer oneself is a necessary prerequisite to the adoption of a genuine commitment to alleviate the suffering of others.[29] The assertion is awkwardly expressed and misleading as it stands. Suffering, or willingness to suffer, is not in fact a prerequisite of charitable action. As we have noted, not even the vivid perception of other people's distress is necessary. But by offering ourselves for the alleviation of other people's suffering, and thus a fortiori by acknowledging the existence of such suffering, we expose our unconscious to its deepest fears. We pose it a direct and profound challenge.

Our tendency to deny and minimize suffering is a formidable obstacle to accurate moral understanding. It leads us to underrate the evilness of suffering, and consequently the urgency of eliminating it. We go about oblivious, blindfolded as it were, to the true moral state of the world and the response that its state requires of us. In order to remove the blindfolds, to see the world as it is, and thus become more fully acquainted with the extent of our duty to relieve suffering, we could strive to preserve a continuous awareness of the meaning of suffering. But such knowledge would be acutely difficult, if not costly, to maintain. Perhaps it is difficult to preserve a realistic view of the world. But at least we can come close to knowing our duty—which is the important thing—if we now and then make an effort to behold the

29. See Dorothee Soelle, *Suffering*, trans. Everett R. Kahn (Philadelphia: Fortress Press, 1975).

true nature of suffering, make a mental note of its utter moral horror, and then, after our perception fades, understand that suffering is a much worse thing than we can presently recollect.[30]

In order to retain an accurate picture of suffering, we must be alert to the unconscious mechanisms that distort its meaning and deny its existence. Our picture of suffering, in order to be accurate, need not be a direct one. It can be, and usually must be, mediated. We can, for example, refer by our memory to some past moment in which we were vividly and uncomfortably aware of what suffering is. (I am thinking of the awareness of another person's suffering, not the experience of suffering itself.) Memory need not reproduce that awareness in its original form. It can represent it in the shorthand form of the consciousness of certain true facts pertaining to it: suffering was immediately felt, and was irrefutably *known*, to be horrible; there was a strong lingering sense of disbelief that anything so utterly hideous and hateful could really exist, could really be true, combined with the unimpugnable certainty that it did exist; there was a powerful need and anxiety to banish that suffering somehow, which if no other method were to be found, might mercifully (though deceitfully) be accomplished by suppressing one's consciousness of it. One can recall these facts without summoning the experience of awareness itself, and the facts are sufficient to inform one of the intrinsic horribleness of suffering. Suffering, like the sun, is not something we can steadily behold. We must look at it, if at all, obliquely, in the form of its own reflection. We must rely for our image of it on fainter likenesses of itself, which serve as indirect testimonies of its nature. In this way, if we know just what we are doing, we can aspire to an accurate intellectual understanding of what suffering is.

We need to become aware of, and to compensate for, the habitual denial of suffering. It is also important to give credit where credit is due, and explicitly acknowledge the evilness of suffering. Often one can decry the evil of a situation that involves suffering without mentioning suffering per se. One can refer to the suffering by its source or the particular form it takes. Or one can limit oneself to a denunciation of other real or imagined evils that are present. Cruelty and humiliation are decried as disrespect, though they also produce acute distress. Failure to prevent disease and undernutrition caused by absolute poverty is criticized as contempt for the basic human dignity of the

---

30. It may be objected that this argument does not account very well for the phenomenon of cruelty. Certainly people who deliberately hurt others are not frightened by the evidence of other people's suffering! But I have not tried to present a comprehensive psychological theory, nor have I tried to offer a description that fits everyone without exception. Rather, I have sought to reveal a certain set of psychological forces that lead most of us to behave and think in a certain way. There may be other psychological forces exerting opposite pressures. And there certainly are outliers, sadists and the like, whom the description does not fit. One can of course wonder whether very cruel and callous people are genuinely aware of the suffering they cause. Perhaps their cruelty is possible only because their ability to block out consciousness of other people's suffering is so much *greater* than ours. They can go so far as to create evidence of other people's suffering without fear of genuinely perceiving it.

victims, though it is also responsible for the persistence of fear and pain. Murder is condemned as a theft of life, though it also leaves a wake of terror and grief. I am not saying that suffering need always be named specifically. If the evil of the situation is recognized and prompts the appropriate response, we may be satisfied. However, there is a particular merit in recalling that suffering is an evil generally. The defect of many attempts to define the scope of evil is that they leave out too much. Attention to suffering, however, can widen our moral horizons. It reminds us that there is evil not only in international and civil war, but also in violence of every kind, not only governmental repression, but also insurrectionary violence, feuds, the violence of protest, the violence of prisons for persons accused of common crimes, and slavery; not only political violence, but the violence of ordinary crime and domestic brutality—child abuse, wife-beating, and abuse of the elderly. Not only physical violence, but all forms of cruelty. Not only the effects of deliberate malice, but also starvation, malnutrition generally, punishing or degrading labor, disease, exposure, and destructive dependency on drugs or alcohol. Not only physical affliction, but also emotional neglect, humiliation, despair, intense shame and guilt, painful separation and bereavement, and the general category of low self-esteem, which includes the conviction of one's own stupidity, dullness, ugliness, deformity, unlovableness, wickedness, worthlessness, or failure. Not only the suffering of humans, but of all animals. Not only suffering that is a "normal" response to external blows, but also the ravages of mental illness. Not only deliberate injury and chronic affliction, but also natural calamities, human accidents, and industrial disasters.

The prevalence of painful mental illness is a good example of an evil that is easily overlooked, unless we make a deliberate search of suffering in all its manifestations. Many people have a hard time crediting that such a thing as mental illness genuinely exists; even if they believe in its existence, they may be insensible, or forgetful, of the grave misfortune that it represents, particularly in those instances where it exacts such extreme pain. This is partly because many people fancy themselves completely immune from the danger of mental illness, partly because our society rigidly represses references to real cases of mental illness, and partly because many of the ordeals experienced—by schizophrenics, for example—are so foreign, so bizarre, and so inexplicable that they are not easily believed or imagined. If we can so easily overlook the pain of the mentally ill and the resulting travail of their families, it seems probable that other afflictions of an evil nature will escape our notice also. I am sure that there are a number of such evils missing from the above list, even though I have tried to make it complete.

5. Suffering and Deprivation

According to some estimates, as many as a fifth of the world's population live below the level of subsistence. These people lack minimal levels of nutrition, housing, education, and medical care. They endure hunger and are easy prey to chronic and disabling diseases. For millions, the deprivation takes extreme forms. In one example reported by *The New York Times*, some two thousand abandoned children live on the streets of the Angolan capital of Luanda: "Dressed in rags, they spend nights in the sandy strip along the bay and their days begging and foraging for food through mounds of garbage."[31]

Amartya Sen and Martha Nussbaum argue that if we focus on psychological suffering, we miss the larger tragedy involved in deprivation. The underlying horror of deprivation is that it robs its victims of the capacity to realize essential human functionings. A functioning is, in Sen's words, "an achievement of a person: what he or she manages to do or be."[32] Both Sen and Nussbaum claim that certain functional capacities are essential conditions of a minimally decent human life. In Nussbaum's provisional account, they include

1. Being able to live to the end of a complete human life, as far as is possible; not dying prematurely, or before one's life is so reduced as to be not worth living.
2. Being able to have good health; to be adequately nourished; to have adequate shelter; having opportunities for sexual satisfaction; being able to move from place to place.
3. Being able to avoid unnecessary and nonbeneficial pain and to have pleasurable experiences.
4. Being able to use the five senses; being able to imagine, to think, and to reason.
5. Being able to have attachments to things and persons outside ourselves; to love those who love and care for us, to grieve at their absence, in general, to love, grieve, to feel longing and gratitude.
6. Being able to form a conception of the good and to engage in critical reflection about the planning of one's own life.
7. Being able to live for and with others, to recognize and show concern for other human beings, to engage in various forms of familial and social interaction.
8. Being able to live with concern for and in relation to animals, plants, and the world of nature.
9. Being able to laugh, to play, to enjoy recreational activities.
10. Being able to live one's own life and nobody else's; being able to live one's own life in one's very own surroundings and context.[33]

In Sen and Nussbaum's view, exclusive concern with suffering misleads us about deprivation for two reasons. First, it misses the underlying reason for deprivation's horror. Second, suffering fails even as a *measure* of the badness of deprivation,

31. "Civil War of Nearly Two Decades Exhausts Resource-Rich Angola," *New York Times*, 9 May 1994.

32. Amartya Sen, *Commodities and Capabilities*, p. 10.

33. Martha Nussbaum, "Human Functioning and Social Justice: In Defense of Aristotelian Essentialism," p. 222.

because victims of extreme deprivation often make psychological adjustments to their condition:

> Considerations of 'feasibility' and of 'practical possibility' enter into what we dare to desire and what we are pained not to get. Our mental reactions to what we actually get and what we can sensibly expect to get may frequently involve compromises with a harsh reality. The destitute thrown into beggary, the vulnerable landless labourer precariously surviving at the edge of subsistence, the overworked domestic servant working round the clock, the subdued and subjugated housewife reconciled to her role and her fate, all tend to come to terms with their respective predicaments. The deprivations are suppressed and muffled in the scale of utilities (reflected by desire-fulfilment and happiness) by the necessity of endurance in uneventful survival.[34]

In other words, people sometimes endure deprivation without suffering, but their deprivation remains a grave moral evil, and we should strive to alleviate it. Perhaps we should sometimes alleviate it at the cost of neglecting the suffering of those who do not face deprivation.

The underlying question raised by Sen and Nussbaum is: To what extent does the evilness of deprivation depend on its tendency to produce suffering? This question is exceedingly difficult. It involves some of the deepest and most puzzling questions about the nature of well-being and misfortune. I shall not offer an answer, but will suggest that Nussbaum and Sen may go too far in separating the badness of deprivation from the badness of suffering.

Both Nussbaum and Sen identify suffering as an evil. They include happiness and exemption from suffering in their list of essential human functionings. But their theoretical framework, especially their use of the Aristotelian term "human functionings," is ill-suited to represent the full horror of suffering. The notion that a good life consists in the exercise of human powers implies that suffering is bad because it hinders people from exercising those powers. But suffering is not evil primarily as an impediment or a limitation. Its evilness is more positive than that. Suffering repels all by itself.

When Nussbaum and Sen distinguish the badness of deprivation from that of suffering, they draw on the claim that people's susceptibility to suffering depends on the standard of living to which they are accustomed. Someone who has led a pampered life may suffer from trivial losses and disappointments, whereas someone who has known only grinding poverty may endure major deprivations without suffering. This claim invites the thought that the pampered person's "plight" matters *less* than the intensity of his suffering would suggest, and that the poor person's misfortune matters *more* than the intensity of his suffering would suggest.

Let us examine these thoughts in turn. Does the rich person's plight matter less than the intensity of his suffering would suggest? If we make sure that we are measuring the intensity of genuine suffering rather than mere dissatisfaction, what grounds could there be for discounting his suffering? Considerations of justice might lead us to give it less moral weight if we have independent reasons to believe that

---

34. Sen, *Commodities and Capabilities*, pp. 21–22.

his life as a whole is better than that of the deprived person. If we think he could have avoided his own suffering—say, by pampering himself less—we may want to give it less attention for the pragmatic reasons outlined earlier, or because we think that self-induced suffering is intrinsically less serious. These are the only legitimate reasons I can see for giving less weight to the rich person's suffering. (Some of us may object morally to his selfish life-style, but that is a separate thought.)

Now for the other side. If people living in absolute poverty adjust to their condition in such a way that they experience major deprivations without suffering—or with suffering of a lower intensity than the rest of us would experience in similar circumstances—does their plight matter more than the intensity of their suffering suggests? First of all, we should not exaggerate the extent to which people *can* endure severe deprivation without suffering. Deprivation means powerlessness and vulnerability—vulnerability to violence, disease, abandonment, humiliation, starvation. Even when deprivation is not accompanied by chronic suffering, it is accompanied by a much higher *risk* of suffering of the greatest intensity. Nor should we exaggerate people's ability to adjust to the routine afflictions of deprivation. There is the incontestable pain and discomfort of untreated disease. There is the agony and desperation of hunger, along with its destructive physical and psychological sequelae. There is the blow of losing ordinary bodily functions. There is the terror of premature death, and the grief of losing loved ones before their time.[35] Absolute poverty contains a deep well of suffering.

However, I agree with Nussbaum and Sen that some destitute people suffer less than we would expect them to, given the extent of their deprivation. (I also suspect that there are important regional and cultural differences.) And where this is so, I agree that these people's condition is worse from a moral point of view than a mere reading of their suffering would suggest. Earlier we saw that pure value hedonism is implausible. We should acknowledge other values that contribute to human well-being besides happiness and the prevention of suffering—values such as longevity, liberty, knowledge, accomplishment, and moral goodness. In addition to these goods, Nussbaum's list rightly emphasizes the importance of basic physical capacities. The extreme curtailment of these goods constitutes an evil that can rival or even surpass great individual suffering. If someone were severely deprived of one or more of these goods, we should consider it a great misfortune, even if the deprivation were not accompanied by great suffering.

Sen and Nussbaum look at deprivation through an Aristotelian lens. This understates the evilness of the suffering that is also part of deprivation. Alternatively, we can look at deprivation through an Epicurean lens. But this understates the importance of the realization of essential human powers and capacities. Neither a purely Aristotelian nor a purely Epicurean standard adequately captures the horrors of extreme deprivation. Both are needed.[36]

---

35. For an eloquent account, see Nancy Scheper-Hughes, *Death Without Weeping: The Violence of Everyday Life in Brazil* (Berkeley: University of California Press, 1992).

36. For a comprehensive and illuminating account of the good on broadly Aristotelian lines, see Thomas Hurka, *Perfectionism.*

FIVE

The Duty to
Relieve Suffering

1. The Source of the Duty To Relieve Suffering

I shall now try to state why we have a prima facie duty to relieve suffering. The explanation I shall give appears obvious to me, but is not the sort of account for which I can supply an argument. Some readers may not accept the picture that I offer here.

We have a prima facie duty to relieve suffering, because suffering is bad and ought not to occur. Suffering is bad (as I said before) not only for the individual whom it afflicts, but bad from an impersonal point of view. Its occurrence makes the world that much worse.

I add the claim that it "ought not to occur," because to identify suffering as a bad understates what is involved. Some things are bad without it being the case that we have a prima facie duty to get rid of them. The badness of suffering is different. Here I need to use somewhat metaphorical language to get across what seems to me to be the heart of the matter. Where there is suffering, there exists a demand or an appeal for the prevention of that suffering. I say "a demand or an appeal," but this demand does not issue from anyone in particular, nor is it addressed to anyone in particular. We might say (again metaphorically) that suffering cries out for its own abolition or cancellation.

Some philosophers, trained to give full vent to their skepticism, may deny the existence of such an appeal. Yet we continually refer to it in our talk. For example, we often say, silently or out loud, of some great tragedy, "It ought never to have been." We do not mean merely, "I wish that it had not happened." We mean something beyond that. We acknowledge an appeal (the best available word) that is prior to our own desires, or those of anyone else, an appeal that says—now, in the past, and in the future—"Avert this tragedy." Common sense refers to the appeal without hesitation, and yet when presented with a statement of what it is referring to, doubts the reality of the appeal. Here I believe is one case in which common sense is more perspicacious when it is not yet self-conscious. It perceives something real which self-consciousness causes it to lose grasp of.

I am here denying the view that a phrase like "X ought not to occur" can have only an evaluative meaning—that it means only that a state of affairs in which X does not occur is better, other things equal, than a state of affairs in which it does. I am claiming that on at least some occasions the thought that "X ought not to occur" carries additional content.

Because suffering ought not to occur, we have a prima facie duty to prevent it. The prevention of suffering is our way of honoring the pre-existing appeal for its cancellation. The appeal for the cancellation of suffering is an appeal for whatever causal sequence will prevent it from happening. If we are instrumental in bringing about such a causal sequence, then it is right to say that we have (to that extent) fulfilled our prima facie duty to prevent suffering. One might say: it is better if we prevent suffering. But that would be incomplete. The moral charge is missing. We need to say: we *should* prevent suffering. In the same way, it is incomplete to say that it is better if suffering does not occur. Once more the moral charge is missing. To supply it, we must say that suffering *ought* not to occur, in the more-than-evaluative sense discussed above. Ultimately, the fact that suffering ought not to occur and the prima facie duty to prevent suffering refer to the same moral phenomenon. They are two sides of the same coin. One the one side, suffering ought not to occur; on the other side, *we* do right by preventing its occurrence.

I believe that my position is close to Thomas Nagel's in *The View from Nowhere*.[1] Nagel writes that pain has objective disvalue and that we have an agent-neutral reason to eliminate it. ("Agent neutral" means that each of us has a reason to eliminate it, regardless of whose pain it is.) The idea that suffering (pain) ought not to occur is, I believe, what connects Nagel's two points. Adequate recognition of the objective badness of suffering involves the recognition that suffering must not be permitted to occur, and it is *because* suffering must not be permitted to occur that we have an agent-neutral reason to eliminate it.

Some people claim to be skeptical about the existence of objective values.[2] We may be skeptical that many moral demands, said to be objective duties, really are; especially since, as Mackie reminds us, their content varies depending on the culture in which we live: this should make us suspect that they are nothing more than social rules internalized through a pattern of punishment and reward—not objective requirements antecedently present in the world. Yet there is at least one suggestion of an objective moral duty that can and ought to quiet our skepticism: namely, the idea that anyone who may experience suffering of any significant duration or intensity must not be permitted to suffer, and that we must (in the absence of counter-

1. *The View from Nowhere* (New York: Oxford University Press, 1986), pp. 156–62.
2. For example, John Mackie, *Ethics: Inventing Right and Wrong* (Harmondsworth: Penguin, 1977), chap. 1.

vailing moral considerations) avert his or her suffering. There is no need to import superstition. We can begin with a mechanistic view of the world, one in which bits of energy and matter interact in various ways perhaps according to certain deterministic or probabilistic laws of causation; and in which people's lives are determined by the interplay of their own desires, goals, commitments, urges, and impulses with those of other people, steered by different beliefs about the world, of varying degrees of falsehood and veracity, all within the limits imposed by nature; but a world that exhibits no transcendent purpose or meaning or design in any of its parts—no purpose, that is, outside the purely contingent (and usually quite powerless) wills of individual people and animals. Nevertheless, surely it would be blindness to fail to see, at the very least, that some things in this purposeless world are objectively bad; that these things ought not to arise; that we are obliged by their very badness to prevent them from arising; and that certainly the experience of suffering in its many forms has this very property of objective badness that I have been describing, even if nothing else has it. It seems to me stranger to deny this than to affirm it.

The claim that the badness of suffering generates a prima facie duty to relieve suffering needs to be qualified in certain ways. First, it must be emphasized that this is a prima facie duty. It holds true in the absence of other moral considerations. When other moral considerations are present—other prima facie duties, or moral permissions not to incur certain costs—the prima facie duty to relieve suffering is sometimes overridden by them.

Second, the prima facie duty to relieve suffering applies only to suffering significant in intensity and duration. Some episodes of individual suffering are so mild in intensity or so very brief that they seem insufficient to found a *duty* on our part to prevent them. An example of such "morally insignificant" suffering would be a pinprick that genuinely distresses a child but is forgotten in an instant, or an episode of frightening but not crushing anxiety—amounting to genuine but moderate suffering—that is dispelled in a matter of a few minutes. At some point, however, as the intensity or duration of suffering increases, it passes a threshold such that its elimination—or at least, its reduction to a degree of intensity and duration below the threshold—becomes the object of our duty. I do not think it takes very much to reach this threshold. Suffering concentrated in a very short period of time can nevertheless be so intense (so-called "micro-depressions," for example) that we must not tolerate its occurrence. And if mild suffering lasts a long enough time, it acquires a degree of cumulative evil that morally obliges us to prevent it also. Certainly vast numbers of individuals experience suffering that is of sufficient magnitude to be called morally significant—suffering that creates in each of us a duty to eliminate it, or at least render it morally insignificant by bringing it below a certain threshold of intensity and duration.

Finally, some people may deny that we have even a prima facie duty to prevent the suffering that criminals experience as punishment for their crimes. I have in mind those who uphold punishment as retribution. People who defend punishment as a means of preventing crime may still believe in a prima facie duty to prevent the criminal's suffering; they just believe that it is overridden by the need to prevent crime. Those who support punishment as a means to the moral education or re-demption of the criminal may also think that the criminal's suffering, in the absence of other considerations, ought to be averted; however, they think that the need to avert his suffering is outweighed by the need to secure his moral reformation through punishment. Retributivists are different, for the criminal's suffering is their goal.[3] As I discussed in the last chapter, we may distinguish between deontological and teleological retributivists. The former emphasize our duty to exact retribution, the latter emphasize the desirability of retributive suffering. In either case, retri-butivism blocks the view that we have even a prima facie duty to prevent the criminal's suffering.

2. Other Explanations of the Duty to Relieve Suffering

There may be other explanations of the prima facie duty to relieve suffering, dif-ferent from the one I have offered. Some people may appeal to the Golden Rule: "Do unto others as you would have them do unto you." On one interpretation, the Golden Rule asks us to evaluate our actions from the standpoint of those affected by them. If we imagine ourselves in the position of those who are suffering, we may well be led to acknowledge a duty to relieve suffering. But this interpretation of the Golden Rule needs to be refined, for different people's standpoints conflict with one another, and there are some points of view by which we don't want to be guided too closely. For example, we don't think that we have a duty to satisfy the demands of sadists or exploiters. Perhaps the idea is that the effort of imagining ourselves in other people's shoes is the *first step* in a process of appropriate moral reasoning that leads to the acknowledgment of a duty to relieve suffering. There could be several different accounts of the form that such moral reasoning would take.

Some people may appeal to Kant's categorical imperative: "Act only according to the maxim that you can at the same time will to be a universal law." Kant claimed that his categorical imperative did imply a duty of beneficence to those in distress.[4] Philosophers have debated how, and if, Kant's derivation succeeds. Without entering this debate, I'll only note that the categorical imperative, like the Golden Rule, is frequently thought of as telling us to act on principles that we could uphold from an impartial perspective—a perspective that attaches no greater weight to our own interests than anyone else's. It may be that the impartial perspective, by distancing ourselves from the egocentric concerns and parochial loyalties that often absorb our attention, brings the impersonal badness of suffering into sharper relief, and therefore encourages us to acknowledge a duty to relieve suffering. I am not claiming

3. This may not be true for all retributivists. Some, for example, may seek the deprivation of the criminal's liberty, and regard his suffering as a neutral or perhaps even regrettable side-effect.

4. Immanuel Kant, *Foundations of the Metaphysics of Morals*, trans. Lewis White Beck (Indianapolis: Bobbs Merrill, 1959), p. 41.

that principles judged acceptable from the impartial perspective require us to *pro-mote* everyone's interests impartially. That may or may not be the case. I am only suggesting that the impartial perspective may give the impersonal badness of suffering more salience than it would otherwise have.

Some people may offer a contractualist justification. John Rawls and Ronald Dworkin have suggested that reasonable moral rules are those that would be chosen by people made temporarily ignorant of their life circumstances.[5] Rawls and Dworkin have used this method to identify principles of justice governing the distribution of basic resources like liberty and wealth, but the same method might be used to derive the duty to relieve suffering. People who could not predict the extent of their vulnerability to suffering in real life might seek protection from the worst eventuality by agreeing on a strong requirement to relieve suffering. T. M. Scanlon, taking the contractualist argument in a somewhat different direction, has proposed that correct rules of right and wrong are those that "no one could reasonably reject as a basis for informed, unforced general agreement."[6] On one interpretation, those with the strongest justification for rejecting a set of rules are those "who would do worst under it."[7] So we look for a set of rules under which the strongest complaint is less than what it would be under any alternative set of rules. Scanlon's theory might be seen as laying the foundation for a strong requirement to relieve suffering, since, in the absence of such a requirement, those whose suffering it would be permissible to neglect would have strong grounds for complaint.

Derivations of the duty to relieve suffering from the Golden Rule, the categorical imperative, and contractualism share certain features that distinguish them from a direct appeal to the badness of suffering. All three derivations locate the source of the duty in the agent's own will or consent. The contractualist argument says that we consent to the duty to relieve suffering when we deliberate under appropriate constraints. Arguments from the Golden Rule and the categorical imperative both claim, more or less, that the relief of suffering is willed by us if we look at matters in a certain way. (Kant, in fact, discards the "if" clause, since he identifies the categorical imperative with our true will, freed from heteronomous impulses.) The direct appeal to the badness of suffering, however, locates the source of the duty to relieve suffering squarely *outside* the agent. The mere fact that others may suffer gives us a reason to prevent their suffering. The disposition of our will has nothing to do with it.

This difference in the direction of justification might be seen as giving a certain advantage to the alternative derivations. By connecting the duty to relieve suffering

---

5. John Rawls, *A Theory of Justice* (Cambridge, Mass.: Harvard University Press, 1971); and Ronald Dworkin, "What is Equality?, Part II: Equality of Resources," *Philosophy and Public Affairs*, 10 (1981): 283–345.

6. T. M. Scanlon, "Contractualism and Utilitarianism," in Amartya Sen and Bernard Williams, eds., *Utilitarianism and Beyond* (Cambridge: Cambridge University Press, 1982), p. 110.

7. Ibid., p. 123.

to the agent's will or consent, they may supply it with stronger motivational backing.[8] The thought that the duty emanates from my will may bolster my determination to comply with it. The alternative derivations may have other advantages. In addition to providing grounds for the duty to relieve suffering, they may have clear things to say about its limits. And the premises on which they are based may appeal strongly to many people.

I shall not, however, rely on any of the alternative justifications in my book. Doubts may be raised about what the alternative justifications actually show: whether they provide a secure basis for the duty to relieve suffering, and whether they give us a duty to relieve suffering of the right kind. I would not like our discussion to become hostage to these uncertainties. Moreover, it seems to me that the impersonal badness of suffering really is the heart of the matter. To replace a direct appeal to the badness of suffering with one of the alternative justifications is, it strikes me, to replace something more certain with something less certain. In any case, the duty to relieve suffering does not *depend* on the alternative justifications. Whether or not other arguments can be mustered, it remains the case that we ought to prevent someone from suffering just because his or her suffering is bad and ought not to happen.

3. Basic Features of the Duty to Relieve Suffering

The duty to relieve suffering, I have suggested, arises from the badness of suffering. This has certain implications for how we should understand the duty to relieve suffering itself, implications that I now wish to explore. (To those who object that the resulting picture does not accommodate enough of their moral convictions, I repeat that the duty to relieve suffering is a prima facie duty, to be supplemented by other moral considerations in a complete account of morality.)

First, the duty to relieve suffering is universal. It is binding on all agents, regardless of historical period or culture. It takes its cue from the badness of suffering, not from cultural acceptance. Someone who is culturally unprepared to acknowledge the duty to relieve suffering is not thereby exempt from its requirements. What rather is the case is that the ignorance for which his culture is responsible may prevent him from acting as the duty requires.

The duty to relieve suffering is universal also in the sense that it applies to all significant suffering. That includes the suffering of people from cultures in which the duty to relieve suffering is unrecognized.

What of non-human animals? Like people, other animals have an interest in avoiding suffering. The duty to relieve suffering must apply with the same vigor to animal suffering as it does to human suffering, unless it is the case that the interest of animals in avoiding suffering carries less moral weight than the similar interest

---

8. The motivational power of contractualist justifications is a main theme of Scanlon's "Contractualism and Utilitarianism."

of humans in avoiding suffering, even where the intensity and duration of suffering are equivalent. This is a much disputed issue, which I cannot properly examine here. As I said in chapter 1, my own view is that the suffering of non-human animals carries no less moral weight than the suffering of humans, and that consequently the duty to relieve suffering applies with equal force to both.[9]

A strong duty to relieve suffering that does not discriminate between species would require radical changes in the ways that we relate to other animals. It would, for example, require an end to the practice of factory farming, in which billions of animals are annually subjected to extreme suffering in order to supply humans with meat and other products at the lowest possible cost. It would also raise difficult questions about the practice of experimenting on animals to obtain medical benefits for humans. These cases, much discussed in the literature on animal ethics, involve suffering that is inflicted by human beings. But a species-blind duty to relieve suffering would also make it a prima facie requirement to save animals from suffering brought upon them by natural conditions and other animals. That seems right to me. (That the idea is unfamiliar to many people does not make it absurd.) There are, however, limits to what we can do. Efforts to teach animals less aggressive behavior or to protect them from a harsh environment would frequently fail, and when successful, would often require heavy-handed forms of intervention that would do more harm than good. The difficulty and expense of these efforts might also raise concerns about the limits of obligatory sacrifice. And there are moral opportunity costs. An equivalent expenditure of resources, directed elsewhere, might do much more to reduce the cumulative badness of suffering in the world. If we are serious about reducing animal suffering, we should start with the suffering that is inflicted by human beings.[10]

In addition to being universal (at least as far as humans are concerned), the duty to relieve suffering is consequentialist in form. That is because it is concerned with what happens in the world. It demands a reduction in the cumulative badness of

9. The view that the relevantly similar interests of humans and other animals should be accorded the same moral weight is powerfully defended by David DeGrazia in *Taking Animals Seriously* (Cambridge: Cambridge University Press, 1996), pp. 49–74, 248–50, 272–78. Some people may want to say that animal suffering matters less because it is of a different *quality*—say, because it occurs in the context of a lower level of mental complexity. But we have to be careful here. If the point is that the intensity is lower, there is no quarrel. But if intensity is the same, why should the level of mental complexity matter? After all, we do not think that the intense suffering of babies or severely retarded people matters less because *their* mental life is less complex.

It may be suggested that other animals are prone to suffer less intensely, because they lead a more primitive mental life and consequently cannot endow pain and affliction with the same negative significance that humans do. But I believe that Judith Jarvis Thomson expresses an equally if not more plausible view when she suggests that "other things being equal it is worse to cause an animal pain than to cause an adult human being pain. An adult human being can, as it were, think his or her way around the pain to what lies beyond it in the future; an animal—like a human baby—cannot do this, so that there is nothing for the animal but the pain itself." Thomson, *The Realm of Rights* (Cambridge, Mass.; Harvard University Press, 1990), pp. 292–93.

10. See DeGrazia, *Taking Animals Seriously*, pp. 276–77.

suffering. By "cumulative badness" I mean the degree of impersonal badness of all the suffering that occurs. The cumulative badness of suffering is determined by factors such as the intensity and duration of individuals' suffering, and the number of victims. It is not exactly the same as the *quantity* of suffering, as we will see in subsequent chapters. The more we reduce the cumulative badness of suffering, the more we comply with the duty to relieve suffering. To put it another way, the outcomes of alternative actions can be ranked in order of the cumulative badness of the suffering that they contain: the greater the cumulative badness of the suffering, the worse the outcome. The duty to relieve suffering requires us to produce the least bad—or if you like, the best—of these outcomes. That gives it a consequentialist form, since consequentialism is the view that we are required to produce the best outcome.

That's not to say that the duty to relieve suffering entails the doctrine of consequentialism in its purest form: the view that we must *always* produce the best possible outcome. The prima facie duty to relieve suffering may be limited by nonconsequentialist considerations, and it is silent on the question of whether we are required to promote other values besides the relief of suffering. However, if the duty to relieve suffering forms a large part of morality, morality will be largely consequentialist in character.

It is often assumed that consequentialism is based on an a priori requirement to promote the good. Many apologists claim that this requirement is self-evident or at least intuitive, or that it is built into the very concept of morality. Many critics think they can defeat consequentialism by knocking down such claims. But the notion of an a priori requirement to promote the good seems to me something of a distraction. What gives consequentialism its force is the quite specific horror of a number of specific evils, and the overwhelming need to avert them. One such evil is suffering. The vast amount of suffering in this world contributes greatly to the plausibility of consequentialism, or something close to it. If there were no suffering, consequentialism would be much less plausible. We could go on improving the world in a variety of ways, but it would be less clear that this was, in most cases, morally required.

It is a reflection of its consequentialist character that the duty to relieve suffering, as I have construed it, makes no distinction between the "active" prevention of suffering and the abstention from inflicting it. The duty to relieve suffering arises from the badness of suffering, so it requires us to behave in *whatever* manner will lead to the cumulatively least bad suffering. From the standpoint of the duty to relieve suffering, therefore, abstaining from the infliction of suffering and failing to prevent it are simply two different forms of "prevention" (the word may need to be stretched a little beyond ordinary usage), and neither is more obligatory than the other.

Many people believe that there is a stronger requirement to abstain from inflicting suffering than to actively prevent it. But this belief can't be based on the badness of suffering itself; it must rest on something else. Whether there is an intrinsic moral difference between inflicting and allowing suffering (or harm, more generally) is a subject of notorious controversy among moral philosophers, which I shall not try to settle here.

Another feature of the duty to relieve suffering is its cumulative character. What I mean is this: the duty to relieve suffering falls out of the badness of suffering, so it requires us to reduce the cumulative badness of suffering. The more we can reduce the cumulative badness of suffering, the better. Eventually, this builds up to a duty to achieve the *greatest possible* reduction in the cumulative badness of suffering. We do not comply fully with the duty to relieve suffering until we achieve the maximum reduction, but if we achieve something less than this, we have *partly* complied with the duty to relieve suffering. Compliance admits of degree. Furthermore, though nothing less than full compliance is required of us, there is nothing significant about taking the final step into full compliance, as distinct from intermediate steps that lead from lesser to greater though not yet maximum compliance.

It is cumbersome to go on referring to "a duty to achieve the greatest possible reduction in the cumulative badness of suffering." So, by way of shorthand, I will often refer to "a duty to prevent the worst cumulative suffering" or "a duty to minimize the cumulative badness of suffering." The latter of these two phrases should not be misunderstood. The only way to reduce the badness of some pattern of suffering is to change the pattern itself—for example, by reducing the intensity or duration of the suffering or the number of people who suffer.

Finally, a word about sanctions. I believe we express matters most clearly when we distinguish the assertion of a duty to relieve suffering from any claim about the appropriateness of negative sanctions—such as guilt, anger, or punishment—for those who fail to relieve suffering. The badness of suffering gives rise to a requirement to prevent suffering. That is the first and most essential point. Negative sanctions for non-compliance are a separate matter. They are not to be inferred directly from the badness of suffering. Rather, they ought to be seen as potential instruments for reducing the cumulative badness of suffering. (There may be additional reasons to apply, or withhold, sanctions.)

How should we apply negative sanctions so as to minimize the cumulative badness of suffering? This is a complex and difficult question, one that we would need a whole other book to address properly. Many different factors need to be taken into account, and these factors can push in contrary directions. Here I shall just mention a few of the most important factors. Obviously, negative sanctions will be more effective, other things being equal, when applied to behaviors that lead to worse suffering rather than less bad suffering. However, we must also be guided by a sound understanding of human motives—an understanding of what people in general are strongly motivated to do, and what they are only weakly motivated to do. That's because negative sanctions will be more effective, other things being equal, when they are applied to behaviors that people are in general less strongly motivated to perform. Another factor is ease of predictability. Negative sanctions will be more effective, other things being equal, when the agent should easily have foreseen that his or her behavior would have led to worse cumulative suffering. Finally, we need to be selective in our use of sanctions. Excessive use can undermine their power. And when sanctions take a severe form—such as the kinds of punishment normally administered by the state—there is a major prima facie moral cost in the use of the sanctions themselves.

4. Indirection

The duty to relieve suffering requires a reduction in the cumulative badness of suffering. It requires us to adopt behaviors, policies, and dispositions that achieve this goal. This may entail a somewhat unfamiliar use of the word *duty*. Normally when we think of morality, we think of simple rules of conduct. What makes them simple is that their practical requirements are made clear to agents; the rules tell the agents in a fairly straightforward manner just what they must *do*. The ordinary conception of morality is one designed for use by human beings. It is meant to illuminate the deliberations of an agent deciding how she must behave.

The duty to relieve suffering is unlike this, however. It is not a rule that has been shaped to give clear instructions to human beings. It requires us to do *whatever* will minimize the cumulative badness of suffering. Figuring out what to do, then, is a matter of reasoning backwards from the need to prevent suffering. And the results of this investigation may not be simple at all.

Here is one complication. The duty to relieve suffering is concerned not only with our behavior, but also with our motives. Motives shape behavior, so the duty to relieve suffering calls for those which lead to behavior that prevents the worst possible suffering. In the case of *moral* motives, this gives rise to a paradox. The duty to relieve suffering calls for certain moral motives that do not have the duty to relieve suffering as their object and that, in some cases, even *contradict* the duty to relieve suffering.

Why should this be the case? The answer is that motives are not made to order. Human beings are limited creatures. So we must choose the most suitable motives from a narrow range of options.

In a more perfect world we could tell people that they were required to minimize the cumulative badness of suffering, give them all the information needed to accomplish this goal, instill in them a capacity to pursue it with unflinching determination, and send them on their way. But in the real world, no one can be this well-equipped. People need help in order to comply with the duty to relieve suffering, and the best available help includes motives that lack the duty to relieve suffering as their content.

Notice that the duty to relieve suffering is not as transparent as, say, the prohibition against killing. We need to calculate what would actually be required to prevent the worst cumulative suffering. Such calculations are difficult, often impossible, to carry out on short notice. So we need secondary principles, or rules of thumb. These principles mandate behaviors that in the great majority of cases are necessary to prevent the worst cumulative suffering. They are likely to include familiar rules of commonsense morality: do not kill; do not inflict pain or injury;

do not humiliate; do not lie; do not break promises; protect close relatives, friends, clients, and patients.

However, these secondary principles need to have a stronger hold on our motivations than mere rules of thumb.[11] We should feel a sincere reluctance to violate them, as though violating them were wrong in itself. Here is why. Though compliance with sound secondary principles is generally necessary to prevent the worst cumulative suffering, exceptions do arise: sometimes prevention of the worst cumulative suffering permits or even requires their violation. An agent who regarded these principles as mere rules of thumb would ignore them whenever she calculated that compliance wasn't necessary to minimize the cumulative badness of suffering. The problem is that it might also be in her own interest to violate these principles, and self-interest could distort her calculations, even when she calculated sincerely. She could thus acquire a pattern of violating the principles even when compliance with them really was necessary to prevent the worst cumulative suffering. To avoid this, we would want her to feel strongly inhibited from violating the principles. Inhibitions of this kind can insulate agents from the effect of biased calculations.[12]

Self-interest is not the only motive that can lead our calculations astray. In politics, for example, people who are anxious to make the world a better place (say, by achieving social justice) often determine that adherence to a particular policy or party or individual leader is the best means to this end. Over time, their allegiance may solidify, and they may become reluctant to admit that adherence to the policy or party or leader does not, in some or even most cases, contribute to the hoped-for outcome. This reluctance has many sources; chief among them, I think, is the reluctance to admit that the hoped-for outcome is less easily attained than one had thought, along with the reluctance to admit that the route to the best possible outcome is less clearly marked than one had thought. There is the fear both of gloom and uncertainty: it is much more comforting to have one's path clearly laid out, and to think that by following it one can achieve great good. For these and other reasons (such as the pain of admitting past error), there will be continuous pressure to believe that adherence to one's chosen policy or party or leader contributes to the best possible outcome. Consequently, one will often believe this when the opposite is in fact true. The internalization of sound secondary principles, many in the form of commonsense inhibitions, can help us withstand this pressure. We

---

11. In this paragraph I follow Jonathan Bennett, *The Act Itself*, (Oxford: Clarendon Press, 1995) pp. 23–24. The idea is most fully developed in the work of R. M. Hare. See his "Ethical Theory and Utilitarianism," in Sen and Williams, eds., *Utilitarianism and Beyond*, and *Moral Thinking* (Oxford: Clarendon Press, 1981). Throughout this section I am indebted to Hare's work. Hare, like Bennett, uses the idea to defend consequentialism, but that is not my agenda here.

12. For an interesting illustration, see Sissela Bok, *Lying: Moral Choice in Public and Private Life* (New York: Vintage, 1978). Bok's main argument against lying is that it causes great harm. However, she warns agents not to use consequentialist reasoning when deciding whether to lie. We are prone to overestimate the immediate benefit of lies to ourselves and to underestimate their harm to others, as well as to ourselves, in the long term. For purposes of moral deliberation, Bok recommends a "principle of veracity" that establishes a strong presumption against the permissibility of lying.

will be reluctant to perform some actions dictated by our chosen policy or party or leader, because we will feel that those actions are wrong in themselves. Such inhibitions will often save us from behavior that would, in fact, lead to a worse outcome. Where our goal is the prevention of the worst cumulative suffering, the inhibitions will often save us from behavior that defeats this goal.

Because the duty to relieve suffering calls for moral motives that do not have the relief of suffering as their object, it creates some complexity. Suppose there is a rule requiring behavior that is almost always necessary for the prevention of the worst cumulative suffering. An unusual case arises in which an agent must *violate* the rule in order to prevent the worst cumulative suffering. However, the agent feels strongly inhibited from violating it. Thinking only in terms of the duty to relieve suffering, we might want to say that the agent is morally required to break the rule, and nevertheless also say that it is desirable that she feel inhibited from doing so. If we fear a weakening of her inhibition, because this could lead to worse cumulative suffering over the long term, we may even think it right to encourage her not to break the rule.

The duty to relieve suffering, we might say, does not always serve as an immediate guide to practice, and therefore needs to be translated for human use. We guide ourselves by the duty in translation so as to achieve maximum compliance with the duty in its original form. If we tried to guide ourselves by the original version instead, we would fall far from the mark.[13] The best translation, moreover, is likely to include several inhibitions that are staples of commonsense morality, such as inhibitions against killing, inflicting pain or injury, lying, coercion, and the abandonment of close relatives, friends, clients, and patients.

We can capture this general phenomenon by saying that the duty to relieve suffering often requires indirect methods for the attainment of its end. Indirection is a recurrent theme in consequentialist moralities. It appears in Mill's plea for "secondary principles," and in Sidgwick's admission that it may be desirable on utilitarian grounds for people to be guided by non-utilitarian principles.[14] Consequentialists are often anxious to emphasize moral indirection, since it makes consequentialist morality seem less foreign to common sense and therefore more plausible; for the same reason, critics of consequentialism often attack the idea. Because moral indirection is typically brought up in debates between consequentialists and their critics, I want to stress that my own purpose in discussing it is not to defend consequentialism, but only to elucidate the duty to relieve suffering. Indirection is required by the duty to relieve suffering; given the duty's consequentialist character, that is not surprising. But the duty to relieve suffering is only one prima facie duty

---

13. As Bennett remarks, "It would be astonishing if our deepest and most careful views about how it is right or wrong to behave were simple enough to be usable in the rush of daily life." *The Act Itself*, p. 24.

14. On the need to internalize rules, often of a non-cosequentialist character, in order to produce the best possilbe outcome in the long term, see the penetrating discussion by James Wood Bailey in *Utilitarianism, Institutions, and Justice* (Oxford: Oxford University Press, 1997).

among others; some of the others could be non-consequentialist duties that give our commonsense moral inhibitions a more direct rationale. In claiming that the duty to relieve suffering authorizes certain commonsense moral inhibitions, I am not denying that these inhibitions could have independent validity. All I am saying is that *even if* commonsense moral inhibitions had no independent validity, many of them would still be authorized by the prima facie duty to relieve suffering.

I do not want to take a stand on the truth of consequentialism (the view that we are *always* required to produce the best possible outcome). So my comments in this section are intended for both consequentialists and non-consequentialists. To consequentialists, the message is that commonsense moral inhibitions are necessary. To non-consequentialists, the message is that commonsense moral inhibitions are even *more* important than non-consequentialist reasons can show. Recognizing this in no way threatens non-consequentialism. I know of no more eloquent condemnation of consequentialism than *Darkness at Noon*, Arthur Koestler's meditation on Stalinism. At the end of the novel, Rubashov reflects,

> It was a mistake in the system; perhaps it lay in the precept which until now he had held to be uncontestable, in whose name he had sacrificed others and was himself being sacrificed: in the precept, that the end justifies the means. It was this sentence which had killed the great fraternity of the Revolution and made them all run amuck. What had he once written in his diary? "We have thrown overboard all conventions, our sole guiding principle is that of consequent logic; we are sailing without ethical ballast."
>
> Perhaps the heart of the evil lay there. Perhaps it did not suit mankind to sail without ballast. And perhaps reason alone was a defective compass, which led one on such a winding, twisted course that the goal finally disappeared in the mist.
>
> Perhaps now would come the time of great darkness.[15]

The lesson of this novel is that consequentialism is false *and* that uninhibited consequentialist reasoning has disastrous consequences.

Our commonsense moral inhibitions may have independent validity. Even if they lacked independent validity, many of them would be authorized by the duty to relieve suffering. At the same time, it would be a mistake to suppose that the duty to relieve suffering authorizes commonsense morality in its entirety. There are several reasons for this.

First, I believe the duty to relieve suffering allows and in fact encourages adult agents to be aware that many commonsense inhibitions fulfill the function of steering them to the prevention of the worst cumulative suffering; in commonsense morality itself this idea is absent or unemphasized. Second, the duty to relieve suffering calls on us to override our commonsense inhibitions more frequently than commonsense morality allows. Of course, the danger of ignoring inhibitions and trusting directly to calculation is that irrelevant motives may interfere with our calculations, prompt-

---

15. *Darkness at Noon*, trans. Daphne Harty (New York: Macmillan, 1941), p. 260.

ing behavior that *does not* prevent the worst cumulative suffering. But if the evidence is quite clear that the prevention of the worst cumulative suffering requires us to override an inhibition—so that it is quite clear that extraneous motives aren't leading us astray—then the duty to relieve suffering suggests that we should override the inhibition. To be sure, knowing when we have the requisite level of certainty is a complex matter. Sorting this out would require a long discussion of individual cases that I cannot take up here. A further point is that in fulfilling the duty to relieve suffering we must beware of overriding useful inhibitions if doing so drains them of the power they need in order to be properly effective. But I assume that the duty to relieve suffering can guard against this danger and still authorize more overridings than common sense permits.

The third reason why we shouldn't expect the duty to relieve suffering to authorize the wholesale adoption of commonsense morality is that it is unlikely to select the same exact collection of moral inhibitions enshrined in common sense. It is likely to discard some and add others. For example, it is likely to prefer something weaker than the commonsense conception of our obligation to close relatives, such as children. By the logic of the duty to relieve suffering, we should still feel obliged to secure their basic needs, but less obliged to provide non-essential goods. On the other hand, we should feel a stronger moral compulsion to sacrifice luxuries in order to relieve the suffering of strangers.[16]

Here I have been asking to what extent commonsense morality is authorized by the duty to relieve suffering. But, to repeat, commonsense morality may have independent sources of validity.

My goal in this section has been to show that the duty to relieve suffering must often be fulfilled in indirect ways. In closing this section, I shall briefly consider some objections to the concept of moral indirection.

Some people think of the concept of moral indirection as a way of arguing for consequentialism and oppose it for that reason. But as I have noted, belief in the importance of moral indirection does not commit us to consequentialism.

Some people fear that indirection counsels a policy of deception: a theoretically sophisticated elite is encouraged to deceive the rest of the population into following certain rules for other than the true reasons.[17] This is a possible but not necessary implication of the indirect method. One can deliberately cultivate commonsense inhibitions in oneself, not just others, as a means of achieving fuller compliance with the duty to relieve suffering. One can even deny that one's commonsense inhibitions have inherent validity, yet feel their motivational force, and be grateful for it.

---

16. Derek Parfit makes the same point in *Reasons and Persons* (Oxford: Oxford University Press, 1984), pp. 40–41.

17. See, for example, Bernard Williams's comments on "Government House Utilitarianism," in *Ethics and the Limits of Philosophy* (Cambridge, Mass.: Harvard University Press, 1985), pp. 106–10.

Some people suggest that indirect action—where we pursue X by pointing our-selves toward Y—is psychologically unmanageable. This is clearly untrue. As Peter Railton reminds us, we practice such indirection quite frequently. There are many situations in which we understand the necessity of directing our minds away from our goal in order to achieve it.[18] Think of rowing across a river with a downward current. You guide your boat to a point upstream, but your real destination is directly across.

I believe one reason why the indirect method provokes irritation is the way in which it uses the concepts of morality and duty. It tells us that the precepts that ought to guide our practice do not contain the final or complete truth about morality, but are (at least in part) indirect means to the achievement of certain other duties that cannot be consulted directly (at least not always) at the level of practice. But, it may be felt, morality properly so called is that which ought to guide practical deliberation. So let us call the most appropriate practical guide our morality, and the background justification of this guide by some other name. Discussion of the most appropriate justification may have intellectual value, but it is not discussion of morality.

In reply to this objection, I shall simply repeat my earlier remark that the duty to relieve suffering may use the terms "morality" and "duty" in a somewhat un-familiar way. But there are good reasons for this usage. To repeat: we are morally required to minimize the cumulative badness of suffering. This requirement emerges from the badness of suffering itself. Unfortunately, the non-transparency of the duty to relieve suffering makes it unworkable as an immediate guide to practice. We need a translation of it that is suited for use by human beings. As it turns out, the best available translation includes moral precepts that differ from, even conflict with, the content of the duty to relieve suffering. *But this translation enables us to prevent worse cumulative suffering than we otherwise could, and that is what we are required to do.*

5. The Relief of Suffering in an Uncertain World

The duty to relieve suffering, I have argued, needs to be translated into a form suitable for human use. Part of the translation takes the form of moral motives that do not have the duty to relieve suffering as their object. Another part, which I discuss here, is required by the fact that we live in an uncertain world.

The duty to relieve suffering requires us to act so as to minimize the cumulative badness of suffering. However, we can never predict all the consequences of our

18. Railton, "Alienation, Consequentialism, and the Demands of Morality," *Philosophy and Public Affairs* 13 (1984): 134–71. On p. 154, Railton gives the following examples: "the timid, put-upon employee who knows that if he deliberates about whether to ask for a raise he will succumb to his timidity and fail to demand what he actually deserves; the self-conscious man who knows that if, at social gatherings, he is forever wondering how he should act, his behavior will be awkward and unnatural, contrary to his goal of acting naturally and appropriately; the tightrope walker who knows he must not reflect on the value of keeping his concentration."

behavior with perfect certainty. Some degree of uncertainty attends even our most solid predictions, an uncertainty that expands as we consider the remoter effects of our actions. Therefore, we can never be completely certain, at the moment of deliberation, which action will in fact prevent the worst cumulative suffering.

Most moral theorists believe that, whenever morality requires us to seek the best possible outcome, we should maximize the *expected goodness* of our conduct. The expected goodness of an action is calculated by multiplying the value of its potential outcomes by the probability of their occurrence and adding these products together. Here is a streamlined example. Suppose we face three potential outcomes: Status Quo, Better, and Best. Compared with Status Quo, Best is twice as good as Better, so we can assign Status Quo, Better, and Best values of 0, 1, and 2 respectively. Now suppose we have a choice between action A, which has a 100 percent chance of producing Better, and action B, which has a 25 percent chance of preserving Status Quo and a 75 percent chance of producing Best. Here the expected goodness of B exceeds that of A. If we believe we ought to maximize the expected goodness of our actions, we should choose B.

Applied to the duty to relieve suffering, this approach would require us to minimize the expected cumulative badness of suffering. This assumes we can assign cardinal values to the cumulative badness of different configurations of suffering. Chapter 7 discusses how to assign such values in certain cases. Even when probability estimates and/or estimates of the cardinal badness of suffering are rough rather than precise, we may still be able, some of the time, to identify the behavior that minimizes the expected cumulative badness of suffering. In the following example, however, I shall assume precise values. If action A has a 100 percent chance of producing suffering with a cumulative badness of 1, while action B has a 50 percent chance of producing no suffering—therefore 0 badness—and a 50 percent chance of producing suffering with a cumulative badness of 4, then the expected badness of B exceeds that of A by a ratio of 2 to 1, so we should choose action A.

When we can't know for certain how to minimize the cumulative badness of suffering, it seems intuitively right that we should act so as to minimize the expected cumulative badness of suffering. But notice that this is not what the duty to relieve suffering asks us to do. The duty to relieve suffering springs from the badness of suffering, from the fact that suffering must not be allowed to occur. Thus it demands whatever behavior will *in fact* minimize the cumulative badness of suffering. It is concerned with the actual, not the probable, effects of our behavior. Sometimes an act that minimizes the expected cumulative badness of suffering does not actually minimize the cumulative badness of suffering. Therefore, the minimization of the expected cumulative badness of suffering sometimes leads us to violate the duty to relieve suffering.[19]

---

19. I think this helps to explain why we may feel *remorse* when our act is reasonably expected to prevent the worst possible suffering but, through bad luck, falls far short of this. Imagine, for example, that in trying to rescue other people from grave danger I seal their doom instead. The remorse I may

We have a perverse state of affairs. An agent, at the moment of deciding, *can never know* what is required by the duty to relieve suffering. An agent can never say, "I am doing this because it is required by the duty to relieve suffering." Such an agent claims knowledge she could not have! The actual duty to relieve suffering seems to offer us no practical guidance.

Therefore, it would seem that if we want a practical guide we must turn elsewhere than the duty to relieve suffering. For example, we might establish a standard of subjective rightness according to which we are required to minimize the expected badness of suffering. The standard couldn't be endorsed by the duty to relieve suffering itself. But even so, it may seem intuitively plausible, even obvious.

However, as it turns out, there is a connection, of an indirect kind, between the actual duty to relieve suffering and the policy of minimizing the expected cumulative badness of suffering. It is this. If we are conscious of the actual duty to relieve suffering, we could do one of the following. We could decide to act randomly. Or we could choose between several rule-governed policies, one of which is the policy of minimizing the expected cumulative badness of suffering. Of these alternatives, the last mentioned policy is almost certain, over the long term, to prevent the worst cumulative suffering. If we repeat the policy frequently enough, the minimization of the *expected* cumulative badness of suffering is almost certain to become the minimization of the *actual* cumulative badness of suffering. So although we can never be sure that the minimization of the expected cumulative badness of suffering complies with the duty to relieve suffering on any particular occasion, it is almost certain that the duty to relieve suffering requires us to adopt a policy of minimizing the expected cumulative badness of suffering. I say "almost certain" throughout, since there is a remote possibility that some other policy rather than this one would in fact lead to the prevention of the worst cumulative suffering over the long run. This is unlikely in the extreme, but the possibility cannot be denied.

In conclusion: though the minimization of the expected badness of suffering is not strictly speaking the same as compliance with the duty to relieve suffering, it is the best translation of the duty to relieve suffering into a form that human beings can use.

---

feel could come from the consciousness that I have violated the *objective* duty to relieve suffering, even though this knowledge wasn't available at the moment of action and could not have guided my deliberation. The remorse that often accompanies bad moral luck is a longstanding puzzle in moral philosophy. For a valuable discussion, see Bennett, *The Act Itself*, pp. 58–61.

SIX

The Moral Asymmetry of Happiness and Suffering

1. Introduction

This chapter begins an inquiry, pursued further in chapter 7, into a class of moral dilemmas posed by the prima facie duty to relieve suffering. These are dilemmas in which we must choose between different ways of benefiting people.

This chapter addresses the relative moral importance of happiness and suffering. In addressing this question, I want to restrict our attention to happiness and suffering in the hedonistic sense of these terms and to set other values aside. I also want to set aside cases (if there are any) in which personal attributes or past actions alter the value of an individual's happiness or suffering. In the cases to be examined, I assume that everyone is equally deserving of happiness and protection from suffering. Finally, I want to keep the analysis focused on the value of *outcomes*. Therefore, I assume that when, in the following examples, we have to choose between different outcomes, there is no morally significant difference in the means used to bring about one outcome rather than the other. (If some readers have intuitions that there is such a difference in the examples discussed, I ask them to set such intuitions temporarily aside.)

Is the relief of suffering more important, or is it not more important, than the promotion of happiness? The classical utilitarians answered that it is not. They believed that we should maximize the total surplus of happiness over suffering, so they were committed to the view that an increase in positive happiness and a reduction of suffering, when equal in magnitude, are equal in value. Their view is well-stated by Henry Sidgwick. Utilitarianism, we are told, instructs us to seek the Greatest Happiness, by which is meant "the greatest possible surplus of pleasure over pain, the pain being conceived as balanced against an equal amount of pleasure, so that the two contrasted amounts annihilate each other for purposes of ethical calculation."[1]

Against this view, Karl Popper famously objected:

> I believe that there is, from the ethical point of view, no symmetry between suffering and happiness, or between pain and pleasure. Both the greatest happiness principle of the Utilitarians and Kant's principle, "Promote other people's happiness . . . ," seem to me (at least in their formulations) fundamentally wrong in this point, which is, however not one for rational argument. . . . In my opinion . . . human suffering makes a direct moral appeal, namely, the appeal for help, while there is no similar call to increase the happiness of a man who is doing well anyway.[2]

Many people agree with Popper that the alleviation of suffering is more urgent than the promotion of happiness. Many people also believe that the reduction of more intense suffering is more urgent than the reduction of less intense suffering.

This chapter looks at the question that pitted Sidgwick against Popper. I shall refer to Sidgwick's claim as the view that happiness and suffering are *morally symmetrical*. I shall refer to Popper's claim (together with the claim that it is more urgent to reduce more intense suffering than less intense suffering) as the view that happiness and suffering are *morally asymmetrical*.

We can distinguish between two different versions of the claim that happiness and suffering are morally asymmetrical.[3] According to the *teleological* version, the reason why we should sometimes reduce suffering by a smaller amount rather than increase happiness by a greater amount is that by doing so we produce a better outcome overall. According to the *deontological* version, the relief of suffering exerts a stronger moral claim on us than the promotion of happiness for reasons independent of the over-all value of alternative outcomes. On the deontological version of the asymmetry view, therefore, we should sometimes give priority to the relief of suffering even when doing so leads to a *worse* outcome overall. In the following discussion I ignore the deontological version of the asymmetry view. I assume that if we should give priority to the relief of suffering, the reason is that by doing so we produce a better outcome overall.

The moral symmetry view holds that we should maximize the total surplus of happiness over suffering; therefore, it is always better (other things being equal) to

1. Henry Sidgwick, *The Methods of Ethics* (London: Macmillan, 1907), p. 413. For a reassertion of this view, see James Griffin, "Is Unhappiness Morally More Important than Happiness?" *Philosophical Quarterly* 29 (1979): 47–59. Sidgwick's view is assumed or defended by several other contemporary utilitarians, such as Richard B. Brandt (*A Theory of the Good and the Right* [Oxford: Clarendon Press, 1979]), R. M. Hare (*Moral Thinking: Its Levels, Method and Point* [Oxford: Clarendon Press, 1981]), Peter Singer (*Practical Ethics*, 2nd ed. [Cambridge: Cambridge University Press, 1993]), and Torbjörn Tännsjö ("Classical Hedonistic Utilitarianism," *Philosophical Studies* 81 [1996]: 97–115).

2. Karl R. Popper, *The Open Society and Its Enemies* (Princeton, N.J.: Princeton University Press, 1950), pp. 570–71 (note 2 to Chapter 9); see also pp. 508–9 (n.6 [2] to chap. 5).

3 Here I follow Derek Parfit, *Equality or Priority?* 1991 Lindley Lecture (University of Kansas, Lawrence, Kan., 1995), pp. 3–4.

bring about a larger increase in positive happiness than a smaller reduction of suffering, and to bring about a greater reduction of less intense suffering than a smaller
reduction of more intense suffering. The moral asymmetry view holds, in contrast,
that it is sometimes better to bring about a smaller reduction of suffering than a
larger increase in happiness, and a smaller reduction of more intense suffering than
a larger reduction of less intense suffering. In order to see what is at stake, we need
to be clear about the notion of quantity. To measure quantity, I propose this un-
surprising formula: number of people experiencing happiness (suffering), multiplied
by the duration of their happiness (suffering), multiplied by the intensity of their
happiness (suffering).

There is nothing mysterious about numbers or duration. Intensity is more difficult to pin down. I spent the bulk of chapter 3 trying to bring it into sharper
focus. The concept is highly elusive. Not only is it unrealistic to expect anything
approaching precision in our estimates of the intensity of happiness and suffering,
but there are at least four different ways of understanding what intensity means.
We can think in terms either of an intuitive measure, a preferential measure, a
global evaluative measure, or a local evaluative measure. Since the measures sometimes diverge, the use of different measures can lead to different estimates of the
quantity of happiness and suffering. Consequently, people who use different measures will have different things in mind when they make claims about the relative
moral importance of happiness and suffering. Verbal agreement may mask substantive disagreement, while verbal disagreement may mask substantive agreement. It is
incumbent on anyone who addresses this topic to make clear which measure of
intensity he or she is using. And when discussing the views of other people, one
should ascertain to the best of one's ability which measure they had in mind.

In chapter 3 I indicated a preference for the intuitive measure. I also argued that
the three other measures labored under serious difficulties. In the following discussion I will have in mind the intuitive measure, unless otherwise noted. But I will
try to say something about how the moral and prudential issues are best seen from
the perspective of the other three measures. I will also address a number of questions
regarding the interpretation of classical utilitarianism. When the classical utilitarians
asserted the moral symmetry of happiness and suffering, which measure of intensity
did they have in mind? And how should this affect our interpretation of what they
said?

The question of the relative moral importance of happiness and suffering is a
question about the trade-off between preventing suffering and promoting happiness.
It asks whether the first is more important than the second. We need to distinguish
between two kinds of these trade-offs. There are trade-offs between happiness and
suffering *within the same person's life,* and there are trade-offs between happiness and
suffering *across different people's lives.* In the first case, the question is whether to
prevent one person's suffering or to promote the *same* person's happiness. For example, we may have to choose between protecting someone from suffering at one
point in her life and providing her with positive happiness at another point in her
life. In the second case, the question is whether to prevent one person's suffering

or to promote *another* person's happiness. It is important to distinguish between these two kinds of trade-offs, because one may hold different views about the relative moral importance of happiness and suffering in each case.

I shall look at the question of relative moral importance first within lives and then across lives. I shall claim that, on the *intuitive* measure of intensity, suffering weighs more than happiness in trade-offs that occur within the same person's life. More confidently, I shall then assert, once more with reference to the intuitive measure, that suffering weighs more than happiness in trade-offs between different people's lives. For a number of reasons, the moral asymmetry of happiness and suffering is more obvious in interpersonal trade-offs than in intrapersonal trade-offs. Fortunately, although the intrapersonal question is harder to judge than the interpersonal question, it is also less important, for reasons discussed later.

I shall also include a discussion of how the relative moral importance of happiness and suffering both within and across lives appears from the perspective of the three alternative measures of intensity. In addition, I shall try to determine just how we should interpret the stated view of classical utilitarianism.

2. The Moral Asymmetry of Happiness and Suffering within Lives

Is there a moral asymmetry between happiness and suffering within lives? Is it more important to reduce someone's suffering than to promote (at another time) the same person's happiness? For the time being, I ask this question in terms of the intuitive measure of intensity. As I noted in chapter 3, this measure equates intensity with the "immediately felt goodness" of happiness and the "immediately felt badness" of suffering respectively.

I believe that the answer to this question is yes. Yet some people may be disposed to answer no. On this question, intuitions are divided and uncertain. Though I cannot provide a conclusive argument for intrapersonal asymmetry, I will try to make it seem more plausible by citing certain feelings and intuitions where a belief in such asymmetry seems to be at work.

Some people may say that there is an easy way to determine the relative moral importance of happiness and suffering within the same life: let each person be the judge. When there is a trade-off between the relief of suffering and the promotion of happiness, or between the reduction of more intense and less intense suffering, the alternative that is favored by the person's well-informed, non-discounting preferences is the alternative that is best for that person. People facing identical trade-offs may prefer different alternatives, but whatever alternative is favored by a person's well-informed preference is best *for that person*, even if other people prefer opposite alternatives. Let us call this the consent view.

I am inclined to reject this view. It initially seems appealing because of the homage it pays to individual liberty. Most of us think that it is wrong, in general, to thwart other people's well-informed desires regarding their own lives. Moreover, most of us think that having such desires thwarted generally counts as a *harm*. Our lives go better, other things being equal, when they conform more closely to our well-informed desires. This might seem especially true with something as intimate as the distribution of happiness and suffering within one's own life. The consent view seems attractive because it taps into these beliefs. But we can hold onto these beliefs without adopting the consent view.

The consent view has the right idea in valuing individual liberty, but it goes astray, I think, in its interpretation of what it *means* to value individual liberty. The value of liberty is best captured, not by saying that people's well-informed preferences concerning the distribution of happiness and suffering alter the value of that distribution itself, but by saying that there is a value in having people lead their own lives, even if they make the wrong choices. Their choosing doesn't make the *content* of their choice better. It is their being able to choose that we value. James Griffin expresses the point nicely when he says that my ability to govern my own affairs is still valuable "even if I constantly made a mess of my life, even if you could do better if you took charge."[4] The value of liberty is not directly reflected onto what we choose to do with it. (For this reason, there is something abstract about the value of liberty.)

There are principled reasons to honor individual liberty. I have emphasized its *value*, though some may prefer a less teleological approach that instead emphasizes the *respect* we owe to other persons as autonomous beings. In addition, there are pragmatic or indirect reasons, well-known to us from Mill's essay on the subject. One reason is that individual choosers will often know better than anyone else what is involved in the alternatives facing them; for example, in choosing between different distributions of happiness and suffering, they will often have a better sense of what the relevant intensities really are. Individuals are also, as a rule, more consistently and wholeheartedly dedicated to their own well-being than onlookers who profess concern. And, as Mill stressed, the experience of having to choose for ourselves is a marvelous teacher—one that strengthens our character, deepens our wisdom, and expands our horizons.

The importance of individual liberty makes it more difficult to assess the relative moral importance of happiness and suffering within the same life. In many situations, people's self-regarding desires are the best indicator of which outcome ought to be pursued. For good reason, we become used to referring to such desires as a proper arbiter for resolving intrapersonal trade-offs. This makes it harder to get past individual desires to weigh the relative importance of happiness and suffering in themselves. Notice that the same problem does not affect our judgments about *interpersonal* trade-offs, since in those trade-offs self-regarding preferences, by definition, do not apply. That is why I earlier said that judgments about the relative moral importance of happiness and suffering are both more difficult and less important in intrapersonal trade-offs than in interpersonal trade-offs.

4. James Griffin, *Well-being* (Oxford: Clarendon Press, 1986), p. 67.

Let us now look at the case involving intrapersonal trade-offs. I will try to present the case for the moral asymmetry of happiness and suffering within lives. In doing so, I am obliged to draw on my own intuitions. I do not know how widely they are shared, though I suspect that they are by no means uncommon.

I believe that, within the same life, the relief of suffering is more important than the promotion of happiness. This appears to me most clearly true in the case of very intense suffering. Imagine an episode of very intense suffering—say, one that involves overwhelming physical pain. Now imagine an episode of happiness of equal intensity. Of course it would be happiness of the most glorious kind. Nevertheless, it seems to me that the intense suffering would not be compensated by an episode of the intense happiness lasting for the same amount of time. In fact, it strikes me that the intense suffering would not be compensated by an episode of the intense happiness lasting for a considerably *longer* amount of time.

We give surgery patients anesthesia to avert the agony they would feel if they remained conscious. Suppose some drug became available that gave people a joy as intense as the pain averted by anesthesia, and suppose that there were no drawbacks in the consumption of this drug. It seems quite clear to me that the provision of this drug would be less important than the administration of anesthesia. It is easy to picture this scenario as a trade-off between different people—anesthesia for some versus euphoria for others—which of course takes us away from the issue at hand. But when I place the example in the context of one person's life, so that the question is whether it is more important to provide the same person with anesthesia at one time or the euphoria pill at another, it seems obvious that providing the anesthesia is more important. The moral badness of the suffering overshadows the moral goodness of the happiness.

Other considerations also suggest the intrapersonal asymmetry of happiness and suffering. A moral imbalance between happiness and suffering is reflected in the attitudes that many of us have toward our own futures. I believe many of us can become indifferent to the thought of our own future happiness in a way that we can't to the thought of our own future suffering. The prospect of future pain disturbs us more than the forfeit of future pleasure.

This attitude is revealed most dramatically, albeit implicitly, in the Epicurean doctrine that death is not a harm. It is worth asking why the Epicureans held this view, and why others have been drawn to it. Death is not a harm, the Epicureans maintained, because the person who has died exists no longer, and what does not exist cannot be harmed. Critics accuse this argument of depending on the questionable assumption that harm must be experienced in order to count as harm. They argue that death, though not something that can be experienced, nevertheless harms us by depriving us of the goods of life. I agree that we ought to challenge the assumption that harm must be experienced in order to count as harm. But I do not think that this assumption is all that is at work in the Epicurean argument. The Epicureans were hedonists. They viewed happiness (pleasure) as the sole good and suffering (pain) as the sole evil. They were able to look with equanimity on the deprivation of future happiness through death. I doubt, however, that they could have looked with equal indifference on the elimination, through death, of extreme suffering. Let us turn the Epicurean teaching around and ask whether death is sometimes a *benefit*. Isn't it a benefit to someone who is otherwise destined to live in agony? Some people may deny this because they connect life to non-hedonistic values; for example, they may believe that life is *sacred*. But since the Epicureans were hedonists, such a view was unavailable to them. I am fairly certain that the Epicureans would have said that death *is* a benefit to someone otherwise destined to live in agony, even though this position contradicts the stated logic of their view that death is never a harm: according to that logic, death cannot benefit anyone, since there is no one around to experience the benefit. Leaving aside what the Epicureans themselves would have said, I believe that many people who have been swayed by the their argument that death does not harm us would *not* be similarly swayed by a parallel argument for the claim that death does not benefit someone living in agony. That some of us may doubt (at least temporarily) that death can harm us by depriving us of happiness but are unable to doubt (even temporarily) that death can benefit us by removing our agony is testimony, I believe, to a feeling that suffering matters more than happiness. This feeling lends support to the thought that, within the same person's life, it is more important to reduce suffering than to increase happiness.

There is a certain resemblance between the view I have described and the view shared by many people that there is no moral obligation to bring happy people into existence, but that there *is* a moral obligation not to bring wretched people into existence. I think that a belief in the moral asymmetry of happiness and suffering is one source of this view, though perhaps not the only one.[5]

I have claimed that the relief of suffering is more important than the promotion of happiness within the same person's life. Should we also say that, within the same person's life, the reduction of more intense suffering is more important than the reduction of less intense suffering? Or to ask the same question in a different way: Should we say that as someone's suffering increases in intensity the urgency of *preventing* that person's suffering increases at a faster rate than its intensity? This is an exceedingly difficult question, principally because of the inescapable roughness and uncertainty of intensity estimates. It is impossible to know whether we have ever estimated the intensity of suffering accurately, and consequently impossible to form a precise view about the relationship between the intensity of suffering and the urgency of preventing it. But for my own part, I believe that as suffering increases in intensity, the urgency of preventing it rises at a faster rate than its intensity. If I think about suffering of a serious, fairly intense kind, and then think about another kind of suffering that is *four times more intense*, I think that it would be better to experience far more than four hours of the less intense suffering than to

---

5. For a different explanation, see Derek Parfit, "Future Generations: Further Problems," *Philosophy and Public Affairs* 11 (1981): 113–72, p. 148–51. The explanation is restated in *Reasons and Persons*, pp. 526–27 (n. 32 to Part 4).

experience just one hour of the more intense suffering. The less intense suffering is preferable to the more intense suffering even though the total quantity involved (intensity multiplied by duration) is greater.[6]

If I think about the unimaginable prospect of twelve hours of severe torture, it seems to me that almost an indefinite extension of low-intensity suffering would be preferable. Think of someone who lives a life of persistent bleakness and deprivation: without close companionship, without diversions to lift up the spirit and gratify the senses, and without either an inward sense of accomplishment or the reception of admiration and recognition from other people to raise her feelings of self-worth. At the same time, let us imagine that this person has a certain bare level of material security, stoicism, and underlying self-esteem that together limit the misery she feels. It seems to me that, as far as suffering is concerned, an entire lifetime spent like this would be less bad than the alternative of twelve hours of extreme torture as experienced by the same person. (This seems especially clear to me if the rest of the torture victim's life is spent at the hedonistic zero.) This is how it seems to me, even though the product of intensity and duration of suffering is likely to be much greater in the first case than in the second case. Reflection on this and other examples leads me to think that the reduction of more intense suffering has priority over the reduction of less intense suffering within lives.[7]

I have claimed, with reference to the intuitive measure of intensity, that it is more important to prevent someone's suffering than to promote the same person's happiness, and that it is more important to reduce someone's more intense suffering than to reduce the same person's less intense suffering. Why should we entertain such claims? If the intuitive measure equates intensity with the "immediately felt goodness" of happiness and the "immediately felt badness" of suffering, why shouldn't we maximize the total surplus of "immediately felt goodness" over "immediately felt badness" that characterizes each person's lifetime experience? Why shouldn't we, in other words, maximize each person's total surplus of happiness over suffering, intuitively understood? I believe the reason why we should not is that suffering possesses greater moral weight than happiness, and that as suffering increases in intensity its moral weight increases at a faster rate than its intensity. Moral weight is not distributed evenly across the happiness-suffering scale; it accumulates toward the bottom (that is, if we picture suffering at the bottom of the scale, and happiness at the top).

There are several ways to express this idea. We can say that suffering is more to be feared than happiness is to be desired, and that as suffering increases in

6. In this chapter and the next, I make the simplifying assumption that we can form precise cardinal estimates of the intensity of happiness and suffering. As noted in chapter 3, it may be that, in some or all cases, only rough estimates are possible. However, the ideas in this chapter and the next one can be stated more easily if we temporarily assume the possibility of precise cardinal estimates.

7. I have suggested that as the intensity of someone's suffering increases, the urgency of preventing it rises at a faster rate than the intensity. Someone might propose a similar claim with regard to duration: namely, that as someone's suffering is prolonged without interruption, the urgency of preventing it increases faster than its duration. I postpone an examination of this question to the next chapter.

intensity its fearsomeness increases at a rate disproportionate to its intensity. We can say that, from a normative perspective, suffering is more bad than happiness is good, and that with increases in intensity its badness (normatively speaking) rises faster than its intensity. The key is to distinguish the phenomenological features of happiness and suffering (how good or bad it feels in an immediate sense) from a higher-order judgment about the degree to which it is worth pursuing or avoiding. The intrinsic moral badness of suffering is distinct from its immediately felt badness, just as the intrinsic moral goodness of happiness is distinct from its immediately felt goodness. (In the case of suffering, I believe the two dimensions actually *diverge;* I suspend judgment on whether they diverge in the case of happiness.)

What I am claiming is that the moral asymmetry between happiness and suffering is, at least in part, a fact about happiness and suffering as such. It reflects certain moral properties directly pertaining to happiness on the one hand and suffering on the other. In this section I have claimed that such an asymmetry is played out in intrapersonal trade-offs. So in this context the claimed asymmetry emerges as the view that there exists a *prudential* asymmetry between happiness and suffering. But the underlying claim is not one about prudence—what makes a person's life go better or worse—nor are its implications confined to prudential dilemmas. The underlying claim, to repeat, is just that suffering is (morally) more bad than happiness is good, and that as suffering increases in intensity its (moral) badness increases at a faster rate than its intensity. I shall refer to this claim as the *intrinsic property view*. The intrinsic property view is at work not only in the view that happiness and suffering are morally asymmetrical within lives, but also in the view that there exists such an asymmetry in trade-offs across lives. However, as I discuss later, there may be more at work in the interpersonal asymmetry of happiness and suffering than the intrinsic property view.

3. Epicurus's Hint

Earlier I suggested that the Epicurean belief in the harmlessness of death seemed to reflect a belief in the intrapersonal asymmetry of happiness and suffering. I think there is additional evidence that the Epicureans may have held such a view. The Epicureans are relevant here not only because they were hedonists, but also because, like other ancient philosophers, they reasoned within a framework of ethical egoism. In their view, the good that each person should seek is his own. Specifically, they taught that each person should maximize his own pleasure, though they emphasized that the highest pitch of pleasure could only be attained by those who formed devoted friendships and scrupulously abstained from wrongdoing.

The clue that the Epicureans may have believed in the intrapersonal asymmetry of happiness and suffering lies in their startling claim that the complete absence of pain constituted "the limit and highest point of pleasure."[8] Many people have been

8. See Cicero, *De Finibus Bonorum et Malorum*, trans. H. Rackham, Loeb Classical Library (Cambridge, Mass.: Harvard University Press, 1983), book I, 38 (original pagination).

troubled by this claim. Cicero was among those most exasperated by it. He insisted that pleasure and absence of pain are two different things; the bliss we sometimes experience in indulging our senses to the utmost, for example, is something quite distinct from the merely negative condition of not feeling pain. In Cicero's view, the Epicurean doctrine allowed its proponents to practice the worst kind of intellectual evasion. Depending on the rhetorical needs of the moment, they could celebrate pleasure itself—the real thing in all its immediate sweetness and charm—or else limit their praise to the more general condition of freedom from pain.[9]

Some have interpreted the Epicurean claim as a celebration of *ataraxia*, their term for a feeling of serenity or mental repose untouched by pain and untroubled by desire.[10] Since the Epicureans spoke frequently in praise of ataraxia, this interpretation has some merit. However, it leaves some unanswered questions. One wants to ask, in the spirit of Cicero, whether ataraxia is or is not pleasurable. If it is pleasurable, why understate its value by classifying it as a painless condition? If it is not pleasurable, why value it as highly as the Epicureans clearly did?

Some may read the Epicurean claim in a psychological vein. The claim, on this interpretation, is that loss of pain gives rise to mental pleasure, and that this pleasure is equal to the highest pleasure that can possibly be experienced. This is one way of understanding the remark of the Epicurean Torquatus, as reported by Cicero:

> We do not agree that when pleasure is withdrawn uneasiness at once ensues, unless the pleasure happens to have been replaced by a pain: while on the other hand one is glad to lose a pain even though no active sensation of pleasure comes in its place; a fact that serves to show how great a pleasure is the mere absence of pain.[11]

Sometimes, it is true, release from pain is followed by a grateful swing into mental pleasure. But this does not always happen. There are times, for example, when we continue to brood over the pain that was lately inflicted on us, and keep on feeling sorry for ourselves. We are not fully conscious that the pain has been withdrawn, and are therefore incapable of feeling gratitude for our release. Only when it is renewed do we realize with a jolt that we had enjoyed a reprieve; then we may chastise ourselves for *not* having appreciated the relief while it lasted. It would be a pity if the Epicureans intended a view so clearly contradicted by experience.

I shall put forward another interpretation, and that is that the Epicureans were groping for words to express the intrapersonal asymmetry of happiness and suffering. They understood that the ethical necessity of avoiding pain somehow transcended the ethical necessity of seeking pleasure. They had a sense that once one had succeeded in escaping and guarding oneself from pain, the important work had been done; an ethical maximum had been achieved. Liberation from pain was the main accomplishment; any pleasure that one could achieve thereafter carried lesser value in comparison. Or to put it another way, happiness and suffering occupied

9. Ibid., book II, 5–20, 28–30.
10. See Geoffrey Scarre, "Epicurus as a Forerunner of Utilitarianism," *Utilitas* 6 (1994): 219–31.
11. Cicero, *De Finibus*, book I, 56.

two different levels of moral importance: from the standpoint of suffering, the contrast of happiness with mere painlessness seemed small and insignificant, whereas from the standpoint of happiness, suffering preserved all its terror.

This interpretation permits a different reading of Torquatus's remark quoted earlier. The point is that release from pain ought always to elicit gladness upon reflection (whether or not it always does so in fact), because nothing could be more important.

Additional support for the view that the Epicureans believed in the intrapersonal asymmetry of pain and pleasure can be found in their classification of human desires. Epicurus divided desires among three kinds: those that are natural and necessary, those that are natural but not necessary, and those that are neither natural nor necessary.[12] Necessary desires are those whose frustration brings pain (No. 26). Unnatural desires are founded on "empty opinion," and their frustration does not bring pain; "that they are not got rid of is because of man's empty opinion, not because of their own nature" (Nos. 29, 30). Between necessary and unnatural desires lies an intermediate category of natural but unnecessary desires. Epicurus himself is not clear what distinguishes this category from the other two, but a comment added by the scholiast on the manuscript explains that unnecessary natural desires, unlike necessary natural ones, cause no pain when frustrated, but instead "give variety to pleasure" (Scholium to No. 29). Presumably they differ from unnatural desires in not being invented by empty opinion, and in receiving some kind of justification in the intrinsic merit of their object. It is revealing that Epicurus distinguishes between desires whose satisfaction averts pain and desires whose satisfaction merely diversifies pleasure, and that he reserves the description "necessary" only for the former. Of unnecessary desires "that do not bring pain if they are not satisfied," he says that "they are easily thrust aside whenever to satisfy them appears difficult or likely to cause injury." The Epicurean restriction of the term "necessary" to those desires whose satisfaction is necessary to avert pain seems to reflect a belief that the relief of pain takes priority over the promotion of pleasure.[13]

The Epicurean doctrines that suggest a moral asymmetry between happiness and suffering might be interpreted as saying that the prevention of suffering has lexical priority over the promotion of happiness—in other words, that we should be pre-

---

12. Epicurus, *Principal Doctrines*, No. 29, in Epicurus, *Letters, Principal Doctrines, and Vatican Sayings*, trans. Russel M. Geer (Indianapolis: Bobbs Merrill, 1964), p. 63.

13. Some readers might reply that Epicurus was not distinguishing between eliminating pain and increasing pleasure. He, or the scholiast, defined unnecessary natural desires as those that *diversify* pleasures, not those that *increase* them. But then, what of the distinction between unnecessary natural desires and unnatural desires? The goal of merely diversifying pleasures without increasing them would appear in the light of Epicurus's own criteria as a quest devoid of value. If increase of pleasure and reduction of pain are the only true goods, then the wish for the diversification of pleasure unaccompanied by increase lacks justification and consequently must join the class of desires that are driven by "empty opinion." Epicurus's impulse to establish a second class of unnecessary desires, called natural, seems to indicate that the desire for increased pleasure, rather than for objects of mere illusory value, was what he had in mind.

pared to sacrifice even the greatest amount of happiness in order to avoid even the smallest amount of suffering. The form in which the doctrines are stated do permit this interpretation, but it is an extravagant and implausible view. A more settled view, which the exaggerated formulations of the Epicureans may help us reach, is that happiness and suffering should be measured on different moral scales, with the moral importance of suffering generally outweighing the moral importance of happiness.

4. The Relative Importance of Happiness and Suffering within Lives, as Viewed in Terms of the Three Alternative Measures of Intensity

I have examined the relative moral importance of happiness and suffering within lives, where intensity is conceived in terms of the intuitive measure. I now look at the same question with reference to the three other measures of intensity: the preferential measure, the global evaluative measure, and the local evaluative measure. For now, instead of referring to the "relative moral importance of happiness and suffering within lives," I shall refer to the "relative prudential importance of happiness and suffering." I assume that both terms mean the same thing. (They may not, if deontological considerations play a role in how we should balance happiness and suffering.)

The preferential measure calculates intensity so that people's well-informed, non-discounting preferences always favor the maximum total surplus of happiness over suffering in their own lives. What is the relative prudential importance of happiness and suffering, according to this measure? To answer this question, we must first decide whether a person's well-informed, non-discounting preferences regarding alternative patterns of happiness and suffering always determine what is best for that person. The claim that prudential value is determined by individual self-regarding preferences is what I earlier called the consent view. If we adopt the preferential measure of intensity together with the consent view regarding prudential value, then happiness and suffering are prudentially symmetrical by definition. It is always best for a person to experience the maximum total surplus of happiness over suffering (other things being equal).

If we reject the consent view, we believe that a person's well-informed preferences regarding alternative patterns of happiness and suffering do not always disclose what is best for that person. If we reject the consent view, then there is, on the preferential measure of intensity, no general rule about the relative prudential importance of happiness and suffering. Everything depends on the pattern of that person's preferences. If a person's preferences happen to assign just the right weight to happiness and suffering at all levels of intensity, then happiness and suffering are prudentially symmetrical in that person's life. If a person's preferences give too little weight to the badness of suffering, then the badness of suffering exceeds its intensity as recorded by this person's preferences. Happiness and suffering are prudentially asymmetrical, inasmuch as it is better to reduce this person's suffering than to promote her happiness by the same amount. If someone's preferences give too *much* weight to the badness of suffering, then the badness of her suffering is *less* than its intensity as recorded by her preferences. Once more, happiness and suffering are asymmetrical, but in a sense opposite to that which we have been discussing so far. In this case, it is sometimes better to increase the person's happiness by a *smaller* amount than to reduce her suffering by a *larger* amount.

It seems to me that the preferential measure exerts less appeal if the consent view is rejected. The measure is of less interest if it does not track the value of alternative outcomes. Now the preferential measure combined with the consent view becomes equivalent to the evaluative measure of intensity. The preferential measure will therefore appear most attractive when it is made to correspond with the evaluative measure. (There is also a disadvantage to this version of the preferential measure if, as I have claimed, the consent view should be rejected. My point is just that people are less likely to be drawn to the preferential measure if they reject the consent view.) On the other hand, the evaluative measure combined with the consent view makes it vulnerable to the same objections that I directed against the preferential measure at the end of chapter 3, section 4. So the evaluative measure becomes most compelling when it does *not* correspond to the preferential measure. All things considered, the evaluative measure seems an improvement over the preferential measure. I now examine the relative prudential weight of happiness and suffering from the standpoint of the evaluative measure.

Recall that the evaluative measure comes in two versions, one global and the other local. The global evaluative measure calculates intensity so that it is always best for a person to experience the greatest total surplus of happiness over suffering (other things being equal). On the global evaluative measure, therefore, happiness and suffering are prudentially symmetrical by definition.

I have previously claimed that, on the intuitive measure, it is more important to prevent someone's suffering than to promote the same person's happiness, and more important to reduce someone's more intense suffering than the same person's less intense suffering. If this claim is true, then the global evaluative measure, correctly used, must diverge from the intuitive measure. It must adjust its estimates to take into account the prudential asymmetry of happiness and suffering as recorded on the intuitive measure. The result is that the global evaluative measure will assign higher estimates of intensity than the intuitive measure to the same kinds of suffering.

In a variation of the global evaluative measure, the local evaluative measure calculates intensity so that it is always best for a person to experience the greatest total surplus of happiness over suffering, but only where relatively short, unvarying, and uninterrupted episodes of happiness and suffering are involved. (This formulation has to be qualified in one respect. Where there are large differences in proportional intensity, the local evaluative measure asks us to compare a short episode of happiness/suffering with a much longer episode of happiness/suffering.) The local evaluative measure was introduced to get around the rigidity of the global evaluative measure. Specifically, it was intended to avoid stipulating in advance that changes in sequence or temporal concentration cannot alter the overall value of a given pattern of happiness and suffering. As I argued in chapter 3, the gain may be less than it appears. The local evaluative measure seems unable to compare the intensity of happiness to suffering without assuming that sequence does not affect value. And it permits the view that the temporal concentration of suffering sometimes makes that suffering worse, but only with the paradoxical result that the badness of suffering sometimes diverges from its intensity. The local evaluative measure has a built-in bias in favor of the global evaluative measure.

Still, the *intent* of the local evaluative measure was to leave open questions about sequence and temporal concentration. In chapter 7, I ask whether changes in sequence and temporal concentration do indeed affect the value of individual patterns of happiness and suffering. These are questions that the global evaluative measure settles (in the negative) by the way it is defined, but that the local evaluative measure tries to leave open for substantive investigation. If substantive investigation tells us that changes in sequence and temporal concentration do not affect overall prudential value, this would show that there is no divergence between the global evaluative measure and the local evaluative measure.

What about the relative prudential weight of happiness and suffering? On the global evaluative measure, happiness and suffering are prudentially symmetrical by definition. The local evaluative measure makes happiness and suffering prudentially symmetrical by definition where relatively short, unvarying, and uninterrupted episodes of happiness and suffering are involved. Are there circumstances under which the local evaluative measure might record a prudential asymmetry between happiness and suffering? For example, might there be a prudential asymmetry between happiness and suffering over the long term, though not in the short term? Offhand, this seems unlikely. It is hard to see how prudential asymmetry that is barred from appearing in the short term would nevertheless creep into the long term.

I believe this could happen only if, over the long term, the badness of suffering is disproportionate to its duration, while the goodness of happiness is *not* similarly disproportionate to its duration, or if, over the long term, the badness of suffering is disproportionate to its duration *by a higher ratio* than the goodness of happiness is disproportionate to its duration. This would allow us to say, for example, that although five minutes of happiness at intensity x together with five minutes of suffering at the same intensity x are equal in value to ten minutes at the hedonistic zero, a month of happiness at intensity x together with a month of suffering at the same intensity x are *worse* than two months at the hedonistic zero. In order for suffering to outweigh happiness over the long term, the effect of prolonging suffering must outweigh the effect of prolonging happiness. Now as I showed in chapter 3, the local evaluative measure rules out this possibility in the domain of shorter time spans. We can't go around saying that five minutes of happiness at intensity x are worth exactly five minutes of suffering at intensity x, while twenty minutes of happiness at intensity x are *not* worth twenty minutes of suffering at intensity x. (When I say that x minutes of happiness are worth exactly x minutes of suffering,

I mean that there is no difference in value between x minutes of happiness with x minutes of suffering, and $2x$ minutes at the hedonistic zero.) Thus if there is to be a prudential asymmetry between happiness and suffering over the long term, the differential effects of prolonging happiness and suffering must arise only in longer time spans but *not* in shorter time spans. This possibility strikes me as unlikely, and therefore I think it is unlikely that there could be prudential asymmetry between happiness and suffering on the local evaluative measure of intensity.

The following example is intended to show further obstacles to the suggestion of such an asymmetry. Suppose we invoke the thesis to say that 496 consecutive hours of happiness at intensity x are not worth 496 consecutive hours of suffering at the same intensity x. (I choose this figure, because there are 496 waking hours in a 31-day month if we assume 8 hours of sleep each day.) Now imagine suffering that is 496 times as intense. According to the local evaluative measure, one should be indifferent between 496 hours of suffering at intensity x and 1 hour of suffering at intensity $496x$. The local evaluative measure also tells us that 1 hour of happiness at intensity $496x$ is worth exactly 1 hour of suffering at intensity $496x$, and that one should be indifferent between 1 hour of happiness at intensity $496x$ and 496 hours of happiness at intensity x. It seems we must therefore say that 496 hours of happiness at intensity x *are* worth, exactly, 496 hours of suffering at intensity x.

I end by reviewing the claims made in this section. I suggested that on the version of the preferential measure that is most likely to attract adherents—the preferential measure combined with the consent view—happiness and suffering are prudentially symmetrical by definition. I observed that the global evaluative measure also makes happiness and suffering prudentially symmetrical by definition. Finally, I argued that a belief in this symmetry is the most plausible view if one uses the local evaluative measure. The three measures converge on the same result: happiness and suffering are morally symmetrical within lives.

5. Where Did the Classical Utilitarians Stand?

Classical utilitarians—here I have in mind Bentham, Mill, and Sidgwick—believed that each person's life went best when it contained the greatest possible surplus of happiness over suffering. They thus believed in the prudential symmetry of happiness and suffering. I have claimed that, on the intuitive measure of intensity, happiness and suffering are prudentially *asymmetrical*. But I have also said that on the global evaluative measure of intensity, happiness and suffering are prudentially symmetrical by definition; that on the local evaluative measure the denial of prudential symmetry is implausible; and that most people drawn to the preferential measure are likely to believe in prudential symmetry as well. If the classical utilitarians had in mind the intuitive measure of intensity, the claims I have advanced thus far contradict classical utilitarianism. If they never had in mind the intuitive measure, the claims I have advanced thus far do not contradict classical utilitarianism.

Which measures did the classical utilitarians have in mind? The texts do not allow us to answer with certainty.[14] Now, it is clear that they *used* both an evaluative and preferential measure. They could depend on the evaluative measure, in either version, to yield accurate estimates of intensity, since they believed it was best for each individual to experience the greatest possible surplus of happiness over suffering—or "greatest happiness" as they dubbed it. Bentham and Mill, since they believed that people desired nothing as an end in itself but their own greatest happiness, could depend on the preferential measure as well. So could Sidgwick, who evidently believed that people desired their own greatest happiness, *other things being equal.*[15]

It is harder to determine whether the classical utilitarians also thought in terms of the intuitive measure. To simplify somewhat, two interpretations are possible. On the first interpretation, the classical utilitarians thought in terms of an intuitive measure at least part of the time. However, they felt no need to distinguish the intuitive measure from either the preferential or the evaluative measure, because they believed that it corresponded with both. In other words, *they believed that, on the intuitive measure of intensity, there is prudential symmetry between happiness and suffering*.

On the second interpretation, the classical utilitarians never had in mind the intuitive measure when discussing the greatest happiness principle. On this interpretation, they give us no indication of what they thought, or what they would have thought, regarding the relative prudential importance of happiness and suffering on the intuitive measure.

Though I do not think the question can be settled definitively, I shall conclude this section by explaining why I am inclined to the first of these two interpretations.

Sometimes the classical utilitarians speak in a manner that suggests to me, at any rate, that they were thinking in terms of an intuitive measure. In chapter 4 of *The Principles of Morals and Legislation*, Bentham writes:

> To a person considered *by himself,* the value of a pleasure or pain considered *by itself,* will be greater or less, according to the four following circumstances:

14. For this reason, people may have been attributing divergent meanings to classical utilitarianism without realizing it. Not long ago I was surprised to learn that Derek Parfit had always assumed that the classical utilitarians primarily intended an evaluative measure of intensity. He was equally surprised to learn that I had always assumed that they primarily intended an intuitive measure.

15. In a passage from *Utilitarianism*, Mill uses a measure that combines preferential and evaluative elements. After stating that the quality of pleasure is measured by the verdict of experienced judges, he adds: "And there needs be the less hesitation to accept this judgment respecting the quality of pleasures, since there is no other tribunal to be referred to even on the question of quantity. What means are there of determining which is the acutest of two pains, or the intensest of two pleasurable sensations, except the general suffrage of those who are familiar with both? Neither pains nor pleasures are homogeneous, and pain is always heterogeneous with pleasure. What is there to decide whether a particular pleasure is worth purchasing at the cost of a particular pain, except the feelings and judgment of the experienced?" (In *Utilitarianism, On Liberty and Considerations on Representative Government* [London: Dent, 1972], p. 11.) Sidgwick uses the evaluative measure in the long paragraph on pp. 123–24 of *Methods of Ethics*.

1. Its *intensity*.
2. Its *duration*.
3. Its *certainty* or *uncertainty*.
4. Its *propinquity* or *remoteness*.[16]

On what I think is the most natural reading of this passage, Bentham meant "intensity" in the intuitive sense. He meant how good a pleasure feels or how bad a pain feels at the moment of its occurrence. This strikes me as the most natural reading, because here Bentham speaks of intensity as an input that helps *determine* the overall value of a pleasure or pain. On the preferential and evaluative measures, the calculation goes the other way: one looks at the overall value of a pleasure or pain in order to determine its intensity.[17] Bentham also classifies intensity with duration, certainty, and propinquity—terms whose meanings are clearly not derived from judgments about the overall value of an individual's pattern of happiness and suffering. This suggests that in Bentham's mind the meaning of intensity was similarly independent of such judgments. It represented an independent dimension of experience.

As I argued in chapter 3, the preferential measure and both versions of the evaluative measure are all burdened with serious disadvantages. Charity makes me reluctant to believe that the classical utilitarians thought exclusively in terms of these measures.

But my main reason for preferring the first of the two interpretations is this. The intuitive measure equates intensity with how good happiness feels or how bad suffering feels at the moment of its occurrence. This seems to me a fairly natural way of understanding intensity, and I find it hard to believe that this sense of the word did not cross the classical utilitarians' minds. If this sense of the word did cross their minds, and if they believed that happiness and suffering were *not* prudentially symmetrical where the intuitive measure was concerned, one would have expected them to point out that they did not have the intuitive measure in mind when they asserted the prudential symmetry of happiness and suffering. Because they did not point this out, I am inclined to think that they believed in the prudential symmetry of happiness and suffering, intuitively measured.

Such a view is in character with the rest of their thought. The general tendency of classical utilitarianism is that good things ought to be maximized. Thus there should be the greatest possible happiness in society as a whole. And thus the value of an outcome is not altered by the order in which happiness and suffering occur, or the degree to which happiness or suffering is temporally concentrated. (Bentham's mention of "propinquity" indicates a bias toward the near future, but this attitude

---

16. Jeremy Bentham, *The Principles of Morals and Legislation* (Buffalo: Prometheus Books, 1988), p. 29. Emphasis in the original.

17. On the preferential measure, the value is construed in terms of the person's well-informed preferences; on the evaluative measure it is construed objectively. As both a psychological and an ethical hedonist, Bentham ran these two kinds of value together.

is firmly rejected by Sidgwick.) Distributive principles other than maximization are generally absent from their thought. One can easily imagine their believing that the "immediately felt goodness" of experience is also something that should be maximized. They may well have looked on a belief in the prudential asymmetry of happiness and suffering, intuitively measured, as reflecting a neurotic fear of suffering, or a confused application of the principle of diminishing marginal returns. (See the following section.) Or they may have believed, dogmatically, that such a view demonstrated a failure to be "rational."

I shall make a final remark. If the classical utilitarians never meant to refer to the intuitive measure, this would mean that their theory was seriously incomplete. The intuitive measure marks a dimension of experience of central significance, and it is of the utmost important to know how happiness and suffering, thus measured, should be distributed both within and across lives.

6. The Moral Asymmetry of Happiness and Suffering across Lives

I now look at the relative importance of happiness and suffering across lives. In this section and the next, I address this question in terms of the intuitive measure, while in section 8 I look at it in terms of the evaluative measure.

Earlier I claimed that, on the intuitive measure of intensity, happiness and suffering are morally asymmetrical within lives. Within the same life it is more important to avoid suffering than to seek happiness, and it is more important to reduce more intense suffering than less intense suffering. Nevertheless, the question of intrapersonal trade-offs is a difficult one and may elicit a fair amount of uncertainty in people's minds.

When we turn to interpersonal trade-offs, the moral landscape becomes much clearer. It is clear, or ought to be clear, that there is a moral asymmetry between happiness and suffering across lives. Imagine that if we do nothing, one person will be in agony for a certain period of time, while another person will be happy for the same period of time. Now imagine that we can either decrease the intensity of the first person's suffering by a significant amount or else increase the intensity of the second person's happiness by a marginally greater amount. If happiness and suffering were morally symmetrical, we should increase the happiness of the second person. But surely this is wrong. Surely the wretched person requires our help first. The relief of his suffering is urgent in a way that the magnification of the other person's happiness is not.

In trade-offs across lives, not only does suffering have priority over happiness, but more intense suffering has priority over less intense suffering. Imagine that if we do nothing two people will suffer during the same period of time, and that the first person is in agony, while the second person's suffering is just half as intense. Suppose that we can either lower the first person's agony by a significant amount, or else lower the second person's suffering by a marginally larger amount. The symmetry view instructs us to reduce the second person's suffering, but surely we should reduce the first person's suffering instead.

Some people appeal to the principle of diminishing marginal returns to claim that, on closer examination, there really is no moral asymmetry between happiness and suffering. In most cases one cannot be certain whether this argument is intended to defend moral symmetry in terms of the intuitive measure of intensity, or only in terms of the evaluative measure. Here I want to look at the version of the argument that defends moral symmetry in terms of the intuitive measure. I believe that the argument is often intended, and often understood, in this way. At any rate, it is worth showing why this version of the argument is unsuccessful. Doing so will allow us to introduce some practical examples of moral asymmetry.

The argument from diminishing marginal returns acknowledges certain intuitions that say we should give priority to the relief of suffering over the promotion of happiness. But it claims that these intuitions are in fact compatible with the moral symmetry of happiness and suffering. Given the way the world is constructed, it just so happens that the maximization of overall happiness (i.e., the surplus of happiness over suffering) is usually achieved by giving priority of assistance to those who are suffering. The general reasoning is as follows. Human beings can succumb to suffering of a very deep kind. It is harder for them to attain happiness equivalent in height to the depth of the suffering to which they are all ultimately vulnerable. Left destitute or undefended, people easily fall into the depths. Consequently, a fixed set of resources generally moves someone suffering very intensely a farther distance up the happiness-suffering continuum than someone who starts out happy, or even someone suffering less intensely. A gift of ten thousand dollars brings more happiness to a pauper than to a millionaire. And so forth.

This argument claims that the symmetry view already accommodates the intuitions that are being cited against it. I think this argument fails for two reasons. First, it begs the question. What it shows at most is that we have two ways of explaining why in practice we should give priority to the relief of suffering. One explanation is that giving priority to the relief of suffering leads to the maximization of overall happiness. Another explanation is that the relief of suffering is morally more important in itself than the promotion of happiness. The diminishing returns argument seems to assume that the first explanation is superior. Not only does this beg the question, but it is opposed by intuition. For intuition tells us not only that we should give priority to the relief of suffering, but that we should do so because the relief of suffering *matters more* than the promotion of happiness.

Second, the law of diminishing marginal returns does not apply in all cases. There are cases where we would maximize overall happiness by increasing some people's happiness rather than reducing other people's suffering. And in many of these cases it seems better to alleviate suffering, though this contributes less to overall happiness. One type of case is that in which it is *harder* to help those who are suffering. Imagine someone who is severely disabled to the point where he endures chronic suffering. Because of his handicap, a large amount of resources is needed to achieve even a moderate reduction of his suffering. (For example, a pro-longed and expensive therapy is necessary to enable him to perform some simple task that will lessen his dependence and moderately improve his self-esteem. Or a very costly medicine is required to gain partial relief from physical pain and dis-comfort.) The same resources, when given to a healthy person, might enable her to realize an important goal or ambition that will increase her happiness by a signifi-cantly greater amount.[18] It is hard to generalize about such a case. If we can achieve only the *tiniest* reduction of the disabled person's suffering, which, let us suppose, is not intolerable, or else a *vast* increase in the healthy person's happiness, where, moreover, this involves the realization of one of her core projects, we may possibly favor the healthy person. But suppose that the increase in the healthy person's happiness is only slightly greater than the decrease of the disabled person's suffering. Then I think it is clear that we should help the suffering person instead. And this is sufficient to show that the relief of suffering and the promotion of happiness are morally asymmetrical.

Just as it is harder to help some people who are suffering, so it is harder to help some countries with suffering populations. Some poor countries, especially those that have been devastated by war or political tyranny, are so lacking in infrastructure that they have a severely limited capacity to benefit from even well-intentioned and well-designed aid efforts. Imagine two different countries. Country A is severely lacking in basic infrastructure, and most of its inhabitants suffer from acute hunger and associated disabilities and diseases. Country B has a solid infrastructure and is relatively but not absolutely poor. The standard of living for most of its inhabitants is quite low, but very few people, if any, suffer acute hunger. Now suppose that a highly competent aid agency is deciding whether to launch assistance projects in country A or B. If it devotes its resources to country B, it can generate a large number of successful and durable development projects. These projects will broaden educational and cultural opportunities, improve economic security, and make life more comfortable for large numbers of people; moreover, these benefits will last several generations. And because these people start out with such a meager standard of living, the improvements will make significant contributions to their happiness. If the aid agency devotes the same set of resources to country A, however, its projects will reach far fewer people, and their staying-power will be in far greater doubt. In the end it will rescue some people from hunger and chronic disease, but the number will be far fewer than those it could help in country B. We can suppose that the aggregate reduction of suffering in country A would be smaller than the aggregate increase of happiness in country B. Nevertheless, we may still want to claim that the agency should assist country A, just because the urgency of relieving the extreme suffering of some of its inhabitants is so much greater.[19]

---

18. I take this example, with adaptations, from Thomas Nagel, "Equality," in *Mortal Questions* (Cambridge: Cambridge University Press, 1979), pp. 123–24.

19. Someone might say that the solution is for the aid agency to build an infrastructure in country A. But suppose that it lacks sufficient resources for this.

Other cases in which the maximization of overall happiness is not achieved through the alleviation of suffering are those that pit a fortunate majority against a vulnerable minority. William James asks us to consider "a world in which Messrs. Fourier's and Bellamy's and Morris's utopias should all be outdone, and millions kept permanently happy on the one simple condition that a certain lost soul on the far-off edge of things should lead a life of lonely torture."[20] In James's description of his example, it might appear that we seek the single person's torture as a means to the happiness of the millions, and there could be a separate deontological objection against intending harm in this way. So let us just imagine that we have a choice between preventing the one person's lifelong torture, and bringing happiness to millions.

Some people think we should ignore an example like this because it is so unlikely.[21] I disagree. I think it is important for us to point out that in this and any parallel cases the bliss of millions cannot justify the lifelong torture of one.

Here is an example closer to home. Imagine that in some country two parties are competing in national elections. If party A wins, it will continue the persecution of a tiny and despised minority. A small handful of these people will wind up in jail being tortured.[22] On the other hand, A's victory will greatly boost the happiness of large numbers of people from the majority. Imagine that for whatever reason (say, the support of powerful economic actors at home and abroad, and access to skilled advisors), it can provide broad-based economic growth that will bring significant improvements in the standard of living for large numbers of people. Party B, on the other hand, will be unable to provide any economic growth, but because of its commitment to human rights, will end the practice of arbitrary imprisonment and torture. It would be best if we could combine the merits of both parties, but in the real word such an option is often lacking. Here we face a trade-off between preventing the suffering of a very small number and increasing the happiness of a much larger number. It is easy to imagine that the latter choice would maximize overall happiness. Nevertheless, we should reject it. Before increasing the happiness of the large number, we should insure that the small number do not suffer torture.

Some people may claim that there exists a well worked-out moral theory supporting the symmetry view, and that such a theory cannot be defeated by mere intuitions. But a theory is only as strong as the premises on which it rests. The challenge for defenders of the symmetry view is to show that our asymmetrical intuitions unavoidably conflict with some premise more deserving of our confidence. I have yet to see this demonstrated.[23]

20. William James, "The Moral Philosopher and the Moral Life," in *Essays in Pragmatism*, ed. Alburey Castell (New York: Hafner, 1958), p. 68.

21. See Russell Hardin, *Morality within the Limits of Reason* (Chicago: University of Chicago Press, 1988), pp. 22–29.

22. In many countries, democratic majorities have acquiesced in the torture of their fellow-citizens. India, Turkey, and Brazil are some prominent examples.

23. The argument from diminishing marginal returns fails to prove that happiness and suffering are morally symmetrical. Nevertheless, the empirical point to which it appeals is an important one. Generally,

7. Explaining Interpersonal Asymmetry

What accounts for the interpersonal asymmetry of happiness and suffering? There are two possible explanations, either or both of which may be true. Earlier I claimed that if we believe in the moral asymmetry of happiness and suffering *within* lives, we should attribute this asymmetry to the intrinsic moral properties of happiness and suffering. Suffering is bad to a greater degree than happiness is good; moreover, as suffering increases in intensity, its moral badness rises at a faster rate than its intensity. I called this the intrinsic property view. If we apply the intrinsic property view to trade-offs within lives, we should apply it no less to trade-offs across lives.

But the intrinsic property view may not be all that is at work in the assertion of interpersonal asymmetry. The assertion may derive some of its support from a different kind of view, one that appeals to distributive justice and focuses its concern on the fate of *persons*. This view holds that in interpersonal trade-offs it is more important to help the person who is worse off with respect to suffering. This view is an application of the claim, which has recently received much attention from moral philosophers, that it is more important to help people who are worse off.[24] Following Derek Parfit, I shall call this the *priority view*. The priority view holds, as Parfit writes, that "benefiting people matters more the worse off these people are."[25]

In this discussion, I examine the priority view only as it applies to suffering, and to trade-offs between happiness and suffering. I leave aside the question what the priority view might imply for goods other than happiness and suffering. I also leave aside the question whether it applies to interpersonal trade-offs that involve only happiness—that is, whether it is more important to increase one person's mild happiness than another person's intense happiness. When applied to suffering, as it is in this discussion, the priority view holds that it is more important to help those persons who are worse off with respect to suffering.

---

though not always, we can move people a greater aggregate distance up the happiness-suffering scale if we devote our efforts to the prevention of suffering rather than the increase of happiness. Positive utilitarians say that we should maximize overall happiness, where "overall happiness" means the total surplus of happiness over suffering. But as Derek Parfit points out, they could just as well say that we should minimize overall suffering, where "overall suffering" means the total surplus of suffering over happiness. If as most utilitarians agree we accomplish more by trying to prevent suffering than by trying to increase happiness, the exhortation to "minimize overall suffering" points us in a more useful direction.

24. Dennis McKerlie, Thomas Nagel, Derek Parfit, and T. M. Scanlon are among those who have done most to elucidate this idea.

25. *Equality or Priority?*, p. 19. Other philosophers have adopted Parfit's term, but it takes on different shades of meaning in different discussions. Given the complexity of the issue, this is not surprising. In "Priority and Time" (*Canadian Journal of Philosophy* 27 [1997]: 287–309), Dennis McKerlie develops a "time-specific priority view" that corresponds to what I am here calling the "intrinsic property view." In my own discussion, however, I intend a conception of the "priority view" that is distinct from the "intrinsic property view." The "priority view" I have in mind might be more precisely described as the "distributive priority view."

When the priority view is applied this narrowly, it may seem hard to distinguish from the intrinsic property view. The difference is that whereas the intrinsic property view emphasizes the *intrinsic awfulness of suffering*, the priority view emphasizes the *harm that suffering does to persons*. It may seem odd that we would want to separate these ideas. For surely anyone who recognizes the intrinsic awfulness of suffering also recognizes that it harms the individuals who experience it. Nevertheless, there is a difference. The intrinsic property view doesn't particularly care *who* is hurt; the identity of the victim is not an issue. In this it resembles utilitarianism, which has been criticized on the grounds that it treats persons as mere vessels of happiness and suffering. For the intrinsic property view, it is the evilness of suffering that counts, not the harm done to a particular person. Thomas Nagel gives voice to this view when he proposes in *The View from Nowhere* that the badness of pain can be recognized in abstraction from the thought that someone in particular is harmed by it.[26] By contrast, the priority view directs its attention, not to the intrinsic evilness of suffering, but to the person affected by it. It says that the urgency of helping this person increases the worse off he or she is. In this way, the priority view is centrally concerned with the identity of the victim. It sets itself apart from both utilitarianism and the intrinsic property view in asserting the moral separateness of persons.

The difference between these two views is made clear when we examine certain kinds of moral dilemmas. One way to illustrate the difference is to compare interpersonal trade-offs with intrapersonal trade-offs. Some people who deny the moral asymmetry of happiness and suffering within lives may accept it across lives. Though they believe that within lives it is always best to maximize the greatest possible surplus of happiness over suffering, they believe that in interpersonal trade-offs we should sometimes reduce some people's suffering by a smaller amount rather than increase other people's happiness by a greater amount. On this combination of views, it becomes difficult to explain the moral asymmetry of happiness and suffering across lives just by claiming that suffering is bad to a greater degree than happiness is good (the intrinsic property view). For within the same life, happiness and suffering are given equal moral weight. What rather seems to be doing the work is the notion that it is more urgent to help those *persons* whose suffering is worse (the priority view).

Another possibility is that we accept the moral asymmetry of happiness and suffering both within and across lives, but hold that it is *steeper* across lives than within lives. That is, we may believe that suffering has greater priority over happiness (and more intense suffering greater priority over less intense suffering) across lives than within lives. The following would be an example of such a view. We may believe that it is bad for someone to experience one day of fairly intense suffering

---

26. *The View from Nowhere* (New York: Oxford University Press, 1986), p. 161. Elsewhere Nagel strongly endorses prioritarian principles (for example, in *Equality and Partiality* [New York: Oxford University Press, 1991]). He thus offers a good illustration of the point that the intrinsic property view and the priority view, though distinct, are by no means incompatible.

even if it is compensated by a day and a half of equally intense happiness. We thus think that there is some asymmetry between happiness and suffering within lives. On the other hand, we may think it is better for this person to experience a day of this suffering if it is compensated by a *week* of equally intense happiness. But in an equivalent trade-off across different lives, we may think that it is more important to spare one person a day of this fairly intense suffering, than to provide *another* person with a week of equally intense happiness. (Assume that the two lives are similar in other respects.) If we hold this set of views, we believe that there is some moral asymmetry of happiness and suffering within lives, but that it is less steep than the moral asymmetry of happiness and suffering across lives. If this is what we believe, it seems that we should invoke *both* explanations for the moral asymmetry of happiness and suffering across lives: suffering is bad to a greater degree than happiness is good, *and* it is more important to help those people whose suffering is worse.

A third outlook holds that there is moral asymmetry neither within nor across lives. This outlook denies both the intrinsic property view and the priority view. This was the position of the classical utilitarians if, as I am inclined to believe, they thought that the prudential symmetry of happiness and suffering held true for the intuitive as well as the evaluative measure of intensity.

A fourth outlook finds that there is moral asymmetry both within and across lives, and holds that it applies to the same degree in each case: suffering should be avoided to the same degree in intrapersonal trade-offs as in interpersonal trade-offs. This outlook accepts the intrinsic property view but denies the priority view. This outlook would be compatible with the teachings of the classical utilitarians if they never meant to refer to the intuitive measure of intensity.

As these remarks indicate, the classical utilitarians may or may not have rejected the intrinsic property view—that is a matter for interpretation. But they definitely rejected the priority view. They rejected it, because they believed that net benefits, however defined, should be maximized not only within each life but across society as a whole. In other words, they believed that the same distributive principles apply across lives as apply within lives.

Another way to bring out the difference between the intrinsic property view and the priority view is to consider trade-offs that pit the longer suffering of a few against the shorter suffering of the many. Some governments torture people for years.[27] Compare two different worlds, exactly alike, except that in world A one person endures five years of torture whereas in world B six people each endure one year of torture. Or to draw a sharper contrast, compare one person's torture lasting five years to the week-long torture of 275 people (the cumulative duration of whose torture would slightly exceed five years).[28] Which would be worse from the imper-

27. See Middle East Watch, *Syria Unmasked: The Suppression of Human Rights by the Asad Regime* (New Haven: Yale University Press, 1991), p. 57.

28. This example is highly artificial in several respects. One is that it asks us to imagine an immediate end to suffering upon the cessation of torture. However, we need to remember that in real life the

sonal perspective: the five-year torture of one person, or the week-long torture of 275 people?

This example must be treated carefully. It is easy to imagine that the prolongation of one person's suffering would make it more intense, by increasing his despair. We need to correct for this somehow: for example, by imagining the lone victim with a more resilient temperament, or imagining severer forms of torture for the 275, or imagining them drained of hope until the moment of release. Another complication is that some people may think that the intrinsic badness of suffering for the sufferer is disproportionate to its duration, so that, for example, five years of continuous suffering are more than five times as bad as one year of suffering of equal intensity.[29] Here I shall assume, however, that the badness of suffering to the sufferer is directly proportional to its duration.

Suppose we make these adjustments and assumptions. Which of the two outcomes is worse? Which ought to be prevented if we could only prevent one? Many people will feel strongly that it is more important to prevent one person's five-year suffering than to prevent 275 people's week-long suffering. What appears to lie behind this judgment is the view that it is more urgent to reduce the suffering of those individuals whose suffering is worse. However, it is also possible to focus on the intrinsic awfulness of suffering at the time of its occurrence. If we think in this way, we may find ourselves leaning toward the judgment that the week-long suffering of 275 people is in fact worse than the five-year suffering of one. (Here I have assumed that the badness of suffering is fully aggregative: that two people's suffering is twice as bad as one person's suffering, and so forth. But I think that an aggregative view becomes more likely when we focus on the intrinsic awfulness of suffering.)

8. The Relative Importance of Happiness and Suffering Across Lives, in Terms of the Evaluative Measure

So far, in addressing the relative moral importance of happiness and suffering across lives, I have presupposed the intuitive measure of intensity. How do matters look if we adopt the evaluative measure? (Here I shall ignore the preferential measure. I

---

suffering of torture victims—just like the suffering of war veterans, kidnapping survivors, and rape and assault victims—does not always end with the termination of violence. People who escape situations of extreme violence are often afflicted with lasting psychological disturbances involving obsessive memories, recurrent panic and terror, incapacity to function normally, and extreme alienation from other people. (See Judith Lewis Herman, *Trauma and Recovery* [New York: Basic Books, 1992].) It is hard for the rest of us to grasp this, since we expect their return to safety to be an occasion for pure psychological relief. But the normal sources of comfort do not bring these people a respite. They are doubly victims: first, in having the bad luck to succumb to extreme violence; and second, in being governed by crueler psychological laws. They seem to be targets of a malevolent fate.

29. I discuss this view in chapter 7.

shall also ignore the differences between the local evaluative measure and the global evaluative measure, which I believe to be irrelevant here.)

On the evaluative measure, happiness and suffering are morally symmetrical within lives, by definition. The question then becomes whether suffering weighs more against happiness in trade-offs across lives than in trade-offs within lives. If the answer is yes, there is, on the evaluative measure of intensity, an interpersonal moral asymmetry between happiness and suffering. If the answer is no, there is not.

The view that there is interpersonal moral asymmetry on the evaluative measure implies that the priority view is correct. We need the priority view to support the claim that suffering weighs more against happiness in interpersonal trade-offs than it does in intrapersonal trade-offs.

It may be considered a virtue of the evaluative measure that it transforms the question about the moral asymmetry of happiness and suffering into a question about the truth of the priority view. The priority view is important and deserves a spotlight. Moreover, the priority view is the one view that the classical utilitarians certainly rejected. We cannot be sure whether they rejected the intrinsic property view, but we know that they rejected the priority view. On the evaluative measure, therefore, the assertion of a moral asymmetry between happiness and suffering is in unambiguous contradiction to utilitarianism. This is not so on the intuitive measure, since moral asymmetry might be explained entirely on the basis of the intrinsic property view, and it is possible that the classical utilitarians did not reject this view. On the evaluative measure, the lines between the main historical camps are more simply drawn.

Against these advantages of using the evaluative measure to discuss moral asymmetry must be set certain disadvantages. The evaluative measure throws the spotlight exclusively on the priority view, but only by making questions about the intrinsic property view disappear. If, as I believe, the intrinsic property view states an important truth and ultimately plays a central role in explaining the interpersonal (not to mention the intrapersonal) asymmetry of happiness and suffering, this is a great loss. The intuitive measure allows us to consider the intrinsic property view *and* the priority view. It permits as careful an inspection of the priority view as the evaluative measure does; it just uses different language to do so. The intuitive measure allows us to ask all the questions that can be asked on the evaluative measure, but the evaluative measure does not allow us to ask all the questions that can be asked on the intuitive measure.

I shall now resume use of the intuitive measure, and return from terminological to substantive matters. Should we (in terms of the intuitive measure) adopt the intrinsic property view or the priority view or either or both? My own thinking is as follows. There can be no doubt that there is a moral asymmetry between happiness and suffering across lives. If the intrinsic property view is false, the priority view must be true. If the priority view is false, the intrinsic property view must be true. Reflection on intrapersonal trade-offs convinces me that the intrinsic property view is true. I therefore think that the intrinsic property view plays an important role in explaining the interpersonal asymmetry of happiness and suffering. When I think about certain cases, my intuitions pull me strongly toward the priority view as well. However, my confidence in the priority view is not quite as strong as it is in the intrinsic property view.

As I note in chapter 7, I believe that the interpersonal asymmetry of happiness and suffering is quite steep. In general we should prevent one person's suffering rather than increase other people's happiness by a much larger amount. To explain this view, either we have to say that the moral asymmetry of happiness and suffering is fully as steep within lives as it is across lives, or we have to supplement the intrinsic property view with the priority view. If we have doubts that the moral asymmetry of happiness and suffering is fully as steep within lives as it is across lives, this becomes a reason to entertain the priority view.

Earlier I said that our intuitions declare the moral asymmetry of happiness and suffering more forcefully in interpersonal trade-offs than in intrapersonal trade-offs. One reason is that our views about intrapersonal trade-offs are complicated and partly obscured by the belief that there is a value in having people realize their well-informed, self-regarding preferences: in intrapersonal trade-offs we may think that well-informed, self-regarding preferences often are a better guide to identifying the best outcome, all things considered, than an objective determination of the relative moral importance of happiness and suffering. But another reason is that our belief in interpersonal asymmetry may draw some of its support from the priority view, which does not apply to intrapersonal trade-offs.

To the extent that I have doubts about the truth of the priority view, I have doubts whether, on the evaluative measure of intensity, there is a moral asymmetry between happiness and suffering. And to that extent, it is not clear whether my views are in contradiction with classical utilitarianism. But it is clear that what I have been saying is very *different* from classical utilitarianism. That is because, depending on how we interpret the classical utilitarians' understanding of intensity, either they rejected the intrinsic property view, or they completely ignored it.

9. The Priority View, the Appropriate Unit of Concern, and Personal Identity

In this section, I turn to some questions concerning the priority view. As Derek Parfit has pointed out, the priority view can be applied in two different ways. When we say that it is more important to help people whose suffering is worse, we may have in mind people whose suffering is worse in their lives as whole, or people whose suffering is worse during the period of time in which we can help.[30] Sometimes this distinction makes a practical difference. Suppose that Dolores has led a

---

30. Parfit discusses this point, though without limiting it to suffering, in *Equality or Priority?* pp. 20–22. The distinction is lucidly developed by Dennis McKerlie in "Priority and Time." However, his analytical framework is somewhat different from Parfit's. In my discussion, I use Parfit's terms of analysis.

hard life filled with significant periods of very intense suffering, whereas Fortunata has led a charmed life with very little suffering. But now Fortunata faces the prospect of very intense suffering during a limited period of time, whereas Dolores faces the prospect of suffering that is only half as intense, though it lasts the same amount of time. Suppose that we can either reduce the intensity of Fortunata's prospective suffering by a certain amount, or reduce the intensity of Dolores's prospective suffering by a somewhat greater amount. According to the priority view, whose suffering should we relieve? If we reduce Dolores's suffering, we give priority to the person whose suffering is worse in her life as a whole. If we reduce Fortunata's suffering, we give priority to the person whose suffering is worse during the time in question.

The priority view applied to particular periods of time might be confused with the intrinsic property view—the view that is concerned only with the intrinsic awfulness of suffering and not, as a separate matter, with helping the person whose suffering is worse. But it would be a mistake to confuse these two views. Return to the example in which we can either reduce Fortunata's very intense suffering by a certain amount, or reduce Dolores's suffering, only half as intense, by a somewhat greater amount. Now imagine an analogous example in which Dolores faces the prospect of both kinds of suffering, the very intense suffering followed by the suffering only half as intense, and that we can reduce either the more intense or the less intense suffering by the same respective amounts as in the two-person trade-off. Some people might say (given certain intensities) that in a trade-off where only Dolores's suffering is concerned, we should reduce the less intense suffering by a greater amount, but that in the equivalent two-person trade-off, we should reduce the more intense suffering by a smaller amount. The difference would be that in the two-person trade-off we are dealing with the suffering of two *different* people, and that we should give priority to the *person* whose suffering is worse. This example shows that the intrinsic property view can diverge from the priority view applied to particular periods of time.

Here is another example. Suppose that we can either prevent Dolores's very intense suffering, lasting a certain period of time, or else the considerably less intense suffering of one hundred other people, lasting the same period of time. Some people might say (given certain intensities) that we should prevent Dolores's more intense suffering rather than the less intense suffering of the hundred people, but that if it were a choice between *Dolores* experiencing the very intense suffering and experiencing the less intense suffering for a period one hundred times as long, we should prevent the longer-lasting, less intense suffering rather than the shorter, more intense suffering. The difference is that in the interpersonal trade-off, but not in its intrapersonal counterpart, we are dealing with a case in which one person's suffering is much worse than *other* people's suffering. As this example also shows, the intrinsic property view can diverge from the priority view applied to particular periods of time.

Notice that the priority view applied to the period of time in which we can help is still predicated on the separateness of persons. To borrow Rawls's phrase, it takes seriously the distinction between persons. If it did not, it would make no distinction between interpersonal and intrapersonal trade-offs.

If we believe in the priority view, should we give priority to people whose suffering is worse in their lives as a whole, or people whose suffering is worse during the period of time in which we can help—or perhaps some combination? I am inclined to think that at least some, if not all, of the priority should be given to people whose suffering is worse during particular periods of time. This has to do, as I see it, with the kind of good that the prevention of suffering is. We have to remember that there are different kinds of goods, and that different goods apply to different temporal units. Some goods may not be present throughout one's life, yet if one's life as a whole contains a sufficient measure of them, there is little to complain of. Such goods, as it were, resonate over time. This is most true of a good like accomplishment, true but to a lesser extent of something like friendship, and true to an even lesser extent of knowledge. The prevention of suffering, however, is not like this. Suffering is an evil that makes its moral impact in small, even minutely divisible, periods of time. Losing one's knowledge for five minutes is not a catastrophe; experiencing five minutes of torture is. Five minutes of torture are a moral catastrophe, even if the rest of one's life is very good. Attention to suffering encourages us to look on a person's life less as a unified entity than as a succession of experiences, in which primary importance attaches to the quality of each experience in turn rather than the quality of the life overall.

The question of whether to give priority to people whose suffering is worse in their lives as a whole, or to people whose suffering is worse during particular periods of time, may be thought to depend on our views concerning personal identity. In *Reasons and Persons*, Derek Parfit argues that personal identity over time just involves certain psychological relations such as the persistence of beliefs, thoughts, and desires; the memory of past experiences; and the performance of past intentions.[31] In his own account, Parfit has argued that what matters rationally and morally is not personal identity per se, but rather these psychological relations. Because these psychological relations tend to fade over time, the reductionist theory of personal identity makes individual lives appear less unified. It therefore encourages the view that we should give priority to people whose suffering is worse during the period of time in which we can help, rather than to people whose suffering is worse in their lives as a whole.[32] But notice that attention to suffering may have an effect similar to that of Parfit's metaphysical arguments. It, too, makes individual lives seem less unified. In *Reasons and Persons*, Parfit proposed that our views about personal identity can alter our moral priorities; however, the influence may also run in the opposite direction.[33]

31. *Reasons and Persons* (Oxford: Clarendon Press, 1984), Part 3.
32. See Ibid., p. 334.
33. Christine Korsgaard presses this point in "Personal Identity and the Unity of Agency: A Kantian Reply to Parfit," *Philosophy and Public Affairs* 18 (1989): 101-32. Reprinted in Korsgaard, *Creating the Kingdom of Ends* (Cambridge: Cambridge University Press, 1996.)

Parfit's reductionist theory of personal identity favors a certain kind of priority view over the other. But it may also have the effect of undermining, or at least diluting, the priority view itself. This is because the reductionist view makes the relation of a person to herself at different stages in her life resemble more closely the relation between separate individuals. It therefore suggests that there is less of a moral difference between interpersonal and intrapersonal trade-offs.

Suppose that we earlier believed in the priority view, but that recently we have been converted from a non-reductionist to a reductionist theory of personal identity. What effect will the reductionist theory have on our views about the moral asymmetry of happiness and suffering? Those views can shift in either of two directions. We could make our current view about interpersonal trade-offs move closer to our previous view about intrapersonal trade-offs. If so, we now believe that the interpersonal asymmetry between happiness and suffering is less steep than we previously thought. Or we could make our current view about *intrapersonal* trade-offs move closer to our previous view about *interpersonal* trade-offs. In that case, we now believe that the *intrapersonal* asymmetry of happiness and suffering is *steeper* than we previously thought.

What underlies these alternative adjustments?[34] If we bring interpersonal trade-offs closer to our previous model of intrapersonal trade-offs, we may be thinking as follows: "Having moved from a non-reductionist to a reductionist view of personal identity, we now believe that individual persons are less unified than we previously thought. Because persons are less unified, they have diminished standing from the point of view of distributive justice. Consequently, distributive principles matter less in interpersonal trade-offs. This makes interpersonal trade-offs more similar to our previous model of intrapersonal trade-offs, where distributive principles do not apply (or apply with less force)."

If on the other hand we bring intrapersonal trade-offs closer to our previous model of interpersonal trade-offs, we may be thinking as follows: "Having moved from a non-reductionist to a reductionist view of personal identity, we now believe that lives are less unified than we previously thought. Because individual lives are less unified, the notion that burdens at one time can be compensated by benefits at another time is called into question. Some such compensation may be possible, but it is more difficult to achieve. It takes more happiness than we previously thought to compensate a given amount of suffering, and it takes a greater reduction of less intense suffering than we previously thought to compensate a given amount of more intense suffering. In other words, the distributive principles that we previously applied to interpersonal trade-offs should be extended to intrapersonal trade-offs."

According to the latter line of thought, distributive principles help to account for the asymmetry of happiness and suffering within lives. This may seem to challenge an assumption that I have made throughout this chapter. That is the assumption that the intrapersonal asymmetry of happiness and suffering reflects something about the intrinsic properties of happiness and suffering—namely, that

34. Here I follow Parfit in *Reasons and Persons*, pp. 329–45.

suffering is bad to a greater degree than happiness is good. It may seem that distributive principles constitute a different explanation for intrapersonal asymmetry. However, the role of distributive principles within lives can be interpreted in two different ways. They can be seen as *giving rise* to the intrapersonal asymmetry of happiness and suffering. Alternatively, they can be seen as a statement of the inadmissibility of overturning an intrinsic asymmetry between happiness and suffering that is already present in the background. In the latter case, there is no conflict with the intrinsic property view. There may not be a significant difference between these two ways of interpreting the role of distributive principles within lives. I think there is no great danger in continuing to explain intrapersonal asymmetry in terms of the intrinsic property view.

10. Life and Death

There is a possibility that by dwelling on the evil of suffering one comes to despise life. Throughout the ages there have been poets and philosophers who, reflecting on the sorrows of life, have said that it is better to die young, and best never to have been born.[35] Schopenhauer pursued this thought to its logical conclusion:

> If you imagine, in so far as it is approximately possible, the sum total of distress, pain and suffering of every kind which the sun shines upon in its course, you will have to admit it would have been much better if the sun had been able to call up the phenomenon of life as little on the earth as on the moon; and if, here as there, the surface were still in a crystalline condition.[36]

Philosophers sometimes call this attitude "pessimism." Nietzsche gave it the more sinister name of "nihilism." He feared its destructive potential, predicted its spread following the decline of Christianity, and devoted all his powers to combating it.

Pessimists sometimes explain their attitude by saying that life is never free from suffering. Life *is* suffering, the Buddhists tell us; their view is echoed by Schopenhauer, who held that we endure pain and frustration for most of our lives, and that when we succeed in overcoming adversity we succumb instantly to boredom, which too is a form of suffering.

But the claim that suffering never lets go of us is an obvious distortion; the most cursory observation reveals that a great many people are happy a great deal of the time, or at least aren't suffering. The claim may stem from the failure to separate suffering from the frustration of desire. Frustration may be close to a constant in our lives, but it need not be accompanied by suffering. We might even say that, for

35. This sentiment receives remarkably similar expression in *Ecclesiastes*, Sophocles' *Oedipus at Colonus*, and the poetry of Theognis. Schopenhauer writes: "Nothing else can be stated as the aim of our existence except the knowledge that it would be better for us not to exist." *The World as Will and Representation*, vol. 2, trans. E. F. J. Payne, (New York: Dover, 1958), p. 605.

36. *Essays and Aphorisms*, ed. and trans. R. J. Hollingdale (Harmondsworth: Penguin, 1970), p. 47.

many people, happiness is characterized by the generation of new desires faster than they can be satisfied.

The real source of pessimism, I believe, is not the thought that suffering is constantly with us, or even the thought that the quantity of suffering in each person's life exceeds the quantity of happiness; rather it is the thought that nothing in our existence can justify the suffering that occurs, The most persuasive pessimism is the moral kind: the view that nothing in our existence compensates or makes up for suffering's evil. Schopenhauer, in an inconsistent moment, alludes to this: "That thousands had lived in happiness and joy would never do away with the anguish and death-agony of one individual."[37]

We can distinguish between two different kinds of moral pessimism. The first is the thought that no one's life, or very few people's lives, are worth living because of the suffering they contain. The second thought is that, whether or not most people's lives are worth living, there are some lives that contain such horrendous suffering, that it would have been better if the world had never existed. If, for example, we think of a small child who dies after prolonged suffering from severe burns, we may think that the non-existence of the world would have been preferable to a world, even a preponderantly happy one, that included this child's suffering. We might refer to the first thought as the thought that life is not worth living, and the second thought as the thought that the world is not worth having. The thought that most people's lives are not worth living may imply that the world is not worth having. But one may think that the world is not worth having without thinking that life is not worth living.

Most pessimists have not thought to draw practical consequences from their view. At most, they have been led (like Hamlet) to ponder suicide, or (like Socrates) not to struggle against death.[38] It has not occurred to them to go around killing people (though perhaps a certain kind of pessimism has helped motivate the violent acts of some terrorists, revolutionaries, and generals).

The thought that the world is not worth having could suggest the idea that we ought to try to destroy all sentient life, or at any rate all of humanity. In an age of nuclear weapons the question is not wholly academic, though it hardly needs pointing out that a nuclear annihilation would spell suffering beyond any imagining. I have sometimes thought that the world is not worth having. But I am sure that it is wrong to seek the destruction of sentient life, even if it could be done painlessly. I am not sure I know how to defend this conviction. Or I should say: I do not think I could articulate the defense it deserves. The right defense may rule out the thought that the world is not worth having. Then again, there may be a crucial difference between thinking that it would have been better if the world had never come into existence, and thinking that we may take it upon ourselves to destroy the life that

37. *The World as Will and Representation*, vol. 2, p. 576.

38. It may be an exaggeration to call Socrates a pessimist. But there are pessimistic strands in his thought. See Plato's *Apology*, in *The Trial and Death of Socrates*, trans. G. M. A. Grube (Indianapolis: Hackett, 1975), 40c–e.

already exists. Or perhaps the earlier thought is also false and is allowed to survive only because its practical irrelevance shelters it from ever being put to the test.[39]

In what remains of this section, I want to say a few words about the wrongness of killing. It may be alleged that I have put the value of life in question, by claiming in this chapter that the relief of suffering is more important than the promotion of happiness. According to classical utilitarianism, one's life is worth living if it contains a surplus, however small, of happiness over suffering. If we amend classical utilitarianism by giving suffering more weight than happiness, the implication is that one's life is not worth living unless it contains a sufficiently *large* surplus of happiness over suffering—and the required surplus may grow larger the longer one is exposed to very intense suffering. Yet it may be that many people's lives do not contain a surplus of happiness over suffering of the required size. It seems, therefore, that according to the asymmetry thesis these people would be better-off dead, and indeed that we would do them a favor by killing them (though preferably in a painless manner and by surprise). Perhaps this implication extends to *most* people.

The short answer to this complaint is that the asymmetry thesis does not have such implications, provided we dissociate it from the hedonistic teaching that suffering is the sole evil and happiness is the sole good. If happiness (in the hedonistic sense) were the only good to be balanced against the evil of suffering, then we would be in trouble. But it is not.

We can cite a number of reasons other than the value of happiness for valuing the preservation of life and fearing death. Life makes possible a wide range of goods besides happiness—all those goods, in addition to happiness, that are involved in experiencing the world and acting in it. We fear death because it deprives us of these goods.[40] We also fear death because (unlike, say, a recoverable coma) it eliminates the very possibility of future existence.[41] And we fear death because the successful completion of our projects depends on our staying alive.[42]

Other reasons can be added. Most people have a deeply rooted desire to go on living. A proper respect for their autonomy requires that we do not thwart their desire to live. Another reason is that *persons* are valuable. Every person represents a unique outlook on the world; the death of that person removes something from the universe that can never be replaced. Finally, many people feel that life should

---

39. For a profound meditation on the possibility of human extinction, see George Kateb's three chapters devoted to the subject in *The Inner Ocean* (Ithaca, N.Y.: Cornell University Press, 1992). Drawing on Nietzsche, Kateb warns against the effort to justify existence on moral grounds only: "From the moral point of view, existence seems unjustifiable because of the pain and ugliness in it, and therefore the moral point of view must be chastened if it is not to block attachment to existence as such" (p. 145).

40. See Thomas Nagel, "Death," in *Mortal Questions* (Cambridge: Cambridge University Press, 1979).

41. See F. M. Kamm, *Morality, Mortality*, vol. 1 (New York: Oxford University Press, 1993), part 1.

42. See Bernard Williams, "The Makropulos Case: Reflections on the Tedium of Immortality," in *Problems of the Self* (Cambridge: Cambridge University Press, 1973).

be preserved because it constitutes a sacred investment of natural, human, and perhaps divine powers.[43]

According to value hedonism, life is worth living so long as it contains a favorable surplus of happiness over suffering. As many people have pointed out, this provides a shaky basis for the value of life, even if we think that happiness and suffering are morally symmetrical. But on reflection, suffering does seem more important than happiness. Therefore, hedonism is not a theory well-suited to the affirmation of the value of life. It is no accident, I think, that the Epicureans flirted with nihilism.

If we preserve an adequate recognition of the evilness of suffering, the degree to which we think death an evil will depend on the degree to which we acknowledge the existence of non-hedonistic values. I have mentioned some non-hedonistic reasons for regarding death as an evil and killing as a crime. This is not to deny that death is in some cases a benefit. Nor is it to deny that there may be irrational elements in our fear of death. The fierce desire of most persons to go on living may not be *fully* backed up by reasons. (But again, even if someone's desire to go on living is irrational, we should generally honor it out of respect for the person's autonomy.)

The asymmetry thesis alone doesn't tell us to stop valuing the lives of people who are already alive. What about bringing people into existence? Some of the reasons I have cited for condemning killing also support the permissibility of procreation, though with less cumulative force. Some of the people we can create will have lives worth living, but some will not. When we bring a person into the world, we expose him or her to the risk—sometimes greater, sometimes smaller—of prolonged suffering, and of extremely intense suffering. Sometimes the person's life will not be worth the suffering experienced in it. And sometimes, even if the person's life is worth living, we may wish that a different person had been brought into existence, one who would have experienced much less suffering.[44] One effect of the asymmetry thesis is to make us weigh the responsibility of procreation more seriously.

43. The last reason is explored in Ronald Dworkin, *Life's Dominion* (New York: Vintage, 1994).
44. For an elaboration of this point, see Parfit, *Reasons and Persons*, chapter 16.

SEVEN

Trade-offs Internal to the Duty to Relieve Suffering

1. Introduction

There is some suffering that we cannot prevent at all. There is also some suffering that we cannot prevent without neglecting other suffering. Sometimes, that is, we may have to choose between preventing one portion of suffering and another. For example, we may be able to save one group of people or another group of people from suffering, but not both. Or we may have to choose between letting a person endure suffering of one kind and suffering of another kind. This chapter asks how we should resolve these kinds of dilemmas. We can think of them as trade-offs internal to the prima facie duty to relieve suffering.

This subject is continuous with the subject of the last chapter. There we asked whether it is more important to relieve suffering than to promote happiness. We also asked whether it is more important to reduce more intense suffering rather than less intense suffering. This chapter looks at additional cases in which we have to choose between different ways of helping people. For the most part, the trade-offs considered are ones in which we must choose between preventing different kinds or patterns of suffering. But in a later section we will take another look at trade-offs between the prevention of suffering and the promotion of happiness.

As in the last chapter, I want to bracket a number of issues. I shall set aside non-hedonistic harms and benefits, and imagine trade-offs in which only happiness and suffering, in the hedonistic sense, are involved. I shall also assume that in the following trade-offs everyone is equally deserving of happiness and protection from suffering. Finally, I shall assume that there are no morally significant differences in the *means* used to prevent one outcome rather than another. Many people believe that inflicting suffering is morally worse than failing to prevent it. They believe, for example, that if we can prevent Prima's suffering only by inflicting suffering on

Secunda, while we can prevent Secunda's suffering merely by neglecting Prima's suffering, this is a reason to prevent Secunda's suffering rather than Prima's. People who hold this view should imagine that in the following examples the prevention of one kind of suffering does not involve the infliction of another kind of suffering.

In the following examples, I shall be comparing trade-offs between outcomes containing different kinds or patterns of suffering. Where the value of happiness is held constant, I shall assume that we ought to choose the outcome containing the least bad sum of suffering—or in other words that we have a prima facie duty to prevent worse cumulative suffering rather than less bad cumulative suffering. Here I mean "worse" and "less bad" from a moral or impersonal point of view.

The claim that we should minimize the cumulative *moral badness* of suffering needs to be distinguished from the claim that we should minimize the *quantity* of suffering. By "quantity" I mean the number of people who suffer, multiplied by the intensity of their suffering, multiplied by the duration of their suffering. How we understand quantity will depend on our conception of intensity. On the intuitive measure, which I shall employ throughout most of this chapter, there are several cases in which the quantity and moral badness of suffering diverge. But even on the alternative measures of intensity, the quantity and moral badness of suffering may sometimes diverge.

In the last chapter I claimed that, on the intuitive measure, it is sometimes more important to save someone from more intense suffering lasting a shorter time than less intense suffering lasting a longer time, even if the product of intensity and duration is less in the first case than in the second. If this claim is true, it shows that suffering that is smaller in quantity can be morally worse. In interpersonal comparisons, the potential divergence between quantity and moral badness of suffering becomes even clearer. It seems clearly better to reduce one person's more intense suffering by a certain amount than to reduce another person's suffering, only half as intense, by a marginally greater amount. If we help the first person rather than the second, there will be *more* suffering left over but it will be *less bad* from a moral point of view.

On the alternative measures of intensity, the moral badness of suffering appears to correspond to its quantity where intrapersonal trade-offs are concerned. Where intrapersonal trade-offs are concerned, the global evaluative measure makes moral badness and quantity correspond by definition, while on the preferential and local evaluative measures belief in such a correspondence is the most plausible view. The most plausible view on each of the alternative measures is that it is always morally better for someone to suffer less.

But even on the alternative measures, quantity and moral badness may diverge in trade-offs between different people. Even on the alternative measures, we may think, as the priority view claims, that it is more important to help those people whose suffering is worse. Consequently, we may think that it can be better to reduce one person's more intense suffering by a smaller amount rather than to reduce another person's less intense suffering by a greater amount. We may also think that one person's intense suffering lasting five years is cumulatively worse than the one-year suffering, equally intense, of six other people. If this view is correct, the suffering that is smaller in quantity is morally worse. As all these examples remind us, our goal is not the prevention of more suffering rather than less, but the prevention of worse (cumulative) suffering rather than less bad (cumulative) suffering.

Often we speak of the value of "reducing" suffering. For example, we praise someone who is motivated to minimize the amount of suffering in the world. But, to echo a remark made in chapter 3, I believe that on these occasions, we are using normally quantitative words in an evaluative sense. One outcome has "less" suffering than another, according to this usage, if the suffering in it is less bad from a global point of view. When on these occasions we use quantitative words like "less" and "more," we do not mean to refer to the product of numbers, intensity, and duration.

I now turn to the examination of particular kinds of trade-offs. I begin by asking how variations in the timing of a person's suffering affect the overall badness of his or her experience. I look next at the impact of duration, and then of numbers. (Intensity was discussed in the last chapter.) I end with two difficult cases: the trade-off between preventing the agony of one and providing the bliss of many, and the trade-off between preventing the agony of one and preventing the less intense suffering of many.

2. Timing

In this section I ask whether differences in the timing of a person's suffering can affect the badness of the overall outcome for that person. I shall look at two variables: the order in which experiences of varying intensities of suffering and experiences without suffering occur; and the chronological concentration of suffering. I shall hold numbers, intensity, and duration constant, and I shall examine only the suffering of single individuals. I also assume that the intensity and duration of happiness does not vary.

2.a. *Sequence*

Suppose that a person will experience a period with suffering and a period without suffering, or a period of more intense suffering and a period of less intense suffering. Does it matter in which order these experiences occur? Does it matter whether (more intense) suffering occurs before or after?

We must be careful how we approach this question. We may be inclined to say that it is better to experience suffering sooner rather than later. But this preference may be simply owing to the fact that, if we expect the suffering, its occurring earlier cuts down on the period of fearful anticipation. Fearful anticipation is something to be avoided; in some cases, it can rise to the level of genuine suffering. But in deciding whether the earlier occurrence of suffering *in itself* makes suffering worse or less bad, we mean to keep other things equal; therefore, we should abstract from the factor of fearful anticipation. One way to do this is to imagine a case in which the suffering arrives without warning.

We also need to abstract from the hopeful anticipation of release from suffering. Suppose there is a choice between (1) suffering followed by happiness and (2) happiness followed by suffering, and that each of these sequences takes one to the end of one's life. In the first case, but not in the second, the sufferer may draw solace from the expectation of future happiness. Indeed, unless we are careful, we may have unwittingly constructed an example between less intense suffering (in the first case) and more intense suffering (in the second case). That is because we may be comparing afflictions that *normally* would occasion the same intensity of suffering, but not in this example, since one is accompanied by hope and the other by despair.

Alterations in the sequence of suffering and nonsuffering can alter the phenomenological features of the experiences themselves. This is *one* way in which a change in the sequence of suffering and non-suffering can alter the value of the overall outcome. But this doesn't show that the sequence *in itself* alters value. To address that question we have to imagine a case in which a change in sequence does not alter the phenomenological features of the experiences. Or if this is difficult to imagine, we have to imagine that any positive or negative impact on the phenomenological features of the relevant experience owing to a change in sequence is balanced by the introduction of a countervailing negative or positive feature. For example, if a change from happiness-then-suffering to suffering-then-happiness makes the suffering easier to bear or the happiness less attended by anxiety, we should imagine that, in the latter sequence, the affliction that causes the suffering is somehow nastier, and that the happiness, though freer from anxiety, is less perfect in some other respect.

When we have whittled the question down in this way, should we say that it matters in itself whether suffering comes before or after? Some people may say that it does matter—that it is better for suffering to come before rather than after.[1] My own feeling is that the sequence does not matter in itself. Yet I am not sure how to argue for this negative claim.

If we sometimes prefer that suffering comes before rather than after, part of the reason may be traced to the difference in our attitude toward the past and future.[2] We tend to care more about the future and less about the past. Suffering that comes before rather than after moves more quickly into the past, where it no longer seems to matter, or seems to matter less. However, though we often favor the future over the past, I don't think we should wholly identify with that attitude. Suffering in the past matters tremendously, no less than it matters in the future. It is true that

1. For example, John Rawls, *A Theory of Justice* (Cambridge, Mass.: Harvard University Press, 1971), p. 421. See also F. M. Kamm, *Morality, Mortality*, vol. 1 (New York: Oxford University Press, 1993), pp. 67–71.

2. There is an extended discussion of our bias toward the future in Derek Parfit, *Reasons and Persons* (Oxford: Clarendon Press, 1984), chap. 8. Drawing on Parfit, Kamm discusses how our bias toward the future may help to explain why we think that death is worse than pre-natal non-existence, in *Morality, Mortality*, vol. 1, chaps. 2 and 3.

we shouldn't try to prevent suffering in the past, but the reason for that is just that we *cannot*.

Also it may be harder than we think to separate our views about the inherent moral significance of sequence from the impact that we imagine sequence having on the felt quality of our experiences. Thus we may have a particular horror of ending our lives in a state of wretchedness. But much of what we really fear is the extinction of hope: the sense of defeat, the sense that we have nothing to look forward to, the sense that we *had* our chance to be happy, but that we have used it up, that it is now unrecoverable, and that what we are suffering through now is all that there is in store for us. And if our plight is the product of shortsightedness in the past, we may also fear being afflicted by the sense that this is what we deserve, by having made the foolish choice to postpone hardship under the illusion that remote suffering was just that—remote, and therefore unreal—so that we have only our shortsightedness to blame.

It is sometimes suggested that past suffering may be redeemed by future outcomes, for instance by the subsequent happiness of the person who has been suffering. When suffering is a prologue to happiness, according to this line of thought, it is not as bad as it would otherwise be.

I believe this view rests on a confusion. The happy sequel of past suffering does not make the former suffering less bad in itself. Rather, it makes the cumulative badness of the overall picture less great than it would have been if past suffering had continued unabated.

It is true that past suffering often appears less grim when we look back on it from the standpoint of the victim's subsequent happiness. But such a standpoint fosters illusion. Too often, we fancy that the victim's past suffering is tightly bound to his present happiness, in order to form a more agreeable unit, as though he were a character in a novel whose present trials lead by the certain authority of the written text to the reward of a happy ending. But just as the fictional victim lacks the luxury that we have of peeking ahead or depending on the merciful intentions of a humane novelist, so the real victim lacks the luxury of regarding his present misery from the perspective of a chimerical future free of troubles. He does not carry the happy conclusion along with him, as does the reader of a novel. If he does not predict his subsequent release, then it is nothing to him. If he does, then the fact that he is still suffering shows how powerless his hope is in the face of his present affliction.

Sometimes former victims partake of the illusion themselves: they forget how bad their past suffering truly was. This may come partly from a general feebleness of memory, partly from the difficulty of recalling suffering in particular, partly from the tendency I have just described of falsely compressing past experience. But it goes deeper than that. When people experience great suffering, they cannot view their wretchedness from the soothing perspective of posterior comfort and retrospective wisdom. All they can do is *want* and *hope* and *pray* that their suffering will give way to happiness. Now after happiness is attained, their prayer often carries over. It echoes and reverberates in the fortunate present. They pray for continued happiness, but they also pray for the happiness they are actually experiencing in the very moment of their prayer. And it goes directly against the deep and powerful current of this prayer to recall ("relive") their past suffering as it was actually experienced. Their prayer for present happiness requires them to rewrite the past as something it never was, as a teleological journey to happiness, as happiness unfolding, in which, to be sure, "suffering" was experienced, but suffering with a purpose, suffering with the foreknowledge of release, suffering steeped in hope—hence, not real suffering at all (certainly nothing like the original), but rather "suffering" bathed in the glow of retrospective happiness.

2.b. Chronological Concentration

Now consider another variable: the chronological concentration of suffering. Imagine some individual suffering, of fixed total duration and unvarying intensity, against a backdrop of no suffering or less intense suffering. This suffering could be concentrated in a shorter period of time, or spread out over a longer period of time. In the latter case it is interspersed with longer periods that are free from suffering, or are characterized by less intense suffering. Can it matter, in itself, whether suffering is temporally concentrated or dispersed?[3]

It seems to me that only two answers can be seriously entertained. Either chronological concentration can make no difference, or it can make the suffering worse. Someone who says that it can make the suffering less bad has forgotten, I think, to abstract from the factor of fearful anticipation. This person is guided by the thought that when suffering is temporally concentrated there is less time to fear the return of suffering. But this factor should not be accorded any influence if we mean to keep everything else equal in our comparison between temporally scattered and concentrated suffering.

The difficult question is whether chronological concentration can make suffering worse. There seem to be strong grounds for going either way. Consider the limiting case in which the temporal concentration of suffering squeezes out all intervals of relief. There is real plausibility in the idea that continuous, uninterrupted suffering over a long period of time is worse than the sum of the short time segments of suffering that make it up. We might say that as the duration of uninterrupted suffering increases, the badness of that suffering increases at a faster rate. When total duration is fixed, suffering may appear worse when there are no islands of relief to break it up, when it assumes the form of a monolith in time, constant, unshakable, and unrelenting.

But we can also imagine a skeptical rejoinder. What makes most examples of prolonged, continuous suffering so frightening, it may be argued, is the crushing

---

3. Here is one example: labor pain typically swells to intolerable levels during contractions and subsides between contractions. Would the suffering of the mother during her contractions be worse, equally bad, or less bad if it were collected into an uninterrupted block of time?

out of hope. Continuous suffering crushes out hope, because it reduces the proportion of our time spent suffering during which we can expect prompt relief. And by crushing out hope in this way, continuous suffering is apt to become more intense. That's because the expectation of prompt relief, even if it is not permanent, can have the effect of mitigating suffering.

This effect is particularly pronounced in the case of afflictions—such as severe bodily pain—that cause us intense suffering. Searching wildly for hope in a condition that is itself the negation, almost the prohibition, of hope, we find that we can fasten it on our anticipation of prompt relief. Imminent relief bears a tantalizing resemblance to, though we know that it is utterly removed from, the all-important now; for this reason, our consciousness of it may bring a small mitigation of present suffering. Relief in the distant future cannot produce the same effect. Thus a severe affliction that is similar in all other respects is likely to be attended by less intense suffering if it is broken up into short time segments separated by moments of relief. Of course, during these moments of relief we may be troubled by the fear of the affliction's return—unless such fear is displaced by the simple euphoria of release.

Thus someone could offer the following argument against the claim that temporal compression, in itself, can make suffering worse. In real life, temporally compressed suffering is often worse suffering, but what makes it worse is not the compression itself, but rather the intensification of suffering caused by such compression. What we may mistakenly see as increased badness stemming from the temporal concentration of suffering is actually increased badness stemming from the greater intensity of suffering.

Once the factor of anticipation is taken into account—the argument continues—it becomes more difficult to see why the badness of my present suffering is increased by the fact that it will be followed without pause by further suffering. What matters, surely, is what I feel at each particular moment. And the badness (or goodness) of what I feel at each particular moment cannot be changed by the badness (or goodness) of what I feel in the future and the past.[4] The mystery comes when we must determine the total disvalue of a string of particular moments during each of which I experience suffering. How can we say something intelligible and true about the overall badness of more than one moment of suffering joined together, let us suppose

4. See Katz's remarks on pleasure: "Some, at least, of the experiential moments of my life seem to be lived in . . . splendid isolation, not only from everything other than myself, but also from my life's other moments. Suppose *this* to be such a moment. But my life can end at any time. That would be a *further* fact, extrinsic to what occurs within this moment, because it involves a relation to *other* moments, and so goes beyond what is internal to 'my life at *this* moment.' My life in this moment is already what it just now is. As nothing external to its own existence could constitute *its* existence or its value, so nothing happening later (or, what some, as we have seen, will find more controversial: earlier) can take this existence or value away. What has (nonrelationally) happened at *one* time cannot later be made not to have happened at that time, or to have had a different intrinsic value at that time, by virtue of what happens somewhere *else*. For these matters are decided only by what happens *just then*. Now, on the hedonist's view, the occurrence or presence of pleasure, and its value, are matters such as these; matters completely decided by what happens in the pleasure's moment or time." Leonard David Katz, "Hedonism as Metaphysics of Mind and Value," (Ph.D. diss., Princeton University, 1986), pp. 89–90.

for the moment, without interruption? What seems most plausible is that the overall badness of the longer stretch is determined by taking the badness of the first particular moment *together with* the badness of the next particular moment *together with* that of the next and so on. And this seems to spell simple addition. It is hard to see what else we could or should include in our measurement of total disvalue.

This argument asserts that all that ultimately matters is what suffering is like at the time it occurs. Isn't this what the experience of suffering tells us? Think of intense suffering brought on by severe pain. When we are racked by pain, we know that the past is nothing, and we know that the future is nothing either, except insofar as we pray and strive and hope to make a future free from pain become the present. We may strive to *deny* our pain, by moving imaginatively to the future where it no longer exists. And if we can bring off this psychological feat, we achieve at least a small mitigation of our present suffering. (We also run the risk that this is followed by a crushing psychological defeat, and intensification of suffering, when reality reasserts itself.) What we certainly do *not* do is look squarely at our present pain with its attendant suffering, recognize it for what it is, and declare it less intrinsically bad because of its temporal proximity to a pain-free existence in the future.

As suffering stretches out in time (the argument continues), its badness accumulates; but this is nothing more than the repetitive addition of the badness associated with each moment of suffering. Each moment of suffering is *so* bad that we look at its badness as if from below. We see the gaping vault of its badness stretching far above us, and we are surprised, almost incredulous, that there could be so much badness. How much more difficult for us to perceive that this awesome badness can be *doubled* when one moment of suffering is joined by another equal in length and intensity! Nevertheless, this is true. And we are simply unable to comprehend the towering badness signified by the succession of, not two, but three, four, or even more moments of suffering. Unable to understand such dimensions, we compensate. We claim that the evil of prolonged, uninterrupted suffering is disproportionate to its duration, and consequently much worse than any of its component parts. But then we lose sight of these parts; we forget the unutterable badness of *actual, present, momentary, now-occurring* suffering; or, if through an improbable feat of memory, we succeed in recalling this badness to mind, we cannot extend it beyond a sample of one. We may represent the longer stretch by placing this one horrible moment side by side with some numerical factor *n*. But this factor has no more than intellectual, notational significance. We see one horrible moment tracking empty time, as though this made any sense. We do not see the horrible moment multiplied. How can we?

Nevertheless, the argument may fail to convince. When all is said and done, we may be unable to relinquish the view that the temporal concentration of suffering may make it worse, possibly much worse. Imagine two equally long periods of very intense suffering, and imagine that we could either run them together (say, in the middle of a person's life), or separate them by thirty or forty years. We may have a stubborn intuition that the second alternative would mark a great improvement. We may continue to believe this, even if the period of separation were narrowed to a year or six months. In the end I am unsure whether the temporal concentration of suffering can or cannot make it worse.

3. Duration

Our discussion of timing has led to the question of duration. I have just examined the claim that the chronological concentration of suffering sometimes makes it worse. As I noted, this is equivalent to the claim that the badness of uninterrupted suffering can be disproportionate to its duration. Such a claim is exemplified in the view that five hours of continuous suffering are *more* than five times as bad as one hour of continuous suffering. As I indicated, I find it difficult to choose between the affirmation and denial of this view.

In chapter 6 I discussed a situation in which we can either prevent the five-year suffering of one person or the one-year suffering, equally intense, of six other people. Many people think that it is more important to prevent the five-year suffering of one person, even though the cumulative duration of the suffering is less. In chapter 6, I said we could explain this judgment by claiming, with the priority view, that it is more important to help those people whose suffering is worse. However, there is another possible explanation for this judgment. We might say that, for the person who suffers, five years of continuous suffering are more than five times as bad as one year of continuous suffering. If five years of continuous suffering are more than *six* times as bad as one year of continuous suffering, this alone could explain why we should prevent the five-year suffering of one person rather than the one-year suffering of six other people.[5]

If we think that it is more important to shorten the longer suffering of the few rather than the briefer suffering of the many, should we explain this in terms of the priority view, or the view that the personal badness of uninterrupted suffering can be disproportionate to its duration? Or are both views part of the correct explanation?[6]

One way to test for this would be to imagine an example in which the longer suffering of the few takes a temporally scattered form. Suppose that we can either

5. I have assumed that the suffering of six people is six times as bad as the suffering of one person. Some people may challenge the assumption that the impersonal badness of suffering is proportional to the number of people who suffer. I take up this issue in the next section.

6. There could also be another explanation, the appeal to *equality*. On egalitarian grounds, it is more important to shorten the longer suffering of the few, because this reduces the disparity between the welfare of different people. The egalitarian perspective is not directly concerned with how well off people are in an absolute sense, but how well off they are *in comparison to others*. I shall ignore the appeal to equality in my discussion. In part, this is because I doubt that egalitarian considerations should apply to the distribution of suffering. On the complexity of equality as an ideal, see Larry S. Temkin, *Inequality* (New York: Oxford University Press, 1993). On the distinction between egalitarianism and the priority view, see Derek Parfit, *Equality or Priority?* The 1991 Lindley Lecture (University of Kansas, 1995). See also Temkin, *Inequality*, chap. 9.

prevent Prima's suffering or the suffering of six other people. Prima's suffering takes the form of five *nonconsecutive* week-long periods of uninterrupted suffering, where each week of suffering is separated from the next by an interval of one year. The six other people's suffering, equal in intensity to Prima's, takes the form of one week of uninterrupted suffering each. The lives of these seven people are in other respects identical.

Now because Prima's five weeks of suffering take a temporally scattered form, I find it hard to believe that they are, for her, over five times worse than one week of suffering. Of course, her five weeks of suffering are *much worse* for her than one week of suffering. But, it seems to me, they are just five times worse.

Our question was how to explain the judgment that it is more important to reduce the longer suffering of the few than to reduce the briefer suffering of the many. So suppose we agree that it would be more important to prevent five *consecutive* uninterrupted weeks of suffering for Prima than the one-week suffering of six other people. Suppose we also agree that the prolongation of suffering over wide intervals does not lead to a disproportionate increase in the personal badness of that suffering. If we think that it is still more important to prevent five weeks of nonconsecutive suffering for Prima than the one-week suffering of six other people, this suggests that we accept the priority view. We give her priority because she faces worse cumulative suffering than any of the others. If we do *not* think it is more important to prevent five weeks of nonconsecutive suffering for Prima than the one-week suffering of six other people, this suggests that we reject the priority view. If, at the same time, we think that it is more important to prevent five weeks of *consecutive* suffering for Prima than the one-week suffering of six other people, our reason appears not to be the priority view, but rather the view that the personal badness of suffering can be disproportionate to its duration.

On this issue, my own views remain uncertain. I find it possible to doubt both the priority view (applied to duration) and the view that the personal badness of uninterrupted suffering is disproportionate to its duration. Yet I am still pulled toward the view that it can be more important to reduce the longer suffering of the few than the shorter suffering of the many. This view is most compelling in extreme cases. If we can prevent either the thirty year-long suffering of Prima or the one hour suffering of many other people whose combined suffering marginally exceeds thirty years, it is hard to deny that the prevention of Prima's suffering is more important.

4. Numbers

How does the badness of suffering vary with the number of those afflicted? I believe the only plausible view is that this relation is a direct one. Imagine one person who endures intense suffering for a certain period of time. This is very bad. Now imagine that a second person also experiences suffering of this intensity and duration. The second person's experience is in itself very bad, as bad as the first person's. But now there are *two* people with this experience. Whereas before there was only one very bad experience, now there are two very bad experiences. It seems clear to me that the suffering of both these people is twice as bad as the suffering of one of them.

This judgment should be extended. Imagine a third person who endures suffering of the same intensity and duration as that of the first two people. We should say that his suffering is as bad as each of theirs, but that their *combined* suffering, which is twice as bad as each of *their* suffering, is twice as bad as his also. In the following trade-off,

Prima	*Secunda*	*Tertia*
(1) suffering of intensity x and duration y	suffering of intensity x and duration y	no suffering
(2) no suffering	no suffering	suffering of intensity x and duration y

we should say that outcome 1 is *twice* as bad as outcome 2.

Some writers have argued against this view. In fact, they deny that there is *any* relation between the number of people who suffer and the badness of the suffering. They deny that the number of people who suffer has any intrinsic moral significance.

The view that numbers don't count can be traced to the simple refusal by the view's proponents to evaluate the combined suffering of two or more people. They are unwilling to step behind the perspective of any particular victim. They may switch from one victim's perspective to that of another, but this change does not broaden their outlook, since they tend to assume that one victim's perspective must exclude all others. As they move from one perspective to another, therefore, they lose the knowledge gained from the earlier one.

Thus John M. Taurek, considering a dilemma between the untimely death of one person and the untimely death of five others, writes that

> I do not wish to say in this situation that it is or would be a worse thing were these five persons to die and David to live than it is or would be were David to die and these five to continue to live. I do not wish to say this unless I am prepared to qualify it by explaining to whom or for whom or relative to what purpose it is or would be a worse thing.[7]

He later adds,

> Should any one of these five lose his life, his loss is no greater a loss to him because, as it happens, four others (or forty-nine others) lose theirs as well. And neither he nor

7. Taurek, "Should the Numbers Count?" *Philosophy and Public Affairs* 6 (1977): 293–316, p. 304. For a probing discussion of Taurek's argument, see Kamm, *Morality, Mortality*, vol. 1, Part 2. For another discussion, with some powerful counterarguments, see Derek Parfit, "Innumerate Ethics," *Philosophy and Public Affairs* 7 (1978): 285–301.

anyone else loses anything of greater value to him than does David, should David lose his life. Five individuals each losing his life does not add up to anyone's experiencing a loss five times greater than the loss suffered by any one of the five.[8]

Taurek concludes from this that there is not a special obligation to spare the suffering or death of the many rather than that of the few.

C. S. Lewis writes something similar:

> Suppose that I have a toothache of intensity x: and suppose that you, who are seated beside me also begin to have a toothache of intensity x. You may, if you choose, say that the total amount of pain in the room is now $2x$. But you must remember that no one is suffering $2x$: search all time and all space and you will not find that composite pain in anyone's consciousness. There is no such thing as a sum of suffering, *for no one suffers it* [my emphasis]. When we have reached the maximum that a single person can suffer, we have, no doubt, reached something very horrible, but we have reached all the suffering there ever can be in the universe. The addition of a million fellow-sufferers adds no more pain.[9]

We might reply to both writers as follows: "You talk as if we only wanted to know what is the most that anyone suffers. But that is not our question. We want to know how much *each and every* person suffers, and we want to know the *cumulative badness* of the suffering *of all of them*." Lewis conspicuously avoids this question. Taurek considers it long enough to conclude that the idea of evaluating the combined suffering of more than one person for comparative purposes is "at best . . . confused" and "typically . . . outrageous."[10]

However, it does not have to be either confused or outrageous. Both Lewis and Taurek can, and frequently do, move imaginatively from one victim's perspective to that of another. Lewis is explicitly interested in finding the person who experiences the most pain in the universe, an effort that requires him to compare the suffering of many different people; and Taurek allows that "for each of [the] six persons [threatened with an untimely death] it is no doubt a terrible thing to die. . . . His loss means something to me only, or chiefly, because of what it means to him."[11] But an imaginative shift from the perspective of one victim to that of another need not be accompanied by amnesia. While learning to view the world as victim Y sees it, we can remember how it was seen by victim X. We can discover that Y's suffering is bad without forgetting that X's suffering is bad, too. We can be aware of the suffering of *all* victims, and know that the suffering of *each* is bad. As a result, we can know that the addition of the suffering of each one makes the world much worse than it would have been otherwise, because if someone's suffering were not added to the total picture, then *that* person would not have suffered.

8. Taurek, "Should the Numbers Count?" p. 307.
9. Lewis, *The Problem of Pain* (New York: Macmillan, 1948), pp. 103–4.
10. Taurek, "Should the Numbers Count?," p. 309.
11. Ibid., p. 307.

It is more difficult when the alternatives under consideration includes both winners and losers: that is, when the suffering of one group of people is prevented in outcome A but permitted in outcome B, while the suffering of another group of people is prevented in outcome B but permitted in outcome A. Even if the number of people whose suffering is prevented in A (call them the A-winners) is larger than the number of people whose suffering is prevented in B (call them the B-winners), and the intensity and duration of suffering faced by each of the A-winners in B is just as great as that faced by each of the B-winners in A, it may be difficult to assert that outcome A is better than outcome B. We might naturally want to say that outcome A is in one way better and in one way worse than outcome B. It is better for the people whose suffering it prevents, and worse for the people whose suffering it permits. Can we say that, overall, A is better (or less bad) than B? I think it is Taurek's basic point that we cannot say this: we can say, perhaps, that A is both better and worse than B—better for those whom it helps, and worse for those whom it harms—but the hypothesis that it is better overall flies in the face of the fact that for at least some people it is just worse.

Taurek might make one exception. In his article he implies that one person's harm may be less bad than another's from a moral point of view, if, but only if, the first person would be *morally required* to undergo his harm in order to spare the second person his. But Taurek thinks there are many situations in which one may refuse to undergo a smaller harm to oneself rather than prevent a greater harm to someone else. For example, he thinks that one is not required to sacrifice one's arm in order to save another person's life.[12] By his logic, therefore, the loss of one person's arm is just as bad, from a moral point of view, as the loss of another person's life. Furthermore, since Taurek denies that numbers count, it doesn't matter how many people endure the greater harm. The loss of my arm is just as bad as the loss of any *number* of other people's lives. To return to the example in the previous paragraph: An outcome in which fewer people suffer is just as bad as an outcome in which more people suffer, and vice versa, unless the suffering of every person in one group would be so minor in comparison to the worst suffering experienced by anyone in the other group that, in a one-on-one trade-off, every person in the first group would be morally required to accept his own suffering in order to prevent the worst individual suffering in the second group.

I believe that Taurek, in denying the significance of numbers, has made a mistake, an extremely serious mistake. The consequence of acting on his view would be morally catastrophic. I cannot prove this, but I can urge him to think again. I would do this by asking him to reflect on the potential suffering of *each* person threatened by suffering in alternative outcomes and to do this without forgetting the potential suffering of all *other* persons who are similarly threatened. In a trade-off between the intense suffering of one person and the equally intense suffering of one thousand other people, we should say that the latter suffering is *very much* worse.

12. Ibid., pp. 301–2.

Disturbing consequences also flow from Taurek's views about one-on-one trade-offs. At one point, Taurek implies that one is not required to endure minor pain in order to save someone else from agony.[13] This would imply, according to Taurek's position, that one person's minor pain is just as bad, from the moral point of view, as another person's agony. Consequently, *it is not more important to prevent one person's agony than another person's minor pain.* Combined with the denial that numbers are morally significant, this yields the view that it is not more important to prevent the agony of millions than the minor pain of one. I would like to think that such a view refutes itself.

Some people might agree with Taurek's denial that numbers count, but disagree with his reluctance to rank the moral significance of individual harms in one-on-one trade-offs. These people can avoid saying that it is no less important to prevent the minor pain of one than the agony of millions. Their view would instead be that all of the suffering in the world is only as bad as the worst suffering experienced by any individual.[14] According to this view, we should always reduce the suffering of the individual whose suffering is worst rather than the suffering of those who individually suffer less, even if they are far more numerous and we can reduce their suffering by a much larger amount. This is a pure version of maximin applied to the relief of suffering (called "maximin" because it instructs us to maximize the well-being of the worst-off individual). Though it is an improvement on Taurek's view, I still find it implausible. It would tell us to reduce one person's intense suffering by a very small amount rather than to *eliminate* the suffering, only slightly less intense, of millions of people. That strikes me as wrong.

Some people may fear that by acknowledging the moral significance of numbers, we open the door to false and unwarranted evaluative judgments based on certain kinds of arithmetic. Taurek writes,

> I would like to combat the apparent tendency of some people to react to the thought of each of fifty individuals suffering a pain of some given intensity in the same way as they might to the thought of some individual suffering a pain many or fifty times more intense. I cannot but think that some such tendency is at work in the minds of those who attribute significance to the numbers in these trade-off situations.[15]

Taurek is right that we should not view the pain of fifty people in the same way that we view the pain, fifty times more intense, of just one person. But we don't

13. On pp. 308–9. Parfit draws attention to this passage in "Innumerate Ethics," p. 288. It is of a piece with Taurek's general reluctance to move beyond the perspective of one person at a time. Recall what he says concerning the dilemma of letting one person die or letting five people die: "I do not wish to say in this situation that it is or would be a worse thing were these five persons to die and David to live than it is or would be were David to die and these five to continue to live. *I do not wish to say this unless I am prepared to qualify it by explaining to whom or for whom or relative to what purpose it is or would be a worse thing.*" ("Should the Numbers Count?" p. 304, emphasis added.)

14. See the passage from C. S. Lewis cited earlier.

15. "Should the Numbers Count?" pp. 309–10

have to deny the moral significance of numbers to claim that the severe pain of the one is morally worse than the fractional pain of all the others. (Interestingly, Taurek's own position may prohibit him from saying this!) There are at least two other explanations. One is that the severe pain, though only fifty times as intense as the more moderate pain, is over fifty times *worse* for the person who suffers it. Another is that it is more important to help those whose suffering is worse, and consequently that suffering becomes *morally worse* as it is concentrated in fewer people's lives. As I said at the beginning of this chapter, the moral badness of suffering is not to be confused with its "quantity," where quantity refers to intensity times duration times the number of victims.

In this section, I have claimed that the numbers *do* count and, more specifically, that the moral badness of suffering is directly proportional to the number of sufferers. Nevertheless, a problem I discuss in section 6 may act to weaken the confidence that some of us place in this claim.

5. The Agony of One Versus the Bliss of Many

I now want to examine a dilemma that arises when we examine trade-offs between the prevention of suffering and the promotion of happiness. In the last chapter I claimed that the relief of suffering has priority over the promotion of happiness. But how *much* priority does it have? On the most extreme view, the relief of morally significant suffering has lexical priority over the promotion of happiness. According to this view, whenever there is a trade-off between the prevention of significant suffering and the promotion of happiness, we should *always* prevent suffering, even when the increase of happiness vastly exceeds the reduction of suffering in size.

Most people will reject this view. It is hardest to accept when the relevant trade-offs occur within the same life. Suppose that at the cost of some barely significant suffering—a few seconds of excruciating suffering, say, or a few minutes of moderately intense suffering—someone who would otherwise spend his entire life close to the hedonistic zero is permitted to spend the rest of his life in extreme bliss. Is his bliss worth the barely significant suffering—say, the few seconds of agony? I can *understand* the view that even a lifetime of bliss is not worth a few seconds of agony, but on due consideration I am inclined to reject it. And most people will reject the view with little hesitation.

The lexical priority view is somewhat more plausible when applied to trade-offs across lives. But many people will also reject it here. If we can either prevent one person from experiencing some barely significant suffering, or provide someone else with a lifetime of bliss, many people will say that we ought to do the latter.

My own view is that even if positing lexical priority is too strong, the moral asymmetry of happiness and suffering across lives is very steep. In general, we should prevent one person's suffering, even at the cost of failing to prevent a much larger amount of other people's happiness. This seems especially clear to me in the case of very intense suffering. Consider the following trade-off:

	Prima	Secunda
(1)	an entire lifetime close to the hedonistic zero	an entire lifetime close to the hedonistic zero
(2)	same as in 1, but with the addition of a period of excruciating suffering	a lifetime of extreme bliss

What duration of excruciating suffering for Prima would be justified by a lifetime of bliss for Secunda? Certainly not a day of such suffering, certainly not an hour. I doubt that even a minute of such suffering would be justified. If we change the example so that Prima's example is acute but not excruciating, I am certain that not even a week of such suffering would be justified by the lifelong bliss of Secunda.

On any view that denies the lexical priority of relieving significant suffering over promoting happiness in interpersonal trade-offs, perplexities arise when we allow numbers to vary. Consider the following trade-off:

	Prima	Secunda
(1)	an entire lifetime close to the hedonistic zero	an entire lifetime close to the hedonistic zero
(2)	same as in 1, but with a slight addition of significant suffering[16]	a lifetime of extreme bliss

Suppose we believe that 2 is better than 1. (This is what we are likely to believe if we deny that the relief of significant suffering has lexical priority over the promotion of happiness.) Now imagine a similar trade-off that includes a third person, called Tertia:

	Prima	Secunda	Tertia
(1)	an entire lifetime close to the hedonistic zero	an entire lifetime close to the hedonistic zero	an entire lifetime close to the hedonistic zero
(2)	same as in 1 but with a slight addition of significant suffering	a lifetime of extreme bliss	same as in 1
(3)	same as in 2 but with a slight addition of significant suffering	a lifetime of extreme bliss	a lifetime of extreme bliss

If we said earlier that 2 is better than 1, we should continue to do so now. Now compare 2 with 3. This trade-off seems quite similar to the one between 1 and 2. The only difference is that Prima starts off with a little more suffering, and that

16. A more exact but less graceful formulation would be "same as in (1), but with an addition of barely significant suffering."

her additional suffering is now being offered as the price for Tertia's extreme bliss rather than Secunda's (which was purchased by an earlier increment in Prima's suffering). These differences do not (at first glance) seem significant. If we believe that 2 is better than 1, it seems that we should also believe that 3 is better than 2. And if we believe that 2 is better than 1 and 3 is better 2, then, from transitivity, we should believe 3 is better than 1.[17]

We can continue this process. Imagine a fourth person, Quarta, who can be moved up from a life close to the hedonistic zero to a life of permanent extreme bliss if we make Prima experience some more significant suffering than she would have experienced in 3. If we agreed to grant a lifetime of bliss to Secunda and Tertia under similar terms, it seems that we should grant a lifetime of bliss to Quarta under these terms. We can keep granting additional persons a lifetime of bliss, by slightly adding to Prima's suffering. If we keep the process up long enough, we wind up with the following outcome:

Prima	*Many other people*
(*n*) a lifetime of torment	a lifetime of extreme bliss

Where the original alternative had been:

Prima	*Many other people*
(1) a lifetime close to the hedonistic zero	a lifetime close to the hedonistic zero

Like William James, I find the conclusion that (*n*) is better than 1 unacceptable.[18] The lifelong bliss of many people, no matter how many, cannot justify our allowing the lifelong torture of one.

How can we avoid this conclusion? There are a number of options. We could decide that the relief of significant suffering has lexical priority over the promotion of happiness in interpersonal trade-offs. We could, in other words, retract our earlier claim that 2 is better than 1, and claim that it is *worse*. Some may find this an implausible view. However, I think it is much less implausible than the claim that *n* is superior to 1.

An alternative to claiming either that 2 is better or that it is worse than 1 is to claim that it is *neither* better *nor* worse than 1. We could then claim that 3 is neither better nor worse than 2, and so on all the way to *n*. This could be seen as having

---

17. Some people may want to question the assumption that "better than" must be transitive. I come to this point later.

18. I refer to his refusal, discussed in chapter 6, to accept "a world in which Messrs. Fourier's and Bellamy's and Morris's utopias should all be outdone, and millions kept permanently happy on the one simple condition that a certain lost soul on the far-off edge of things should lead a life of lonely torture." "The Moral Philosopher and the Moral Life," in *Essays in Pragmatism*, ed. Alburey Castell (New York: Hafner, 1958), p. 68.

the implication that n is neither better nor worse than 1. That implication, by denying that n is worse than 1, would also strike me as unacceptable. But it may be the wrong implication to draw. That is because "neither better nor worse than" is not always transitive.[19] "Neither better nor worse than" describes a rougher relation than "equal in value to," which *is* transitive. Larry Temkin offers a nice example.[20] We may think that Kant is neither better nor worse as a philosopher than Aristotle, Hume neither better nor worse than Kant, and Descartes neither better nor worse than Hume, and nevertheless think that Descartes is a worse philosopher than Aristotle. The same holds true for our present example. So long as we understand by "neither better nor worse than" something rougher than "equal in value to," we may judge 2 as neither better nor worse than 1, 3 as neither better nor worse than 2, and so on all the way to n, and *still* claim that n is worse than 1.

I have mentioned two ways of avoiding the conclusion that n is better than 1. We can claim that 2 is worse than 1, or that it is neither better nor worse than 1. Alternatively, we could claim that 2 is *better* than 1, but try to block the chain of reasoning that leads from this claim to the claim that n is better than 1. We might do this by claiming that the threshold of lexical priority lies, not between happiness and suffering, but somewhere *within* the zone of suffering. On this claim, there is a certain amount of significant individual suffering, specified in terms of intensity or duration or both, beyond which we may never advance, even for the sake of the largest imaginable increase of other people's happiness. To put it another way, as an individual's suffering is increased, there comes a point where the prevention of further suffering has lexical priority over the promotion of other people's happiness. I find this a plausible claim. Perhaps we should add that, as one draws near the threshold of lexical priority, it takes ever larger numbers of people receiving lifetimes of bliss to permit equally small additions of significant suffering.[21]

If we try to locate the threshold of lexical priority within suffering, we might try to do it at a certain level of intensity. Intensity of suffering matters a lot. A sophisticated moral understanding requires a knowledge of the moral significance of each level of intensity of suffering. We might want to say of a certain intensity level that it is morally significant in this way. This intensity level must never be crossed if the only purpose is to bring happiness to others.

It would be implausible, however, to specify the threshold of lexical priority *only* in terms of intensity. Doing so would imply that immediately above the threshold-level intensity, no individual suffering, however brief, can be justified by even the largest gain in other people's happiness, while immediately below the threshold-level intensity an *indefinitely long* period of suffering can be justified by a sufficiently large gain in other people's happiness. That can't be right. It is more plausible to

19. See Parfit, *Reasons and Persons*, p. 431; and Larry S. Temkin, "Intransitivity and the Mere Addition Paradox," *Philosophy and Public Affairs* 16 (1987): 138–87, pp. 145–46.

20. Ibid.

21. The point that as we approach the threshold it might become harder to justify equally small additions of suffering I owe to Derek Parfit.

have the threshold of lexical priority specify both intensity and duration, with a different duration for each level of intensity: no more than this duration at this level of intensity, no more than this (longer) duration at this (lower) level of intensity, etc.[22] Now it might be suggested that there is a level of intensity beneath which duration may be indefinitely prolonged if the gain in other people's happiness is sufficiently large. I find this implausible. It seems to me that we should never consign anyone to a lifetime of genuine suffering for the sake of other people's happiness, even if the suffering does not belong to the higher reaches of intensity.

There is another way of avoiding the implication that William James and I find unacceptable. We can claim that in a dilemma between the reduction of one person's suffering and the increase of other people's happiness, the *number* of people whose happiness would be increased has no moral weight. Which is to say: against the suffering of one person, the happiness of two or three or three billion people has no greater weight than the happiness of one person.

Recall the above example. We were led to the conclusion that n is better than 1, because we balanced the suffering of Prima against the happiness of *many* other people. But under the present claim, the happiness of many other people can have no greater weight against Prima's suffering than the happiness of just one person, say Secunda. If we believe that a lifetime of bliss for Secunda can only justify a slight increase of significant suffering for Prima, we should similarly believe that a lifetime of bliss for the greatest possible number can only justify a slight increase of significant suffering for Prima.

But, it might be objected, we were led to the unacceptable implication by balancing Prima's suffering against the happiness of separate individuals, one at a time. Numbers were not involved. This is not true. When we concluded, for example, that 3 was better than 1, this followed from the claim that 2 was better than 1 *and* the claim that 3 was better than 2. The bliss of Secunda was the justification for a certain increase in Prima's suffering, and the bliss of Tertia was the justification for a certain *additional* increase in Prima's suffering. The bliss of two people, so it was implied, justified a larger increase in Prima's suffering than the bliss of one person. This implicit view made possible the eventual conclusion that n was better than 1. This implicit view is what we are now rejecting. The rejection of this view implies that if Secunda's bliss had been purchased with the maximally allowable increase of Prima's suffering, no additional suffering on Prima's part could be used to purchase a lifetime of bliss for Tertia. If under 2 Prima's suffering had been increased by the maximally allowable amount, then 3 was *worse* than 2.

Suppose we accept the claim advanced here: against the suffering of one person the happiness of the greatest number has no more weight than the happiness of one person. This claim, if true, suggests a striking difference in the moral properties of happiness on the one hand and suffering on the other hand. This is because the equivalent claim with regard to suffering is highly implausible. Suppose that we

22. This is an oversimplification, since it implies suffering of unvarying intensity, and the individual's suffering need not take this form.

could either prevent the intense suffering of one person, or else the slightly less intense suffering of n other people, where n could be one or any number larger than one. It is hard to believe that the value of n doesn't matter. If n is one, we should of course prevent the first person's suffering. But if n is some very large number, it seems clear that we should prevent the suffering of the larger number.

I have listed what I think are the most plausible means of blocking the unacceptable conclusion. There may be other ways that involve certain variations and combinations of the proposals described here. However, I shall not discuss these variants.

Throughout this discussion I have assumed that "better than" is a transitive relation. For that reason, I claimed that if 2 was better than 1, 3 was better than 2, and so on all the way to n, we were forced to conclude that n was better than 1. Some people may suggest that the right way to block that conclusion is to *deny* the transitivity of "better than." Then we can claim that 2 is better than 1, and so on all the way to n, and nevertheless claim that n is *worse* than 1.

In "Counterexamples to the Transitivity of Better Than," Stuart Rachels presents an example that seems to provide powerful evidence for intransitivity.[23] I cannot think of a satisfactory response to Rachels's example that allows me to preserve the transitivity of "better than." But at the same time, I am reluctant to accept the intransitivity of "better than." It doesn't seem to make sense. To put it another way, "better than" doesn't seem like the kind of relation that *could* be intransitive; if we insist that "better than" is intransitive, it seems that the proper meaning of "better than" is forced to drop out.[24]

In any event, I believe there are better ways of resolving the problem discussed in this section than to allow the intransitivity of "better than." Moreover, I fear the consequences of introducing intransitivity into this particular set of trade-offs. Suppose we introduced intransitivity by claiming that 2 is better than 1, 3 is better than 2, . . . , n is better than n-1, and that n is *worse* than 1. We would then have the following circle, in which "$x < y$" means that x is worse than y and y is better than x (fig. 7.1).

Suppose we could choose from among *all* these outcomes. Which one should we choose? There seems to be no reason for choosing any one rather than another. Therefore, there doesn't seem to be any reason not to choose n. It is true that n is worse than 1. But n is better than n-1, which is better than n-2, and so on all

23. *Australasian Journal of Philosophy* 76 (1998): 71–83. Rachels asks us to compare an extremely intense pain, with a pain that is very much longer but only slightly less intense, then to compare the second pain with a third pain that is very much longer still but again only slightly less intense, until we arrive at a tremendously long pain of the very mildest intensity. As Rachels plausibly suggests, the pain keeps getting worse until it gets better. For an excellent discussion, see Larry S. Temkin, "A Continuum Argument for Intransitivity," *Philosophy and Public Affairs* 3 (1996): 175–210. For a defense of transitivity in response to Rachels and Temkin, see Alastair Norcross, "Comparing Harms: Headaches and Human Lives," *Philosophy and Public Affairs* 26 (1997): 135–67.

24. Temkin discusses these kinds of misgivings in "A Continuum Argument for Intransitivity," pp. 178, 207–10.

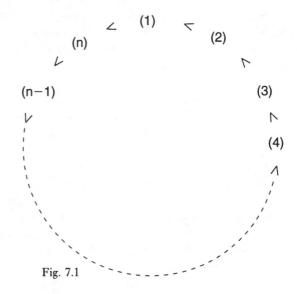

Fig. 7.1

around the circle. If we introduce intransitivity, it seems that *we would be permitted to choose* n *when one of the alternatives had been 1.* This strikes me as a sufficiently good reason to reject intransitivity, at least in this case.

6. The Agony of One Versus the Less Intense Suffering of Many

I now turn to a different kind of trade-off. Sometimes we may have to choose between preventing the more intense suffering of fewer people and the less intense suffering of more people. We can refer to this as a trade-off between numbers and intensity, for short. (To simplify matters, I shall imagine cases in which the duration of suffering is held constant and the suffering takes an uninterrupted form.) As we shall see, this kind of trade-off raises extremely difficult problems.

When we can either reduce the number of sufferers, or else reduce the intensity of suffering of those who suffer, should we reduce numbers or intensity? When the difference in intensity between the more intense suffering of the few and the less intense suffering of the many is very small, we are more likely to favor a reduction in numbers. For example, in a trade-off between the intense suffering of one person and the suffering, only slightly less intense, of a million other people, it seems obvious that we should prefer the more intense suffering of the one. And even in a trade-off between the intense suffering of one person and the slightly less intense suffering of *two* other people, the more intense suffering of one person may seem preferable, if the difference in intensity is small enough.

However, if the difference in intensity is large, we are likely to resist a reduction in numbers at the cost of greater intensity. Imagine that we could either let a million people suffer the sharp sting of disappointment or the grinding rage of accumulated frustration (that is, when these things are genuinely painful) or else let one person undergo severe torture for the same period of time. Many people would say that we should let even one million people suffer acute and painful frustration rather than permit one person to undergo severe torture. My intuitions favor this claim.

If this claim is right, it does not imply that the pain of such torture is over one million times more intense than the pain of acute and painful frustration. On the intuitive measure of intensity I employ here, that is an absurd estimate—unless the pain of the frustration is vanishingly small and virtually non-existent, to the point of imperceptibility, which we are supposing that it is not. I do not know by what proportion the pain of the extreme torture would exceed that of the acute frustration. It might be a factor of about four, or even six, or indeed even ten. It is unlikely that it could be much greater than twenty. Suppose for the moment—what seems to me probably an exaggeration—that the intensity of suffering felt by the torture victim is as much as twenty times greater than the intensity of suffering of the person ravaged by frustration. Then although the torture victim's suffering is only twenty times as intense as the suffering of the other person ravaged by frustration, it appears to be over one million times worse from a moral point of view. In trade-offs between intensity and numbers, increases in intensity can give rise to *much* greater increases in the moral badness of suffering.

I said that my intuitions favor the claim that we should prevent one person from experiencing the pain of torture rather than prevent a million others from experiencing the pain of acute frustration. But in fact my intuitions favor an even stronger claim. It seems to me that when the difference in intensity is this large, *no* difference in the number of sufferers can justify the more intense suffering. The severe torture of one person seems worse than the painful frustration of *any* number of people. The prevention of 20-degree suffering appears to have lexical priority over the prevention of 1-degree suffering. Or, as I shall find it convenient to say: in trade-offs between intensity and numbers, these intensity levels appear to be incommensurable.[25]

So intuition tells me, and I believe I am not alone. But it turns out that it is very difficult to defend this claim. The incommensurability claim (as I shall call it) is hard to deny, but it also has implications that are hard to accept. This presents a dilemma that I am not sure how to resolve.

To see the difficulties involved, let us imagine an intensity scale in which 20 and its vicinity represent suffering of *unimaginably* horrible intensity; while 10 and its vicinity represent suffering of extreme and horrible intensity, though not *quite* so unimaginable; while the neighborhood of 1 indicates suffering that is much lower

---

25. My use of the term "incommensurable" here should not be misunderstood. I use it not to signal the impossibility of ranking different options, but to indicate an unbridgeable gap in value. It is the same use that appears in phrases like "incomparably better" and "incomparably worse," or in a remark such as the following: "You can't compare your trivial disappointment to my tragedy." If its intended meaning is kept in mind, the term need not spark misunderstanding, and it will save us a great deal of breath.

in intensity but still terrible, and from which most people would flee with great relief; and 2, 3, and 4 mark out the stages of suffering as it grows increasingly unbearable. An incommensurabilist would claim, with apparent plausibility, that 20-degree suffering can never be traded off against 1-degree suffering. We should never allow one person to endure 20-degree suffering, even if that were necessary to rescue the greatest *possible* number of people from 1-degree suffering.

But what if we compare 20-degree suffering and 19.8-degree suffering? The difference is real, but nevertheless small.[26] It would be hard to deny that these intensities are commensurable. Surely there must be some number x, such that if x people were threatened with 19.8-degree suffering it would be our duty to spare the suffering of *all of them*, rather than the 20-degree suffering of just one person. In fact, it seems clear that the 19.8-degree suffering of *two* people is cumulatively worse than the 20-degree suffering of one person. The same must be said for 19.8-degree suffering and 19.6-degree suffering: there must be some number of people y, such that if y people were threatened with 19.6-degree suffering it would be our duty to spare their suffering rather than the 19.8-degree suffering of just one person. Again, it seems clear that if only two people were threatened with 19.6-degree suffering, we should spare them rather than one person threatened with 19.8-degree suffering.

If 20-degree suffering is commensurable with 19.8-degree suffering, and 19.8-degree suffering is commensurable with 19.6-degree suffering, then, if we assume transitivity, 20-degree suffering and 19.6-degree suffering are *necessarily* commensurable. If there is some number x such that the 19.8-degree of suffering of x people is worse than the 20-degree suffering of one person, and there is some number y such that the 19.6-degree suffering of y people is worse than the 19.8-degree suffering of one person, then the 19.6-degree suffering of $(x)(y)$ people is worse than the 20-degree suffering of one person. (Compared to the 19.8-degree suffering of *each* of the x people, the 19.6 degree suffering of y people is worse. Compared to the 19.8-degree suffering of *all* x people, the 19.6-degree suffering of $[x][y]$ people is worse. From transitivity, the 19.6-degree suffering of $[x][y]$ people is worse than the 20-degree suffering of one person.)

The rest of the argument is easy to predict. Just as 19.8- and 19.6-degree suffering are commensurable, so are 19.6- and 19.4-degree suffering. Likewise 19.4- and 19.2-degree suffering. We continue this sequence of observations, without break, until the final observation that 1.2-degree suffering and 1-degree suffering are com-

---

26. On the other hand, the difference is not infinitesimal. One has to remember that 20-degree suffering is *extremely intense*. The difference between 20-degree suffering and 19.8-degree suffering, though minuscule in proportional terms, is not minuscule in absolute terms. Think of it this way. The difference between 1-degree suffering and 0.8-degree suffering does not appear minuscule; the difference between 20-degree suffering and 19.8-degree suffering is at least as significant.

I add these remarks to forestall the objection that the argument that follows in the text is a kind of Sorites argument, and unsound for that reason. Despite my remarks, some people may still believe that I use a Sorites argument. I do not think I do, for reasons ably stated by Temkin in "A Continuum Argument for Transitivity," pp. 197–202.

mensurable. Consequently, 20-degree and 1-degree suffering are commensurable. The number of people whose combined 1-degree suffering is morally worse than the 20-degree suffering of one person may turn out to be *very large*. Nevertheless, it is a finite number.

There are various ways to respond to this argument, none of which seems satisfactory. One response is to preserve the incommensurability thesis by invoking maximin. But, as I have noted before, maximin applied to the reduction of suffering seems unacceptable. In this case, it instructs us, among other things, to prefer the 19.6-degree suffering of 10 billion people to the 19.8-degree suffering of just one person. Surely this is intolerable. There must always be a certain narrow *range* of intensities that are commensurable with each other—a range in which it is possible for numerical differences to morally outweigh differences of intensity. And if anywhere on the intensity scale we may (if the ratio is right) purchase a certain reduction in the number of people suffering at the price of a slight increment in the intensity of suffering of the few who will suffer, then it appears that *sufficiently large* reductions in the number of people suffering may justify (if there is no other choice) even the *largest* increments in intensity of suffering for the few who will suffer.

Commensurability over the entire range of intensity of suffering could be blocked if we determined that for at least some points on the intensity scale, no margin of commensurability exists whatsoever. This brings us to a second possible alternative to full commensurability (the first having been maximin). This is to identify a certain finite number of *incommensurability points*. These points correspond to certain absolute points on the cardinal intensity scale. *Between* two consecutive incommensurability points, there is moral commensurability: that is, it is possible for an excess of numbers on the side of lower intensity to tilt the moral balance in favor of permitting the higher-intensity suffering of the few. However, if two different intensities of suffering *straddle* an incommensurability point, then moral commensurability is ruled out: suffering more intense than the incommensurability-point intensity is *always* morally worse than suffering less intense than the incommensurability-point intensity, *regardless* of the disparity of numbers and the closeness of intensity between the two unequally intense sets of suffering.

The merit of this proposal is that it saves us from full commensurability. In itself, however, it is hard to accept. Where could we plausibly locate an incommensurability point? We would not want to locate it anywhere in the zone of intolerable suffering—anywhere, say, on or above 1. If we fixed it at 1.0, we would implicitly be willing to consign 10 billion people to 0.9-degree suffering in order to spare the 1.1-degree suffering of only one person. But surely the improvement of moving from 1.1-degree suffering to 0.9-degree suffering is not so great that we would want to impose suffering in this range of intensity on an additional 9,999,999,999 people. And if we want to avoid such a catastrophe at the level of 1-degree suffering, then surely we want to avoid it at levels of higher intensity as well. But then we permit commensurability between 1-degree suffering and suffering of the greatest possible intensity.

I find it hard to accept that an incommensurability point could lie anywhere but in the most relatively moderate range of intensity of suffering. I find it a *little* less difficult to conceive that an incommensurability point may lie somewhere on the suffering-intensity scale close to the hedonistic zero—somewhere approximately between 0.5 and 0 on the scale we have been using. But I cannot support this proposal with any degree of confidence, nor do I think that many other people would support it unhesitatingly.

Another way to block the commensurability between 20-degree suffering and 1-degree suffering would be to deny the transitivity of "better than." This would allow us to say the following. It is better to permit the 20-degree suffering of one person than the suffering of a larger number of people whose intensity of suffering is somewhat lower. It is better to permit these people's suffering than the suffering of an even larger number of people whose intensity of suffering is somewhat lower still. And so on, until it would be better to permit the suffering of some large number of people whose intensity of suffering is greater than 1, than to permit the 1-degree suffering of an even larger number of people. Nevertheless, it would *not* be better to permit the 20-degree suffering of one person than the 1-degree suffering of this much larger number of people.[27]

However, as I said before, I find it difficult to accept that "better than" could be intransitive. The idea is highly paradoxical, and I don't know how to make sense of it. And as before, I fear the consequences it may have.

Suppose that 8-degree suffering represents suffering of an extreme, though not *unimaginably* extreme, intensity. Now suppose that there is a higher intensity level y and an even higher intensity level x, such that if we had a choice between the following four outcomes,

(1) one person at x
(2) some larger number of people at y
(3) some even larger number of people at 8
(4) twice this even larger number of people at 7.8

the intransitivity proposal would tell us (given the right numbers) that 1 is better than 2, which is better than 3, which is better than 4, which, however, is better than 1. Which of these outcomes should we choose? As far as I can see, the intransitivity proposal wouldn't give us a good reason not to choose 4. It is true that 4 is worse than 3, but it is also better than 1, which is better than 2, and so on around the circle. That the intransitivity proposal would allow us to choose 4, when one of the alternatives had been 3, strikes me as a good reason to resist it.

Perhaps there is another way to block the commensurability of 20-degree suffering and 1-degree suffering. We might want to deny the assumption that the moral badness of suffering is directly proportional to the number of people who suffer. This denial could take different forms. We could deny that the numbers count at all. On this view, since the 1-degree suffering of many can't be worse than the 1-

---

27. This example bears resemblances to the one that Rachels uses to argue for intransitivity.

degree suffering of one, it can't be worse than the 20-degree suffering of one. But this view would have what I think is the disturbing implication that it is more important to prevent the 20-degree suffering of one person than the 19.8-degree suffering of a million. Or we could admit that the numbers count, but claim that they count for less than their proportional weight. On this view, the suffering of two people is worse than the suffering of one, but not *twice* as bad. This view would save us from the implication that the 20-degree suffering is worse than then 19.8-degree suffering of a million. However, it is hard to identify a positive motivation for this compromise position. More to the point, it might not save us from the commensurability of 20-degree suffering and 1-degree suffering. For if the numbers always count for something, then by continually adding to the number of 1-degree sufferers, we *eventually* make their suffering worse, from a moral point of view, than the 20-degree suffering of one. (But perhaps the growth in numbers ceases to matter altogether after a certain number is reached.) Finally, we might try to deny that the numbers count at certain lower intensities of suffering. On this view, the numbers count where 20-degree suffering is concerned, but not where 1-degree suffering is concerned. But this would imply that as we decrease the intensity of suffering, there is a point where the numbers go from having some moral significance to having none at all, and that seems peculiar. (And it seems strange to say, in any event, that the 1-degree suffering of a million is not worse than the 1-degree suffering of one.)

Finally, if none of the previous responses seems satisfactory, we could accept the view that there is full commensurability with respect to numbers throughout the entire range of intensity of suffering—except, just possibly, when the less intense suffering of the greater number is a very moderate intensity, not far in absolute terms from, hence not dissimilar to, the hedonistic zero.

If this conclusion seems troubling, perhaps we could reconcile ourselves to it in the following way. Twenty-degree suffering and 1-degree suffering are not *literally* incommensurable, but they are *virtually* incommensurable. There may be some truly vast number z such that the 20-degree suffering of one person would be preferable to the 1-degree suffering of z people. But the number z is too big for us to comprehend. From where we stand, it will seem an infinity. For this reason, it is understandable that we view 1-degree suffering as incommensurable with 20-degree suffering. Moreover, it may even be desirable for us to believe and say that the distance is incommensurable. This way we are reminded of how truly great the distance is, and we will avoid the dangerous error of thinking that the minimum value of z (where z is the number of potential 1-degree sufferers the prevention of whose suffering justifies the 20-degree suffering of one person) is smaller than it in fact is.

This defense of commensurability tries to overcome our misgivings. But it doesn't succeed in overcoming mine. It still seems wrong to consign just one person to 20-degree suffering in order to save even the largest imaginable number of people from 1-degree suffering. I remain unsure how to think about trade-offs between the very intense suffering of one person and the considerably less intense suffering of a much larger number.

ᴄᴄ

The Limits of the Duty
to Relieve Suffering

1. Introduction

This chapter looks at the limits of the prima facie duty to relieve suffering. It asks, When is it the case that we do *not* have a duty to relieve suffering? More precisely, When are we not required to prevent the worst cumulative suffering?

This is an enormous question. A full answer would require nothing less than a complete theory of morality. Having nothing that even approaches such a theory, I can only take a few broad swipes at the issue, and I shall leave many more questions than answers. This chapter can be seen as a statement of the work that remains to be done.

We can distinguish between four kinds of possible limits on the duty to relieve suffering. First, the value of relieving suffering may sometimes be outweighed by its cost from an impersonal point of view. Second, the relief of suffering might sometimes require the use of impermissible means. Third, compliance with an unlimited duty to relieve suffering might sometimes entail an unreasonable level of sacrifice. Fourth, the prevention of the worst cumulative suffering in the world as a whole might sometimes violate obligations we owe to individuals who are related to us in special ways, such as our children, spouses, friends, clients, patients, and compatriots. We can refer to these four kinds of limits, respectively, as *consequentialist limits*, *deontological constraints*, *limits on obligatory sacrifice*, and *special obligations*. These different kinds of reasons may often blend in with each other; however, I shall set aside a separate discussion for each of the four categories.

I should say a few words about the tone of the following discussion. I grant from the start that there are consequentialist limits on the duty to relieve suffering. However, my attitude toward the existence of other limits remains agnostic. The short explanation for this is as follows. Consequentialist limits are compatible with the truth of consequentialism—the view that we are morally required to bring about the best possible outcome. Each of the other three limits denies the truth of consequentialism. Very few people if any would deny that there are consequentialist limits on the duty to relieve suffering—that is, that the value of preventing suffering is sometimes outweighed by its cost. But a number of people, including some distinguished philosophers, believe that consequentialism is true. My agnosticism regarding non-consequentialist limits reflects a desire to remain neutral on this controversial question.

2. Underestimating the Duty to Relieve Suffering

Identifying the limits of the duty to relieve suffering ultimately involves comparing its force to that of rival moral considerations. We ask when, if ever, it is morally defeated, or morally outweighed. To answer correctly, we must have an accurate sense of its inherent force.

My task throughout the book has been to emphasize its force. Beyond minor levels of intensity and duration, suffering soon becomes appalling. Not too far beyond that, its horror becomes inconceivable. The mind shuts down before the task of comprehending the suffering that individuals, let alone multitudes, have endured. The badness of suffering is immense. Now, our duty to relieve suffering is tied directly to its badness. This has nothing to do with the general properties of the word *bad*, or an a priori requirement to promote the good, or anything like that. It has to do with the nature of suffering. Suffering must not be borne, it must not be allowed to occur. This is to say, on the one hand, that suffering is bad; and on the other hand, that everyone must act so as to eliminate suffering. The badness of suffering and the duty to relieve suffering refer to the same moral phenomenon. Or, if you like, they are two different sides of the same moral phenomenon. So the force of the duty to relieve suffering keeps pace with the badness of suffering. This implies, of course, that the force of the duty to relieve suffering varies depending on the cumulative badness of the suffering in question.

The prima facie duty to relieve suffering is in general quite strong. Other moral considerations must be at least as strong to override its dictates. But in our ordinary thinking, we rarely allow a fair contest to take place. Instead, we routinely underestimate the inherent force of the duty to relieve suffering. We pit it against its competitors in an already weakened and diminished state. (Note that the duty to relieve suffering comes in two parts: a prohibition against inflicting suffering, and a requirement to prevent it. What we tend to underestimate is less the former than the latter.) We do so because of three deeply rooted habits: a tendency to forget the meaning of suffering, to forget the existence of suffering, and to forget or underestimate our ability to prevent suffering. These three habits are mutually reinforcing.

2.a. Forgetting the Meaning of Suffering

It is extremely difficult, except when we are suffering ourselves, to preserve more than a fleeting awareness of what suffering is. There seems almost to be a reflexive reaction against genuine awareness. (See the discussion in chapter 4.) Consequently, what we typically have in mind when we talk about "suffering" is no more than a pale imitation of the original. Sometimes, not content to dilute suffering, we alchemize it. In place of the real thing, we construct something beautiful or stirring; we dwell on the heroic qualities it elicits, or the anger in which it becomes enveloped—anything but the suffering itself. If the meaning of suffering continually eludes us, whether through dilution or falsification, so too does an adequate comprehension of its badness. And the perceived strength of the duty to relieve suffering diminishes in exact proportion to its perceived badness.

2.b. Forgetting the Existence of Suffering

The same powerful reluctance to be aware of suffering that causes us to distort its meaning also causes us to deny its existence. Of course, distortion of its meaning *is* a way to deny its existence. But there are other ways, too. One is straightforward forgetting: there are few things from which we are more easily distracted than the contemplation of other people's suffering. Another means of denial, far subtler but no less effective, is our habit of blaming the victim—a habit much more universal and automatic than typical use of the phrase implies. (Again, see chapter 4.)

Another cause of forgetfulness is the general weakness of our memory: recollection of our own suffering, on which our understanding of suffering is primarily based, fades with our recollection of everything else. Yet another cause, of enormous importance, is the phenomenon that Shelly Kagan has labeled paleness of belief.[1] Pale beliefs are those that do not register fully on us. In Kagan's words, "They are displayed to the mind in such a way that the individual does not fully appreciate their import."[2] Paleness of belief perfectly describes the manner in which we receive news of most of the suffering in the world. We hear of bombing, torture, starvation; but the information registers dimly. It is not absorbed. If by some chance we should become a witness to these horrors, we will no doubt feel surprised, and think to ourselves, "Hey, this really does happen!" It is not because we denied it before, but because our previous acknowledgment had something of an abstract quality. In Kagan's words, our perception of the victims and their suffering lacked flesh and blood. We saw the victims as stick figures (to borrow another image from Kagan), not as individuals with their richly distinguishing characteristics. And we failed to imagine in concrete, sensuous detail the circumstances of their suffering.

Paleness of belief in other people's suffering is not the same as denial, but it has a similar effect. Suffering that is only palely believed does not seem fully real. If it

1 Shelly Kagan, *The Limits of Morality* (Oxford: Clarendon Press, 1989), pp. 283–300.
2. Ibid., p. 283.

does not seem quite real, it cannot seem very bad. And the less bad it appears, the less force we will ascribe to the duty to relieve it.

Paleness of belief is a general phenomenon, not limited to the belief in other people's suffering. But in the case of suffering, it is exacerbated by our general fear of the awareness of suffering. Such reluctance discourages attempts to make our belief in other people's suffering more vivid.

The influence also runs the other way. The fact that palely believed suffering seems less *real* makes it easier to deny. The fact that it seems less *bad* makes it easier to distort. Paleness of belief helps us avoid the awareness of suffering.

2.c. Forgetting Our Ability to Prevent Suffering

How much the prima facie duty to relieve suffering demands of us depends on how much we can do—that is, the cumulative badness of suffering we can actually prevent. If we underestimate our preventive powers, we will shrink the duty to relieve suffering to less than its true scope. We will ignore many of its demands out of the mistaken opinion that we cannot satisfy them.

I believe that we tend to underestimate our preventive capacity: we tend to imagine that opportunities for preventing worse cumulative suffering run out much sooner than they actually do. This error has many sources. People often confuse mere desire, or habit voluntarily preserved, with unalterable obstacles that define the limit of their capacities. "I can't do any more" often simply means "I don't want to do any more," or "I am not used to doing any more, and I don't feel like changing my ways."[3] Often, too, people underestimate their capacity to relieve suf-

---

3. In his inaugural speech, President George Bush declared, "My friends, we have work to do. There are the homeless, lost and roaming. There are the children who have nothing—no love, no normalcy. There are those who cannot free themselves of enslavement to whatever addiction—drugs, welfare, the demoralization that rules the slums. There is crime to be conquered, the rough crime of the streets. There are young women to be helped who are about to become mothers of children they can't care for and might not love. They need our care, our guidance and our education, though we bless them for choosing life.

"The old solution, the old way, was to think that public money alone could end these problems. But we have learned that that is not so. And in any case, our funds are low. We have a deficit to bring down. *We have more will than wallet;* [italics added] but will is all we need.

"We will make the hard choices, looking at what we have, perhaps allocating it differently, making our decisions based on honest need and prudent safety." (*New York Times*, 21 January 1989.)

"*We have more will than wallet*" is a masterful inversion in words of the President's true message, tacitly conveyed: "The wallet that we have set aside for ending these tragedies, a wallet whose size is determined *solely* by our will, and could be multiplied several times over *simply if* our will so determined, is smaller than the wallet that would be needed to end, or at least greatly diminish, these tragedies. We will an end to these tragedies only in the sense that we *would* will their end *if* it cost us a negligible amount. But this is a hypothetical and not a real will. We include it in our fantasies, and discard it in real life. Our *actual* will is for these tragedies to continue since we prefer the continuation of these tragedies to our own monetary loss, which would be necessary for their diminution.

"In other words, we have a lot more wallet than the wallet we are willing to spend on these problems. And the wallet we are willing to spend is far less than the wallet needed to address them satisfactorily. *We have more wallet than will.*"

fering because some effective methods are unknown to them; this is the case either because they fail to search for these methods, or their search is unsuccessful. In addition, it is often assumed that the limits to our capacities are fixed, when in fact they may be highly flexible: what was impossible in the past may be possible now, owing to new technology, greater expertise, improved organizational capacity, more collaboration, or a chance combination of factors that present us with an unusual opportunity to terminate or ward off a great portion of suffering. By imagining that the limits to our capacities are fixed, we will be less alert to these possibilities.

Admittedly, the last factor may also cause us to *overestimate* our beneficent capacity: if our powers can expand unexpectedly, they can also contract unexpectedly. However, if we want to prevent the worst cumulative suffering, we should err on the side of optimism. We should be distrustful of purported obstacles and credulous of possibilities. That way, we will come close to relieving the worst cumulative suffering we can, since we will move with maximum energy and drive.

Another source of error is the frequent confusion of improbability with impossibility. Sometimes people remark, "It is unlikely that I could make any difference." From here they slide, sometimes unconsciously, into another opinion: ". . . So there is nothing I can do to help." But there is a world of difference between the two. That my action has only a small chance of preventing suffering means that it *might* do so. If I perform such actions sufficiently often, the prevention of suffering will eventually become *likely*.

Sometimes whole categories of prevention are overlooked. We may forget, for example, that one form of prevention is to stop other people from inflicting suffering, to keep torturers and their like from having their way. Too often, our minds become fixated on the wickedness of the malefactors themselves, so that we forget that we may be able to prevent their plans from taking effect. It is sometimes suggested that our prima facie responsibility to prevent suffering is reduced if the immediate source of the suffering lies in the malevolent will of another person, rather than, say, human accident or natural disaster.[4] But there is, I believe, no convincing reason why the involvement of other people's wickedness should get us off the hook morally. It doesn't make the suffering less bad; and it doesn't, through some sort of conceptual magic, reduce our capacity to prevent the suffering. Perhaps what is invoked is the thought that we shouldn't be pushed around morally: we shouldn't let our obligations become hostage to other people's good behavior. But then, why is it worse to be morally pushed around by persons than natural forces? It is not as though, in the vast majority of cases, the malefactors have us in their sights, or devote any thought to us whatsoever. Even when they do, as in the moral blackmail cases that philosophers are fond of discussing, it isn't clear why their manipulation of us should affect our responsibility to the *victims*. The prima facie

---

4. See Bernard Williams, "A Critique of Utilitarianism," in J. J. C. Smart and Bernard Williams, *Utilitarianism: For and Against* (Cambridge: Cambridge University Press, 1973), p. 109. For a reply, see Jonathan Bennett, *The Act Itself* (Oxford: Clarendon Press, 1995), pp. 186–89.

duty to relieve suffering is not suspended or diminished when we can prevent suffering by blocking the malevolent designs of other people.

Our tendency to underestimate the suffering we can prevent and our tendency, earlier remarked, to deny or distort suffering are mutually reinforcing. If I am oblivious to other people's suffering, or do not comprehend its true badness, I will expend less energy to locate all my causal ties to it with the aim of using those ties to eliminate the worst cumulative suffering I possibly can. That is, if I am unaware of ongoing and threatened suffering, or unaware of what such suffering *means*, I will not be motivated to carry out the detective work necessary to reveal the true extent of my capacity to avert suffering. On the other hand, if I am blind to the possibility of preventing other people's suffering, I can place moral distance between it and myself. I can afford not to think about it. I can leave it in the far-off domain of "things that do not have to do with me," where it gradually fades from view and becomes a mere wisp of reality.

It is easy to slip into a charmed world where the prima facie duty to relieve suffering becomes a distant echo of itself—where suffering is rarely allowed to make an appearance and our ability to prevent it goes unnoticed. To preserve an adequate sense of the inherent force of the prima facie duty to relieve suffering, we must avoid falling into the make believe and keep our feet firmly planted in reality. We must remember the real meaning and real extent of suffering, and the degree to which we can actually prevent it. This is difficult to do. If we succeed, I believe we will recognize a prima facie duty to relieve suffering of much greater force than is ordinarily acknowledged.

3. Consequentialist Limits

Here I must be very brief. The point is to acknowledge that the cost of preventing suffering is sometimes worse, from an impersonal perspective, than the suffering prevented. Though the prevention of suffering usually makes things better, it some-times makes things worse. When this happens, we have a consequentialist reason *not* to prevent suffering.[5] Beyond this, I can say very little. A full discussion of this issue presupposes a complete theory of value—a theory that tells us not only what counts as a harm or benefit to individuals, but also how such harms and benefits ought to be distributed, whether there are values that cannot be cashed out in terms of individual interests, and if so what they are, and finally how different values should be balanced or ranked against each other. I do not pretend to have anything close to such a theory.

In this section I look only at the value of outcomes. Moreover, I look at their value from an *impersonal* perspective—what we see, as Nagel says, when we look at

---

5. The consequentialist reason may be overridden in turn by non-consequentialist reasons—for ex-ample, if the suffering is my own, and I am allowed to attach disproportionate weight to my own interests.

the world from no particular point of view. I therefore ignore agent-relative reasons—that is, reasons for acting that depend on the identity of the agent—and postpone their consideration until subsequent sections. This means ignoring the agent's particular role in the causal processes that lead to better or worse outcomes—whether, for example the agent's role is an active or a passive one—and the agent's particular relation to the people who may be harmed or benefited by different outcomes. In a sense I am not interested here in the agent at all; or rather, I am interested in the agent only as an instrument for producing better outcomes.

Some moral philosophers have questioned whether the impersonal perspective should be consulted at all.[6] However, the duty to relieve suffering makes some such consultation necessary. Intelligent contemplation of suffering yields the thought that suffering *is* bad from no particular point of view and that its impersonal badness powerfully obligates us to prevent it. But if suffering is an impersonal bad, there may be other impersonal goods and bads capable of outweighing it.

It is clear that the impersonal value of preventing suffering is sometimes outweighed by its cost. Sometimes the value of preventing someone's suffering is outweighed by the cost *to that person*. The cost may be a sufficiently large loss of happiness, hedonistically understood. Or it may be the deprivation of any of a number of non-hedonistic goods. As I said in chapter 4, a list of such goods should include (among other things) longevity, liberty, accomplishment, knowledge, moral goodness, and basic physical capacities. Too zealous a protection against suffering can deprive a person of non-hedonistic goods that would be worth their price in suffering. For example (as we saw in chapter 4), suffering is sometimes justified by its educative value. At the same time, it would be a mistake to suppose that happiness (or avoidance of suffering) is *typically* in conflict with appropriately sought non-hedonistic goods. Philosophers sometimes play up these conflicts to point out the inadequacy of value hedonism, but they are not the norm. Non-hedonistic goods that are worth seeking usually buttress a person's happiness in the long term.

Of the non-hedonistic goods I have mentioned, liberty deserves special notice. For reasons suggested in chapter 6, we should often allow people to choose for themselves, even if they choose to incur greater suffering, indeed even if their choice is all things considered a bad one. Liberty is valuable, even when we do not make good use of it.

Sometimes the value of preventing someone's suffering is outweighed by the cost *to other people*, not in the form of their suffering. For example, it can be more important to teach one person to read and write than to prevent another person's mild and transient suffering. The cost to other people may be the loss of positive happiness, or the deprivation of any of the catalog of non-hedonistic goods.

When we consider the non-hedonistic costs that the prevention of some people's suffering can exact from other people, most attention should be given to what I will

---

6. See, for example, Christine M. Korsgaard, "The Reasons We Can Share: An Attack on the Distinction between Agent-Relative and Agent-Neutral Values," in Ellen Franken Paul, Fred D. Miller, Jr., and Jeffrey Paul, eds., *Altruism* (Cambridge: Cambridge University Press, 1993).

call people's vital interests. Vital interests refer to a certain morally significant minimum level of attainments; they include staying alive, decent health, adequate nutrition, basic socialization and education, elementary moral understanding, and a certain degree of freedom from other people's interference. In interpersonal trade-offs, it is vital interests that carry the greatest weight against the prevention of suffering. This doesn't mean of course that vital interests always win. Everything depends on the gravity of the threatened interests and the scale of the potential suffering.

The enjoyment of non-hedonistic goods beyond the level of vital interests is morally less important. Just as the vital interests of some are more important than the non-vital interests of others, so vital interests weigh more in interpersonal trade-offs against the prevention of suffering than non-vital interests do. For my part, I doubt whether any amount of non-vital interests for one set of people can ever justify the prolonged agony of another individual.

There may be interpersonal trade-offs where the value of preventing some people's suffering is outweighed by the value of promoting other people's non-vital interests. This is likeliest when the non-vital interests at stake are highly significant and widely shared (say, college educations for many), and the suffering is relatively minor (say, an afternoon of moderate depression for one). We live in a world of such pronounced inequality, however, that resources that could be used to prevent the extreme suffering of large numbers of people are routinely used to purchase minor increments in the fulfillment of the non-vital interests of a fortunate few (when they are not used merely to provide pleasure). This imbalance cannot be justified on consequentialist grounds.

The prevention of some people's suffering may come into conflict with the vital or non-vital interests of other people. It can also come into conflict with goals whose value may be thought to be partly independent of individual interests. Works of art and cultural achievements, for example, are sometimes thought to possess a value that transcends the benefits that individuals derive from them. Art and culture also absorb abundant resources that could be used to prevent suffering. Resources that could be used to prevent hunger, disease, and torture are instead used to promote literature, the fine arts, academic research lacking practical application, public beautification, historical restoration, and so forth.

Some people may object to the assumption of a conflict between the promotion of culture and the prevention of suffering. It may be claimed that some cultural and aesthetic achievements have the effect of reducing or preventing suffering. They console people in times of distress, for example, or teach them to be more humane. I doubt that the truth is this simple. Beautiful art can also distract us from the business of relieving suffering; it may even have the potential to nourish projects of evil. Were not the Nazis refreshed and reinvigorated by the music of Beethoven? Even if art sometimes prevents or reduces suffering, it is doubtful that it is the most *efficient* means of eliminating suffering. So long as it is not, there remains a conflict between the promotion of culture and the prevention of suffering.

I think that the promotion of culture can sometimes justify a certain amount of suffering. But, as in the case of non-vital interests, I doubt whether even a cultural achievement of immense value can justify the long-lived agony of one individual, or anything worse.[7] I end this section with the following, admittedly controversial, thought experiment.

Jane Austen was a contemporary of William Wilberforce, the great parliamentarian who led the fight for the abolition of the British slave trade and the practice of slavery in the British Empire. Austen chose to live with her sister and mother and complete six great novels that have brought delight to generations of readers. However, she had an alternative. She could have devoted her life to the cause of abolition—as a propagandist, for example.[8] Let us suppose that if she had chosen this path, she would have hastened the end of the legal traffic and ownership of slaves, and that, as a result of her contribution, there would have been one less shipment of Africans across the Middle Passage, with all the unspeakable suffering endured by the victims in their seizure, transit, and subsequent captivity. Would the loss of Austen's novels be outweighed by the prevention of one shipment of slaves?

Beethoven was another contemporary of Wilberforce. Imagine that if Beethoven had devoted his life to abolition instead of composing, he too could have prevented one shipment of Africans across the Middle Passage. Would the loss of Beethoven's music be outweighed by the prevention of one shipment of slaves?

The cultural loss in either case would be enormous, yet when I try to preserve an accurate sense of the suffering involved I am inclined to think that the answer to both these questions is yes.

4. Deontological Constraints

One objection to an unlimited duty to relieve suffering is that it sometimes leads to a worse outcome overall. Another objection is that, even if it doesn't lead to a worse outcome overall, it sometimes requires impermissible means. It sometimes requires illegitimate violations of moral rules against killing, injuring, lying, cheating, and stealing. We may regard these rules as absolute prohibitions or prima facie prohibitions of varying degrees of force. But even if we regard them as prima facie prohibitions, and hence potentially overridable, we may believe that it is wrong on

7. "No play by Racine is worth a Bastille, no Mandelstam poem an hour of Stalinism." George Steiner, *No Passion Spent* (London: Faber and Faber, 1996), p. 300.

8. I here set aside Austen's apparent tolerance of slavery in her novels. In *Emma* pro-abolition sentiments are put in the mouth of the odious Mrs. Elton. In *Mansfield Park* the heroine's uncle and guardian draws substantial income from a sugar plantation in Antigua, and Fanny even discusses the slave trade with Sir Thomas upon his return from the plantation. The novel celebrates Fanny's virtue, but does not show her having any qualms about living off other people's slavery. In *Persuasion* we are expected to admire Captain Wentworth for helping Mrs. Smith regain valuable property in the West Indies. The property probably derives its value from slave labor.

at least some occasions to violate them in order to achieve a better outcome through the reduction of suffering.

In other words, the duty to relieve suffering may be limited by deontological constraints. Here we need to distinguish between deontological constraints and the broader category of moral constraints. A moral constraint is a general constraint on action. Almost all of us believe in moral constraints against killing, injuring, inflicting pain, lying, cheating, and stealing. This includes most consequentialists, who understand that compliance with these constraints is usually necessary to bring about the best outcome. According to most consequentialists, we should usually abstain from killing, injuring, and other such acts because these acts usually lead to worse outcomes. In that sense, most consequentialists (sensible ones, anyway) believe in moral constraints. Deontological constraints, unlike consequentialist constraints, prohibit certain actions even if they bring about a *better* outcome. For example, a deontological constraint forbids killing one person, even if doing so is necessary to save two other people from being killed.

One of the most contested debates in moral philosophy is whether deontological constraints really exist. From a certain distance, it seems as though they should not. How can an act be wrong if it produces a *better* outcome? In the abstract, this question seems to answer itself: such an act cannot be wrong. Yet, as an examination of particular cases reminds us, deontological constraints have a strong hold on our intuitions. Intuition tells us that it is wrong to kill one person to prevent two others from being killed, wrong to torture one person to prevent another from being tortured more severely, and so forth.

In the philosophical literature there are powerful arguments for and against the existence of deontological constraints.[9] Now, those who are persuaded that deontological constraints do not exist should nonetheless recognize the usefulness of deontological *inhibitions*. Such inhibitions are desirable from a consequentialist perspective, for reasons examined in chapter 5. It is often dangerous for agents to trust their own consequentialist calculations in deciding what to do, because such calculations are prone to the distortions of irrelevant motives. To avoid this danger, it is desirable that agents feel a kind of reverence for certain simple rules that are essential in the vast majority of cases to the avoidance of worse, often disastrously worse, outcomes. Specifically, it is desirable for agents to feel that there is something inherently wrong in the violation of these rules, apart from the consequentialist value of complying with them.

To say that people who deny the reality of deontological constraints should nonetheless cultivate deontological inhibitions may seem an intolerable paradox. How-

9. Arguments in favor of deontological constraints can be found in Judith Jarvis Thomson, *The Realm of Rights* (Cambridge, Mass.: Harvard University Press, 1990); and F. M. Kamm, *Morality, Mortality*, vol. 2 (New York: Oxford University Press, 1996). Arguments against can be found in Samuel Scheffler, *The Rejection of Consequentialism* (Oxford: Clarendon Press, 1982); Shelly Kagan, *The Limits of Morality* (Oxford: Clarendon Press, 1989); Jonathan Bennett, *The Act Itself* (Oxford: Clarendon Press, 1995); and Peter Unger, *Living High and Letting Die: Our Illusion of Innocence* (New York: Oxford University Press, 1996).

ever, we can resolve the paradox if we follow R. M. Hare in distinguishing between two levels of moral thinking.[10] The *critical level* concerns what it is actually right to do. The *practical level* comprises the rules and precepts that are chosen on grounds supplied by the critical level to guide us in real-life situations when we are confronted with a choice and must decide what to do without benefit of perfect calculative powers.[11] Even if deontological constraints are absent from the critical level, they need to be present at the practical level. Consequentialism at the critical level authorizes the incorporation of deontological inhibitions at the practical level, since they steer people in real-life situations to the production of better outcomes. Obedience to deontological inhibitions of the right kind will not lead to a better outcome every time, but rather a better outcome over the long term.

Someone who adopts this two-level view concerning deontological inhibitions will experience a kind of internal division. If she is like most of us, she will discover that her deontological inhibitions are deeply ingrained. She will believe that some of these inhibitions are desirable for consequentialist reasons. She will not, in the ultimate appeals court of her mind, believe what these inhibitions tell her (that certain ways of acting are wrong in themselves). But she will not try to get rid of them, *and* she will let them guide her actions. So, in a sense, she will lead her life *as though* she believed in them.

Suppose we adopt the two-level view concerning deontological constraints. If we are asked whether the duty to relieve suffering is limited by deontological constraints, we should say that the answer depends on the level of moral thinking. On the critical level, the duty to relieve suffering is not limited by deontological constraints; on the practical level, however, it is. So at the level of practice there is not so great a divide between a deontological view and a sensible non-deontological view. I say "not so great a divide" rather than "no divide whatsoever," because a non-deontological, two-level justification of deontological inhibitions is likely to affect which of those inhibitions are deemed appropriate, and what criteria are deemed appropriate for overriding them.

In the following discussion I look at three areas in which deontological constraints may be thought to place major restrictions on the duty to relieve suffering. I shall be asking whether there are deontological constraints on the *practical* level of morality, or in other words, whether there are general moral constraints on the means used to prevent suffering. I want to sidestep the question whether deontological constraints genuinely exist (that is, whether they belong at the critical level of moral thinking). Some readers may find this inconsistent with my general policy of con-

10. *Moral Thinking* (Oxford: Clarendon Press, 1981). See also Bennett, *The Act Itself*, pp. 22–26.

11. I call the second level "practical" rather than "intuitive," as Hare does, because I disagree with Hare about the role of intuitions in moral theory. Hare believes that intuitions should play no role in moral justification, and that their only legitimate function is to guide our motives according to the dictates of critical moral thinking. I believe instead that all moral views, including those that occupy the critical level of moral thinking, ultimately rest on intuition.

sulting intuition. We have deontological intuitions—why not accept them as true? I believe that all moral knowledge ultimately rests on some kind of intuition, but I do not think that intuitions are infallible. Intuitions should be rejected if they are unable to withstand critical reflection. The skeptics argue that deontological intuitions fail this test. I want to leave open the possibility that they are right.

4.a. *Violence*

Violence can sometimes produce a better outcome by, among other things, reducing suffering. This often takes the form of using violence to minimize violence. States resort to violence to preserve public order and prevent crime. Revolutions and interventions are organized to overthrow regimes that are unjustifiably violent or exploitative towards their own citizens. States launch military campaigns to deter other states from international aggression. On at least some of these occasions, the resort to violence successfully reduces suffering and improves the overall outcome. I should make it clear that when I speak of an improved outcome, I mean one that is better from an impersonal perspective—*not* from the perspective of national or group interest, which is the perspective usually assumed by those seeking to justify wars and revolutions.

Many people believe that there are deontological constraints on the use of violence to improve the overall outcome. There is considerable disagreement about the scope of these constraints. Anarchist pacifists oppose violence on all (or almost all?) occasions, even for the purpose of enforcing the law. Non-anarchist pacifists permit the use of violence to preserve domestic order, but not to overthrow unjust regimes or to fight wars. Few people, however, subscribe to pacifism. More common is the view that some wars and revolutions may be justified, but that even in a just armed struggle there are rules prohibiting violence against non-combatants. Some people think that we are forbidden to inflict violent harm on non-combatants, period. Other people think that only the *intentional* infliction of such harm is forbidden. Harm is "intentional," in this context, when it is pursued as a means to one's end, and not merely foreseen as a side-effect of one's actions. The most notorious example of intentionally inflicting harm on non-combatants arguably for the purpose of averting a worse outcome overall is the dropping of the atom bomb on Hiroshima and Nagasaki. A number of historians deny that dropping the bomb really was necessary (or could reasonably be expected to be necessary) to avert a worse outcome overall. But even if it were shown that it *was* necessary to avoid a worse outcome, many people would persist in calling it a crime, perhaps one of the greatest crimes in history.

In addition to prohibitions against harming non-combatants, many people support deontological restrictions on the methods used to fight enemy combatants. In many people's view, we should abstain from using certain weapons, and we should not kill or torture prisoners of war, even in order to achieve a better outcome. (For example, we should not torture a prisoner even if we were certain that doing so would prevent two or more other people from being tortured.)

These restrictions can be justified on deontological grounds.[12] But they can also be justified in terms of a non-deontological, two-level conception of morality. The thread that runs through most deontological restrictions against using violence is the notion that it is *in general* wrong to intentionally inflict violent harm. (By "violent harm" I mean injury, torture, or violent death.) Now, it is desirable for consequentialist reasons to cultivate strong inhibitions against the intentional infliction of violent harm. The intentional infliction of violent harm tends to wreak such terrible damage that it is unwise to allow people to resort to it whenever they calculate that doing so would produce a better outcome overall. Such calculations can go astray, and it only takes a few mistaken calculations in favor of inflicting violent harm for the general practice of employing such calculations to produce a worse outcome overall. Deontological inhibitions guard us against this danger. On the other hand, it may also be desirable, from a consequentialist perspective, to suspend the deontological inhibition against violent harm when the harm is directed against those who use force of arms to perpetrate great evil. The reasoning would be that this is a sharply delineated category of violent action that offers unusually frequent opportunities to prevent worse outcomes in general, and *horrifically* worse outcomes in particular. Even here, however, we would want a powerful restraint against the resort to extreme measures: people in the thick of conflict would be apt to overestimate the long-term impersonal benefits of such measures, and underestimate the long-term impersonal harms. For this reason, we would want a deontological inhibition against using certain methods of war.

Any enlightened consequentialist who is attuned to the real world must place a high value on deontological inhibitions against the infliction of violent harm.[13] Consider the practice of torture. Governments often justify it on consequentialist grounds: they say it is necessary to avert a much greater catastrophe.[14] But an enlightened consequentialism utterly condemns what these governments do, which is another way of saying that their own consequentialist reasoning is misapplied. It either makes use of a false theory of value (e.g., that the glory of our country is worth some individual suffering), or it draws on groundless empirical beliefs (e.g., that unless we torture these witches, the Devil will take control of the world and

---

12. See G. E. M. Anscombe, "War and Murder" and "Mr. Truman's Degree" in *The Collected Philosophical Papers of G. E. M. Anscombe*, vol. 3, *Ethics, Religion and Politics* (Minneapolis: University of Minnesota Press, 1981); Thomas Nagel, "War and Massacre," in Nagel, *Mortal Questions* (Cambridge: Cambridge University Press, 1979); and Richard Norman, *Ethics, Killing, and War* (Cambridge: Cambridge University Press, 1995).

13. "The world has known all too many people whose zeal for killing has not been matched by any great talent for accurately predicting the consequences of their actions, and all too many killers whose judgements about what ends are valuable have been deranged, biased, self-serving or otherwise misguided." Scheffler, *The Rejection of Consequentialism*, p. 110.

14. See the excellent account by Malise Ruthven in *Torture: The Grand Conspiracy* (London: Weidenfeld and Nicolson, 1978).

inflict much greater suffering on us all), or it transforms remote possibilities into near certainties (e.g., that unless we torture this prisoner, the communists will seize power and inflict torture more widely than we ever will), or it serves as a cover for selfish interests (e.g., the repression that is justified as a preventive against communism is in fact undertaken to protect the wealth and power of a vulnerable elite). We need to be aware that consequentialist reasoning can be, and has been, misapplied in this way. A powerful deontological inhibition against inflicting torture will protect us from this kind of mischief.

I think that a consequentialist requirement to produce better outcomes—if nothing else, a consequentialist requirement to minimize the occurrence of violent harm—would support the cultivation of deontological inhibitions against the intentional infliction of violent harm. I won't, however, try to determine in detail the form that such inhibitions would take. Nor is it my intention in this section to argue that the possibility of defending certain deontological inhibitions on consequentialist grounds renders more purely deontological explanations invalid. We may support deontological inhibitions against the intentional infliction of violence for deontological or consequentialist reasons, or for a combination of the two. Whichever explanation we prefer, it is clear that such inhibitions will place significant limits on the methods that can legitimately be used for the purpose of reducing suffering.

4.b. The Right to Private Property

The prevention and alleviation of suffering often requires resources that can be collected most effectively through compulsory state taxes. Tax-based revenues can enable governments to offer food, housing, and medical care to those who would otherwise go without; to fund programs that lift people out of poverty and unemployment; to support education that equips people to manage their own lives better and contribute to other people's well-being; to invest in research and infrastructure that will increase our future ability to counteract old and new sources of suffering; to prevent environmental catastrophes; to provide emergency relief to victims of famine and other large-scale disasters; to support development projects that enable poor third-world communities to become economically self-sufficient; to fund peace-keeping forces in war-torn areas; to support judicial reform and economic stability abroad as a preventive against government repression, social breakdown, and the seizure of power by murderous regimes.

Libertarians believe that legitimate taxation is sharply limited by the right of citizens to private property. Strict libertarians, such as Robert Nozick in *Anarchy, State, and Utopia*, believe that no taxes may be levied for purposes other than the punishment of crime, the arbitration of disputes, and military defense against external enemies.[15] More flexible libertarians permit a few additional functions such as public education and the public provision of basic needs to citizens who live

15. *Anarchy, State, and Utopia* (New York: Basic Books, 1974). Nozick has subsequently recanted libertarianism.

below subsistence. But libertarians who vary in their degree of doctrinal purity are generally opposed to ambitious social policies. They are therefore likely to oppose the use of compulsory taxes to prevent the worst cumulative suffering.

To make their position stick, libertarians have to defend two highly contestable claims. The first is that, despite all the random factors that help determine the unequal distribution of property, individuals have a strong prima facie right to maximum control over the holdings in their possession (provided the holdings were not acquired through a process that violated the property rights of others). The second is that this right to maximal control over one's private property regularly overrides the moral urgency of preventing suffering. It lies beyond the scope of this study to examine all the possible arguments for these claims. My own view is that they cannot be successfully defended.

It is important to remember that we can preserve the right to property without insisting on a right to keep everything: "The right to own is absolute, but not the right to keep every dollar. One's personhood is not present in every dollar one presently has, or at stake whenever one is asked to part with a dollar in taxes."[16] Because governments tax many people together, the contribution drawn from each taxpayer typically generates a much larger collective payoff on the other end. Even a small tax can eliminate a great deal of suffering. The challenge to the libertarian is to show that the inherent objectionableness of taxing people's private property outweighs the moral urgency of preventing large amounts of suffering. I doubt the challenge can be met.[17]

4.c. Democratic Constraints

The two previous examples of alleged deontological constraints on the duty to relieve suffering have focused on political actors: agents of the state or agents of armed movements not recognized as states. This is no accident. Political actors have the greatest capacity to increase and decrease suffering. It is in politics that deontological inhibitions against certain methods of relieving suffering have the greatest impact, for good or ill.

Common sense supports a long list of deontological prohibitions that I have so far ignored, such as rules against lying, cheating, and promise-breaking. I shall not pause to discuss the violation of these prohibitions by private individuals, since I believe that private individuals rarely have an occasion to reduce suffering through these means, and that when they do, common sense is often inclined to waive the prohibition anyway. Very few people accept Kant's assertion that you should never

---

16. George Kateb, *The Inner Ocean* (Ithaca, N.Y.: Cornell University Press, 1992), p. 20.

17. For a powerful criticism of a wide range of libertarian arguments, see Will Kymlicka, *Contemporary Political Philosophy* (Oxford: Clarendon Press, 1974), chap. 4. For an argument that property rights should not get in the way of relieving other people's suffering, see Unger, *Living High and Letting Die*, chap. 3.

lie, even to divert a would-be murderer who chases his intended victim to your house and then asks you if he is hiding there.[18] Where private conduct is concerned, common sense generally allows lying, cheating, and promise-breaking in case of emergency, and it is amenable to recognizing the opportunity to relieve suffering as constituting such an emergency. If it sometimes refuses to do so, the intelligent contemplation of suffering may cause it to relent. I won't say this happens every time. Sometimes common sense may refuse to lift the prohibition against lying, cheating, and promise-breaking even for the sake of relieving suffering. But I think that such occasions are rare, and that they are unlikely to involve large amounts of suffering.

The picture changes dramatically when we shift to the sphere of politics, especially politics in a democracy. First, public officials will have more opportunities than private individuals to prevent suffering   and to prevent suffering on a large scale—through methods normally regarded as illicit. Second, the use of these methods to prevent suffering will generally be condemned. The methods I have in mind include lying to the public; lying to legislators and other government officials; the use of violence, blackmail, surveillance, sabotage, and smearing to weaken one's political opponents; electoral fraud; and breaking the law. There are various moral grounds for repudiating each of these methods. What they all have in common, however, is their anti-democratic character. They seek to circumvent the arrangement whereby people with clashing political values and opinions agree to obey laws that emerge from a process of open deliberation and fair electoral competition, subject to appropriate constitutional constraints.

Although such methods violate democratic principles, one can imagine situations in which they would appear necessary to prevent suffering. Suppose that you are a head of state and must lie to the public to obtain its permission to pursue a policy that you are certain will greatly reduce suffering. If told the truth, the public would oppose the policy either because they have the wrong priorities and do not assign to the relief of suffering the importance it deserves, or because they are empirically confused and would not, from a straightforward presentation of the facts, recognize the policy's true effectiveness. Or suppose that a law has already been passed prohibiting your favored policy, but that you can still pursue it in secret. In these cases it appears that you can prevent great suffering only by deliberately deceiving the public or secretly violating the law. These remarks, I hasten to add, are not intended as a general comment on anti-democratic practices: politicians have almost always used anti-democratic methods for purposes other than the relief of suffering.

Ignore the usual purposes of anti-democratic methods. Should a politician refrain from using them to prevent suffering? Now it is important to remember how dangerous these methods are. A politician who attempts them and is detected may find his career and his cause damaged, even ruined, with the result that his ability to

18. Immanuel Kant, "On a Supposed Right To Lie from Altruistic Motives," reprinted in Sissela Bok, *Lying: Moral Choice in Public and Private Life* (New York: Vintage, 1978).

prevent suffering is much less than it otherwise would have been. If on the other hand he avoids public detection, his anti-democratic maneuvers may undermine the long-term strength and survival of democracy by contributing to a culture of illegality among the politically powerful. If his maneuvers are publicly revealed and he pays no penalty, the example of his success poses an even greater threat to democracy. Democracy should be preserved because the costs of losing it are great—beginning with the drastic contraction of individual liberty and what is likely to be a vast increase in the cumulative badness of suffering. If the use of anti-democratic methods to prevent suffering has the long-term effect of eroding or destroying democracy, the costs are likely to outweigh the benefits.

But suppose that a public official successfully used anti-democratic methods to prevent suffering without causing the eventual deterioration of democracy or making the long-term outcome worse in some other way. Many people would remain opposed to such methods in some or all cases. They might object on grounds of fairness, or in the name of democracy itself, or in specific repudiation of deception and coercion, which are judged all the more heinous when committed by officials acting in the public trust. The objectors believe that anti-democratic methods on the part of public officials can be wrong even when they make the outcome better overall.[19]

Even if we don't believe that anti-democratic methods are wrong in themselves, we may find it desirable for public officials to feel deontologically inhibited from practicing them. Without such inhibitions, we are at the mercy of their consequentialist calculations, and those calculations can go astray for a variety of reasons. Public officials contemplating anti-democratic tactics may underestimate the dangers of detection, or the dangers to the long-term survival of democracy if they avoid detection. They may overestimate the degree to which anti-democratically implemented policies will prevent suffering, and one reason is that the goal of relieving suffering may become a rationalization for policies really guided by self-interest. Party loyalty, ideological rigidity, and the pain of admitting error or uncertainty can also blind them to the deficiencies of their plans. They may also underestimate what can be achieved in the way of preventing suffering through fair and open debate. Powerful people make horrendous mistakes. Democracy requires public officials to submit their proposals to public scrutiny, where dangerous errors can be exposed before wreaking their damage. We can remind public officials of these benefits of democratic consultation. But to be safe we may also want to instill in them a deontological inhibition against evading democratic procedures—a feeling that democratic conduct is morally required for its own sake.

I shall not delve any deeper into this issue. I have tried to make two points. First, there may be deontological constraints against what I have called "anti-democratic" actions by public officials. Second, even if, strictly speaking, there are no deontological constraints against such actions, it may be desirable on consequen-

---

19. See Amy Gutmann and Dennis Thomson, *Democracy and Disagreement* (Cambridge, Mass.: Harvard University Press, 1996).

tialist grounds for public officials to harbor a deontological inhibition against performing them. I am not claiming that deontological inhibitions justified on appropriate consequentialist grounds would perfectly coincide with those justified on the most compelling deontological grounds. They probably would not, but that is not a question I shall address here. Whichever explanation we prefer, it seems likely that some such inhibitions should place a constraint on the legitimate means of relieving suffering.

5. The Limits of Obligatory Sacrifice

As we have seen, the duty to relieve suffering needs to be limited in particular ways. First, it seems clear that on certain occasions the prevention of worse cumulative suffering would result in a worse outcome overall. When that occurs, we should not reduce the cumulative badness of suffering. Second, even when the prevention of worse cumulative suffering does not result in a worse outcome overall, it may be forbidden on the grounds that it requires the use of morally impermissible means. I remain agnostic whether this ever occurs, but I discussed the possibility in the last section.

A third possible limit takes the form, not of a competing moral requirement, but a prima facie moral permission. The idea is that a duty to relieve suffering limited only by the appropriate consequentialist and deontological constraints may be too demanding. It may require the agent to incur too great a sacrifice, to pay too high a cost. When the cost exceeds a certain level, the agent may be allowed to cite her own interests and concerns as a reason not to comply with a maximal duty to relieve suffering. (By a "maximal" duty to relieve suffering, I shall mean one that is limited only by the appropriate consequentialist and deontological constraints.)

In this section I ask how great a sacrifice I am morally required to bear. That is different from asking how great a sacrifice other people may impose on me. An agent may be morally required to bear some sacrifice, yet it would be wrong for other people to impose that sacrifice on the agent. There could be many reasons for this: imposing the sacrifice could violate deontological constraints, or it could lead to a worse outcome overall.[20]

20. See Kagan, *The Limits of Morality*, p. 208: "The impermissibility of one or more individuals *imposing* a sacrifice upon another is completely compatible with that other person's nonetheless being morally *required* to make the sacrifice herself." See also J. S. Mill's discussion in *On Liberty*: "In all things which regard the external relations of the individual, he is *de jure* amenable to those whose interests are concerned, and if need be, to society as their protector. There are often good reasons for not holding him to the responsibility; but these reasons must arise from the special expediences of the case: either because it is a kind of case in which he is on the whole likely to act better, when left to his own discretion, than when controlled in any way in which society have it in their power to control him; or because the attempt to exercise control would produce other evils, greater than those which it would prevent. When such reasons as these preclude the enforcement of responsibility, the conscience of the agent himself should step into the vacant judgment seat, and protect those interests of others which have no external

Does a maximal duty to relieve suffering demand too much? Let us start by asking what sacrifices it is likely to require. The answer to this question depends largely on the overall level of compliance. Suppose the entire adult population of the world committed itself to achieve the greatest possible reduction in the cumulative badness of suffering (subject to appropriate constraints). To reach this goal, we would have to harness an enormous amount of resources, time, and energy. But if we divided the burden equitably, it would be shared by so many people that the ordinary demands placed on each individual would not be severe. Through an equitable system of taxation, we could extract sufficient resources without requiring the affluent to sacrifice every luxury. And we could secure the necessary application of human effort through an appropriate division of labor, under which many people would perform tasks directly related to the relief of suffering—in careers such as medicine, counseling, and disaster relief as well as research, engineering, and administration in the relevant areas—but most people would go on performing the diverse tasks necessary to the functioning of a complex economy. We could even allow some people to pursue non-essential careers—in sports, fine arts, and literary criticism, for example—because there would be more than enough people to cover the essential occupations. Of course, we would need some mechanism to insure that the appropriate division of labor was actually observed, but I assume that in a world where every one was committed to the prevention of the worst cumulative suffering, this would not be an insurmountable problem.

Some people would be needed to perform dangerous and onerous tasks, such as fire-fighting and emergency rescue. And in a world where not quite everyone was committed to the relief of suffering we would also need some people to risk their own death and injury by deterring violent aggressors. I assume, however, that a sufficient number of generous souls would volunteer for these activities, especially if we took care to shower them with honors and rewards. This is not a far-fetched assumption, since many people already volunteer for these activities now.

As the reference to violent aggressors indicates, we could fall short of 100 percent compliance and still keep from imposing severe sacrifices on those collectively committed to the prevention of the worst cumulative suffering. The basic point is that if a sufficiently large number of people join together to prevent the worst cumulative suffering, they can divide the burden among themselves in such a way that the demands normally placed on the resources, time, and energy of each individual do not become extreme.

Matters change when the number of those committed to the prevention of the worst cumulative suffering shrinks below a certain size. When there are too few benefactors, the demands on each begin to rise. That, of course, is the situation in which we find ourselves now, since what is currently done to eliminate suffering falls dismally short of our collective potential. If under the current state of af-

---

protection; judging himself all the more rigidly, because the case does not admit of his being made accountable to the judgment of his fellow-creatures." (Mill, *On Liberty* in *Utilitarianism, On Liberty and Considerations on Representative Government*, ed. H. B. Acton [London: Dent, 1972], p. 80.)

fairs you resolve to minimize the cumulative badness of suffering, you will need to give much more of yourself than you would in a world of widespread benefi- cence. You will not have minimized the cumulative badness of suffering, unless you channel all of your resources, energies, and time toward that end. Under a maximal duty to relieve suffering, then, you must devote all your time, resources, and energies to the prevention of the worst cumulative suffering, so long as this does not produce a worse outcome overall and does not require the use of imper- missible means.

This means that you cannot pursue any career you want, but only one that will allow you to prevent the worst cumulative suffering. It means that you should not devote your free time to pursuits other than the elimination of suffering. It also means that you cannot spend money on luxuries for yourself, or those dear to you, since the same money could be used to prevent other people's suffering. Indeed you should devote all your money to the relief of other people's suffering until the deprivation you impose on yourself and those dear to you becomes worse, from an impersonal standpoint, than the suffering you prevent. This point is reached when any additional sacrifice imposes suffering on yourself and your loved ones that is cumulatively worse than the suffering you prevent, or deprives you and your loved ones of some other good the impersonal value of which outweighs the value of preventing the other people's suffering.[21]

In a world of low compliance, then, the demands of the maximal duty to relieve suffering are severe. We should not exaggerate their severity, however. The remarks in the last paragraph are easily misinterpreted. First, the obligation to choose a career that prevents the worst cumulative suffering is not as constraining as it may sound, since there are many ways in which people can strive to minimize the cumulative badness of suffering. Almost every field of human endeavor offers an opportunity for beneficent action (even though many or most practitioners fail to pursue it): medicine, counseling, law, law enforcement, politics, natural science, social science, engineering, manufacture, psychology, administration, fund-raising, arbitration, ed- ucation, and undoubtedly others. Literature and the fine arts do not appear on this list, but in certain forms they, too, may contribute to the relief of suffering. A novelist, for example, may be able to raise people's consciousness about a certain form of preventable suffering and strengthen their determination to eliminate it. And an artist may be able to earn a great deal of money through her work, which, if she donates it toward the relief of suffering, may accomplish more good than anything else she could do.

It may be argued that I have exaggerated the scope for choice. Though many career choices may enable a person to prevent suffering, only one will enable her to prevent the *worst* cumulative suffering. That may be true. But we should keep in mind that one's effectiveness in any task depends largely on the enthusiasm and

21. For now, I ignore the possibility that you have an *obligation* to set the interests of those dear to you ahead of the prevention of the worst cumulative suffering in the world as whole. I address this possibility in the next section.

talent one brings to it, and these tend to be correlated with how much one likes the task. So we should allow people's preferences some role in determining which beneficent career to pursue. There is also the factor of uncertainty. Though only one career choice may enable a person to prevent the worst cumulative suffering at the end of the day, it is often impossible to know ahead of time which one that will be. From the standpoint of the deliberating agent, several different careers may offer equal prospects of minimizing the cumulative badness of suffering.

As for demands on our time, while it is true that we should use all our free time to minimize the cumulative badness of suffering, we may find that we use our time most effectively when we take occasional breaks for inexpensive relaxation and recreation. Finally, the maximal duty to relieve suffering does not require an attitude of complete impartiality between yourself and those dear to you, on the one hand, and every one else on the other. As has often been pointed out, people are generally in a better position to understand and respond to their own needs and the needs of those in their immediate circle than the needs of mere acquaintances or people unknown to them. For this reason, some degree of preference in favor of yourself, your family, and close friends is generally consistent with, in fact necessary for, maximum effectiveness in eliminating suffering overall.

I emphasized the obligation to spend money on the relief of other people's suffering rather than luxuries for yourself. This does not mean responding to the first charitable solicitation that comes in the mail, but instead taking some time to learn how your money can be used most effectively. You should study particular kinds of suffering, seek to understand what causes them and how they can be most effectively prevented, and then determine how your money can best aid such prevention—whether by funding beneficent efforts of your own or by contributing to an organization engaged in the right kind of work. The more you learn about your area of concern, the more you will care about it. As Frank Jackson has pointed out, it will soon take on the character of a *personal project*.[22] (In fact it will often be related to the career you have chosen.) We therefore have some reason to discount the frequent complaint against strong requirements of beneficence that they alienate people from their projects. That does not carry much weight if people have shaped their projects around beneficent requirements. Shelly Kagan offers a salutary reminder when he writes that it would be a mistake to

> think of the agent who is in pursuit of the good as frantically running around, pushing himself in every direction, until he drops from exhaustion. . . . Most likely such a person would not actually be making his greatest possible contribution to the good. . . . In contrast, an individual who shapes and carries out a life plan with an eye to promoting the good is likely to make a greater contribution in the long run.[23]

Indeed it may be misleading to characterize the normal demands of the maximal duty to relieve suffering in a world of low compliance as *severe*. They certainly are

---

22. Frank Jackson, "Decision-theoretic Consequentialism and the Nearest and Dearest Objection," *Ethics*, vol. 101 (1991): 461–82, pp. 477–78.

23. *The Limits of Morality*, p. 368. For "promoting the good" we can substitute "relieving suffering."

stiff. But they need not be experienced as severe by an agent who has made the relief of suffering her chief goal in life.

So far I have spoken of the *normal* demands of the maximal duty to relieve suffering, which are moderate (though not minimal) in a world of high compliance and considerably stiffer in a world of low compliance. But the maximal duty to relieve suffering is also capable of making extraordinary demands. There may be occasions, under conditions of both high and low compliance, when I have to incur some awful sacrifice in order to comply with the maximal duty to relieve suffering. I may have to give up my life to prevent other people from enduring suffering that is cumulatively worse, from an impersonal perspective, than my premature death. Or I may have to submit to torture to prevent two other people from being subjected to equally horrible torture. I like to think that such occasions are exceptional, but I may be deluding myself.

I have tried to indicate the range of demands—some more likely, some less—that could be imposed by a maximal duty to relieve suffering. It would be a grave mistake, however, to believe that compliance with the duty to relieve suffering is correlated with the severity of the agent's sacrifice. What the duty to relieve suffering demands is quite simply the prevention of worse cumulative suffering. It does not call for sacrifice, except insofar as such sacrifice is necessary to the prevention of worse suffering. There are many other factors that contribute to the relief of suffering, and sometimes these factors count for much more.

Suppose that my life could follow one of the following trajectories.

The Austere Life. I get a job that pays $20,000 after taxes. The work I do at my job does not affect the amount of suffering in the world. By practicing extreme frugality I manage to live on $4,000 a year and give the other $16,000 to organizations that work to prevent suffering.

I use all my spare time to sew blankets for refugees. This augments the supplies handled by various refugee organizations, but achieves only a small reduction in the cumulative badness of suffering.

The Productive Life. I invest more time and money in obtaining the right job, and find one that pays $200,000 after taxes. The work I do at my job prevents a substantial amount of suffering. By indulging in some luxuries and extra comforts, I spend $35,000 on myself every year, while $5,000 go to pay off student loans. The remaining $160,000 go to organizations that work to prevent suffering. Because I direct my charitable giving with a great deal of care, the cumulative badness of suffering it prevents is considerably more than ten times greater than that prevented by the $16,000 of donations in the Austere Life.

I use some of my spare time for pure recreation, such as skiing in the Rockies and sun-bathing in the Caribbean. I use the rest of it to lead and collaborate in carefully designed beneficent projects, through which I prevent an enormous amount of suffering.

The point is obvious. Though I would sacrifice a great deal more by leading the Austere Life, I would comply much more fully with the duty to relieve suffering by leading the Productive Life. This is not to deny the possibility of a third alternative that would achieve even greater compliance than the Productive Life. Let us call this alternative the Austere Productive Life. It is the same as the Productive Life, except that I deny myself the luxuries, extra comforts, and extended recreation; and I use the time and money saved to prevent additional suffering.

We can be led astray if we fail to distinguish carefully between the extent of compliance with the duty to relieve suffering and proper grounds for assigning praise and blame. Suppose that although I devote considerable effort to finding a more lucrative and beneficial job, I wind up with the employment described in the Austere Life, and that this is the life I lead. Now contrast my life with the following.

> *The Prodigal Life.* Millicent is an heiress who doesn't work, but enjoys an annual income from interest and dividends of over $500,000 after taxes. Millicent spends almost all her time and money on personal amusement. But once a year, at Christmas, she writes a check for $32,000 to an organization that is as effective at relieving suffering as the organizations that receive my annual donation of $16,000. In addition, Millicent delivers the fund-raising pitch at an annual charitable event. Millicent's fame and lively personality inspire a collective contribution that does a lot more to prevent suffering than my annual production of blankets.

Millicent prevents much more suffering than I do, and in that sense she complies much more fully with the duty to relieve suffering. But from the standpoint of the duty to relieve suffering, it seems that my life is much more praiseworthy than hers, and that hers merits blame rather than praise. The reason for this is that it is extremely easy and relatively uncostly for Millicent, while it is exceedingly difficult for me, to achieve an enormously greater reduction in the cumulative badness of suffering.

I now return to the original question. Am I sometimes entitled not to comply with the maximal duty to relieve suffering because the sacrifice demanded of me is too high? Of course, the maximal duty to relieve suffering often makes demands I don't *want* to fulfill, but that is beside the point. Suffering is so bad that it generates a moral requirement to eliminate suffering. Suffering must not be allowed to occur, and if we find ourselves in a position to honor this "must," then we must honor it. The mere opposition of our desires is not a sufficient excuse. We need some reason capable of showing that, notwithstanding the prima facie moral requirement to eliminate suffering, we sometimes are entitled not to eliminate it. The burden of proof rests on those who claim that there is such an entitlement.

There is, as we have seen, at least one legitimate excuse. If the cost to myself of eliminating other people's suffering is greater in impersonal terms than the cumulative badness of their suffering, then I am under no obligation to eliminate their suffering. I do not have to lay down my life to prevent other people's suffering that is less bad, in impersonal terms, than my premature death. I do not have to abandon a lifelong project in which I have invested decades of work in order to prevent other people's suffering that is less bad, in impersonal terms, than the sacrifice of my project. No sacrifice is required if it leads to a worse outcome overall.

Now to the harder question. May I be excused from preventing suffering when the cost to myself, from an impersonal perspective, is less than the cumulative badness of suffering I could prevent? If we adopt an impersonal perspective, the answer is no. However, some philosophers have claimed, with the backing of common sense, that morality does not require the adoption of the impersonal perspective. I shall look at the argument of Samuel Scheffler, perhaps the most eloquent exponent of this view. Scheffler points out that a person naturally attaches weight to his or her own commitments and concerns that is "out of proportion to their importance from an impersonal standpoint."[24] We can put this by saying that people give disproportionate weight to their own interests, but "interests" should be understood in the broad sense, to include "our fundamental human needs as well as the major activities and commitments around which our lives are organized."[25] Our "interests" may thus include the well-being and success of family members and friends. Because, in Scheffler's view, "morality is addressed from the outset to human beings as they are,"[26] it should accommodate "not only the equal value or worth of all people, but also the individual moral agent's naturally disproportionate concern with his or her own life and interests."[27]

Scheffler believes that we may depart from the impersonal standpoint to a certain degree. In deciding what to do, we may give our own interests a weight disproportionate to their impersonal significance. Because morality also recognizes the equal worth of all people, it will sometimes issue requirements that are opposed to self-interest. But the requirements must not become too demanding, lest they fail to recognize our naturally disproportionate regard for our own interests. Scheffler calls for a balance between the impersonal and personal standpoints, and he believes that the proper balance will support a conception of morality as moderate, not stringent.[28] He writes:

> On this way of thinking, it is a crucial feature of morality that it is motivationally accessible to normal moral agents: that living morally is a serious if not always easy option for normally constituted agents under reasonably favorable conditions.[29]

24. *Human Morality* (New York: Oxford University Press, 1992), p. 122.
25. Ibid., p. 122.
26. Ibid., p. 125.
27. Ibid., p. 123.
28. Ibid., pp. 126, 125.
29. Ibid., p. 125. Thomas Nagel's *Equality and Partiality* (New York: Oxford University Press, 1991) has as its central theme the conflict between the personal and impersonal standpoints. Like Scheffler, Nagel believes we should seek some sort of balance or accommodation between the two.

I shall use the term "intermediate standpoint" to refer to this notion of a standpoint that is appropriately balanced between the impersonal and personal standpoints.

If Scheffler is right, we are sometimes excused from complying with the maximal duty to relieve suffering. Suppose that I must incur a sacrifice to prevent other people's suffering, and that my sacrifice is less bad than the suffering I could prevent. From the impersonal standpoint, I should prevent the other people's suffering. But from an intermediate standpoint, I may not be required to prevent their suffering. The intermediate standpoint magnifies the significance of my sacrifice, to the point that it may be allowed to outweigh the badness of the other people's suffering. This is not to say that I would be *forbidden* to prevent the other people's suffering. On the contrary, doing so would be regarded as an act of exceptional merit, a "supererogatory" act deserving extra praise, though not actually required.

Let us adopt the terms of Scheffler's discussion. May we attach disproportionate weight to our own interests when determining how great a sacrifice can be legitimately demanded of us by the duty to relieve suffering? If the answer is yes, how much disproportionality is acceptable?

Some philosophers argue that morality should make no concession to the personal standpoint. Shelly Kagan has argued that the appeal to the independent moral weight of the personal standpoint is ambiguous, and that on either of two alternative interpretations it does not succeed in supporting the moderate view.[30] The appeal could be read as saying that human nature *prevents* us from adopting an impersonal point of view; but we can, in fact, be motivated to adopt the impersonal perspective.[31] Or the appeal could constitute a claim that a moral theory that partly accommodates our natural tendency to care more about our own interests is, from some independent vantage point, *more attractive* than one that refuses to do so; but, Kagan argues, there is no compelling reason to accept this claim, and ample reason to condemn it.[32]

Kagan's other argument is that unless we can uphold a distinction between the infliction of suffering and the failure to prevent it, an accommodation to the personal perspective would license us to inflict suffering on others for personal benefit even when the harm to others outweighs the gain to ourselves from an impersonal perspective. Kagan argues in detail that the moral distinction between inflicting suffering and failing to prevent it *cannot* be upheld; since, for this reason, the personal perspective would allow us to inflict harm on others for personal gain, we should make no concession to the personal point of view.[33] Though this argument of Kagan's is controversial, it needs to be taken seriously. It presents each of us with the following challenge. Are we *sure* that allowing suffering is less wrong than inflicting

30. In *The Limits of Morality*, Kagan addresses his critique to Scheffler's earlier book, *The Rejection of Consequentialism*, but I think that the same arguments apply to *Human Morality*.

31. *Limits of Morality*, chap. 8.

32. Ibid., chap. 9.

33. Ibid., especially chaps. 3 and 4. Kagan's arguments against the alleged moral distinction between inflicting and failing to prevent suffering are reinforced by Bennett in *The Act Itself*.

it? If we are not quite sure, we should avoid the moral risk of acting as though we were sure. If (regardless of what we *prefer* to think) we suspect that allowing suffering is no less wrong than inflicting it, we should commit ourselves to preventing the worst cumulative suffering we can, and we should not be held back by the claim that our naturally disproportionate regard for our own interests entitles us to avoid large personal costs.

I shall not, however, lean on Kagan's arguments. Instead I want to suggest, quite simply, that the intelligent contemplation of suffering forces us to move in the direction of adopting an impersonal perspective. To put it another way, suffering demands that we respond to it from an impersonal perspective, or something close to it. If matters were otherwise, we might have settled comfortably into a perspective that gives more weight to our own interests. But an adequate recognition of the badness of suffering wrenches us out of such a perspective. Perhaps an adequate recognition of the badness of suffering permits *some* bias in favor of our interests. But if so, the bias permitted is much less than what is permitted by commonsense morality.

I can offer no tidy demonstration of this claim. But one of the principal aims of this book has been to render it more plausible. It is worth recalling the warning I made at the start of this chapter. We rarely if ever allow ourselves a clear view of the prima facie duty to relieve suffering. Instead, by distorting the meaning of suffering and denying its existence, and by overlooking our capacity to prevent it, we interpose a series of screens that permit no more than a faint image of the duty to relieve suffering to come before us. We should not be surprised if this attenuated image corresponds nicely to the deemphasis of other people's suffering, relative to our own interests, that is permitted by commonsense morality. Indeed, it may be that the degree of disproportionate regard for our own interests permitted by commonsense morality is dependent on a prior concealment of the full force of the prima facie duty to relieve suffering. But we should not, like ostriches, hide ourselves from the available evidence. We should look steadily at the evidence concerning the prima facie power of the duty to relieve suffering. Having done so, we may conclude that the prima facie duty to relieve suffering will not tolerate anything more than a marginal bias in favor of our own interests, if it tolerates any bias at all.[34]

The idea that suffering demands a response from the impersonal perspective, or something very close, is frequently overlooked by critics of demanding moral views.

34. For other arguments supporting a strong duty to prevent suffering, see Garrett Cullity, "International Aid and the Scope of Kindness," *Ethics* 105 (1994): 99–127; Jonathan Glover, *Causing Deaths and Saving Lives* (Harmondsworth: Penguin, 1977); John Harris, "The Marxist Conception of Violence," *Philosophy and Public Affairs* 3 (1974): 192–220; Shelly Kagan, *The Limits of Morality*; Onora O'Neill, *Faces of Hunger: An Essay on Poverty, Justice and Development* (London: Allen and Unwin, 1986); James Rachels, "Killing and Starving To Death," *Philosophy* 54 (1979): 159–71; Henry Shue, *Basic Rights: Subsistence, Affluence, and U.S. Foreign Policy* (Princeton, N.J.: Princeton University Press, 1980); Peter Singer, *Practical Ethics*, 2nd ed. (Cambridge: Cambridge University Press, 1993); and Peter Unger, *Living High and Letting Die*. An early discussion that inspired many of these arguments was Peter Singer's "Famine, Affluence, and Morality," *Philosophy and Public Affairs* 1 (1972): 229–43.

Such critics often assume that stringent moral requirements are derived from a higher-order conception of the ideal moral agent. Thus Susan Wolf takes it for granted that someone who devotes her life to helping those in the greatest need is motivated by the desire to be "as morally good as possible."[35] This permits Wolf to argue that maximum beneficence is not compulsory, because there are more admirable ideals than a life of moral perfection. In *Human Morality*, Scheffler conjectures that impersonal morality answers to an ideal of purity or radical self-transcendence, against which he offers an "ideal of humanity" that allows people to integrate their recognition of the equal worth of all people with their disproportionate concern for their own interests.[36] However, there is a more direct route to impersonal morality than either of these philosophers consider: namely, a belief that suffering is so bad that the prima facie duty to achieve the greatest possible reduction in the cumulative badness of suffering morally overrides our natural tendency to give disproportionate weight to our own interests.

The confusion is especially striking in Wolf's essay. Wolf's view seems to be that we should first judge what kinds of life are more or less admirable, and then act so as to attain a more admirable life. But this gets the order all wrong. We should *first* look to see if there are any moral requirements that are binding on our behavior, and *then* make our notions of what is more or less admirable conform to those requirements. Wolf thinks that someone who reads Victorian novels, plays the oboe, or improves his backhand leads a more admirable life than someone who devotes all his time to the alleviation of suffering.[37] I think that while the first life possesses a kind of superficial attractiveness, the second life is ultimately more admirable (other things being equal), because (other things being equal) it conforms more closely to the duty to relieve suffering. Wolf may reply that I am ignoring her main point, which is that we need to put morality in its place. But I think this attitude is harder to adopt if we pay due regard to the moral significance of suffering.[38]

35. Susan Wolf, "Moral Saints," *Journal of Philosophy* 79 (1982): 419–39, p. 421. This may explain Wolf's puzzling caricature of the moral saint as someone who eschews "a cynical or sarcastic wit, or a sense of humor that appreciates this kind of wit in others," who "should try to look for the best in people, give them the benefit of the doubt as long as possible," who "may not in good conscience be able to laugh at a Marx Brothers movie or enjoy a play by George Bernard Shaw," and who "will have to be very, very nice" (p. 422). Perhaps there are some conceptions of moral sainthood that require these qualities, but they certainly are not essential to a life of maximum beneficence. On the contrary, we should expect that a life of maximum beneficence is *unlikely* to exhibit these qualities. A benefactor who hopes to rival the accomplishments of someone like the late Frederick Cuny needs extraordinary courage, determination, imagination, and energy, as well as a certain indifference to other people's opinions. He must wage a continual battle against human selfishness and stupidity, and may have to knock heads together to get things done. Such traits and experiences will tend to breed a certain degree of toughness, shrewdness, and cynicism that even Wolf could admire.

36. *Human Morality*, pp. 6, 120–25.

37. "Moral Saints," p. 421.

38. In a recent article ("The Demands of Beneficence," *Philosophy and Public Affairs* 22 [1993]: 267–92), Liam Murphy has suggested that the limits of obligation are set by a Cooperative Principle. According to this principle, my obligatory sacrifice is no higher than what it would take for me to achieve the best outcome (prevent the worst suffering) if everyone cooperated on fair terms to achieve this goal. In other

I have claimed that, where the duty to relieve suffering is concerned, we are permitted much less of a bias in favor of our own interests than commonsense morality would have us believe. But perhaps we are not permitted *any* self-interested bias where the duty to relieve suffering is concerned. Perhaps we are required to respond to suffering from a standpoint that is completely impersonal.

What would lead us to this view? The intelligent contemplation of suffering may compel it directly. Or we may reach it in other ways. For example, we may come to think that the badness of suffering occupies an altogether higher level of moral importance than our natural tendency to give weight to our own interests. We may deny that our natural partiality has *any* moral importance in comparison to the badness of suffering. It is true that partiality is fundamental to our characters; natural selection has made it so. We may deny, however, that a trait owing to natural selection has any weight in the moral scales against the badness of suffering.

Scheffler proposes that

> morality is addressed from the outset to human beings as they are. It affords them the prospect of integrating two different motivational tendencies, and it has no "prior" content that must be "reduced" or "modified" when it is brought into contact with human nature.[39]

We can reject this. We can deny that morality is addressed from the outset to human beings as they are. We can even deny that morality, from the outset, addresses human beings at all. Contrary to this, we may hold that the duty to relieve suffering is objectively rooted in the badness of suffering, and that this fact is entirely independent of the disposition or even the existence of human beings. If so, we may come to view our natural partiality, not as something that should be accommodated in some measure by morality, but as an obstacle to correct moral understanding, at least where the relief of suffering is concerned.[40]

---

words, my obligatory sacrifice is determined by my optimal contribution in a world of full compliance. This suggestion is interesting, but resistible. Murphy runs into trouble with the example of another adult and myself who could rescue two toddlers drowning at either end of a shallow pond (pp. 290–92). If the other adult refuses to do anything, and the cost of rescuing both children is higher than the cost of rescuing only one, the Cooperative Principle implies that I have to rescue only one child, though clearly I should rescue both. Murphy replies that the Cooperative Principle does not apply in this case, and that I am governed here by a *special obligation* to rescue both children. But one very much wants to know why this special obligation doesn't extend to the suffering of all people everywhere. Is it because the children are geographically closer, or within my immediate field of vision? Many people, including myself, will be unwilling to concede that this makes a difference.

39. *Human Morality*, p. 125.

40. It is possible to view commonsense morality as the result of a compromise between self-interest and the demands of impersonal morality. We implicitly recognize the truth of impersonal morality, but our self-interest growls at its more extreme demands. To avoid an outright rejection of morality, a bargain is struck. Non-compliance with the more extreme demands of morality is "permitted" in the name of "morality," in return for an agreement to honor the less extreme demands of impersonal morality. An illusion is thereby created that some exemptions from the demands of impersonal morality are authorized by morality itself. What authorizes such exemptions, however, is a sham morality imposed at the behest of our own self-interest.

I waver on the question whether the duty to relieve suffering permits a small degree of self-interested bias, or none at all. But I tend to the view that it permits none at all. Part of me resists this view, but I am inclined to interpret this resistance as the expression of a deeply rooted self-interest that carries no moral weight against the impersonal badness of suffering.

This position is hard to accept. I would to like to focus on its difficulty a little while longer.

If we believe there is a limit to the sacrifice that the prima facie duty to relieve suffering can legitimately demand of us, we can conceive of this limit in different ways. We may believe that the agent is allowed to multiply the impersonal significance of his sacrifice by some constant greater than one when weighing it against the badness of the suffering he could prevent.[41] We may also think that as the sacrifice demanded of the agent increases in severity, new or stronger limits on obligatory sacrifice apply. For example, we may think that at lower levels of sacrifice a bias in favor of the agent's interests is not permitted, while at higher levels of sacrifice it is. Or we may think that the constant by which an agent is allowed to multiply the impersonal significance of his interests *increases* with the severity of the contemplated sacrifice. Finally, we may think that there are some sacrifices so great that they are never morally required, no matter how great the cumulative badness of suffering that would be prevented by means of them.[42]

Now consider the kinds of sacrifice the prima facie duty to relieve suffering might require. Here is a partial list, in rough order of increasing severity.

> *Sacrifice of Economic Assets.* I have in mind assets beyond what is necessary for future needs and the future completion of core projects. I particularly have in mind assets that provide one with an abstract sense of power and future possibilities. Assets of this kind are a characteristic possession of wealthy people. To prevent worse suffering, we may be required to part with these assets.
>
> *Sacrifice of Pleasures.* By "pleasures" I do not mean pleasure in general, much less happiness, but rather those activities and acquisitions that we turn to with the specific purpose of deriving pleasure—anything from seeing a movie or attending a football game to vacationing in the Caribbean or purchasing a Ming vase. These things consume time and money that can often be used to prevent suffering.
>
> *Sacrifice of Projects.* I have in mind "the major activities and commitments around which our lives are organized."[43] Examples would include the pursuit of an artistic career, a commitment to providing a better life for one's

41. Scheffler proposes such a limit in *The Rejection of Consequentialism*.

42. For an interesting effort to probe the limits of obligatory sacrifice, see Tim Mulgan, "A Non-Proportional Hybrid Moral Theory," *Utilitas* 9 (1997): 291–306.

43. Scheffler, *Human Morality*, p. 122.

children, a plan to live in the country and train horses. The duty to relieve
suffering asks us to choose that project or set of projects that will prevent
the worst cumulative suffering. This may require us to choose a project
different from the one we most preferred, or even to abandon a project in
which we have invested years or decades of work.

Sacrifice to our Relationships. It is possible that the prevention of the worst
cumulative suffering would require us to forego or abandon close relationships. It could also place a limit on the time and resources that we may
invest in our most important relationships, and this could limit their du-
rability, richness, and depth.

Sacrifice of Happiness. The duty to relieve suffering might require measures
that would deprive us of happiness during substantial periods of our lives.
It could require us to lead a joyless or even grim existence, without plunging
us into actual suffering.

Sacrifice of Liberty. (An example would be becoming someone's slave.)

Sacrifice of Normal Intelligence.

Sacrifice of Body Parts.

Sacrifice of Basic Physical Abilities. The last four are self-explanatory. I think
the prevention of the worst cumulative suffering is generally unlikely to
require any of these sacrifices. An exception may be the requirement to
surrender some of my organs for transplant if this prevents worse suffering
and leads to a better outcome overall.

Incurrence of Suffering. A clear though extremely unlikely example would be
a situation in which I would have to submit to torture to prevent two other
people from experiencing torture that is equally horrible.

Sacrifice of Life. This is required by the maximal duty to relieve suffering
only if my premature death is less bad from an impersonal standpoint than
the suffering I could thereby prevent.

Resistance to a maximal duty to relieve suffering is likely to increase as one moves
down this list. (Recall that a maximal duty to relieve suffering is one that allows no
bias in favor of the agent's interests.) Different people will begin to rebel at different
points. For my part, I can accept the requirement to sacrifice assets and pleasures.
And unlike several philosophers who object strenuously to principles demanding
the sacrifice of projects, I find myself able to accept the view that an agent should
sacrifice her projects if doing so is necessary to prevent suffering that is worse than
her sacrifice from an impersonal standpoint. But I begin to struggle at the thought
that happiness or normal intelligence or freedom may have to be sacrificed, and the
struggle becomes more intense when we get to body parts and basic physical abilities.
As for personal relationships, I can accept the sacrifices demanded by the maximal
duty to relieve suffering, until one is asked to sacrifice the happiness, or any other
interest at least as important, of the people with whom one has close relations; from
that point on, I begin to feel a resistance that roughly parallels the resistance to
equivalent sacrifices demanded of the agent him- or herself.

Suppose it turned out that by giving up my leg, I could prevent a large amount of suffering that is worse from an impersonal perspective than the loss of my leg. Should I, in that case, give up my leg? Something within me asserts that I do not *have* to do this, and the thought of being asked to do it for the sake of averting a worse outcome inspires in me a grim determination to stand ground. I think to myself that if I did give up my leg, I would afterward curl up and withdraw, that in a world that required this kind of self-sacrifice, indeed self-betrayal, there would no longer be any reason to strive or look ahead or form plans—in short, no longer any reason to go on living. At bottom, I believe this is the same reaction that finds expression in the complaint of philosophers like Bernard Williams that life is no longer worth living if we must be prepared to sacrifice our core projects for the sake of the greater good.[44]

It is possible to stand back from this feeling, however, and to view it as the outraged protest of our own self-interest, a self-interest that is not above threatening extreme retaliation to the psyche (e.g., in the form of a permanent sulk) if it perceives itself subjected to a major attack. What I find difficult to decide is whether, for the purpose of determining the limits of the duty to relieve suffering, I should identify with these powerful self-protective instincts, or dissociate myself from them. Sometimes, at least, I think I should dissociate myself from them. Dissociation from these feelings, needless to say, does not mean getting rid of them. Even if I thought that I should, if necessary, incur the most extreme sacrifices to prevent worse cumulative suffering—that is, surrender body parts, or submit to torture, or sacrifice my life—I suspect that I would not incur them if called on to do so. I already shirk morally obligatory sacrifices that are much less costly than these. What I am suggesting is that my avoidance of these sacrifices may not reflect a moral entitlement to avoid them, but rather the force of powerful self-protective feelings that prevent me from doing what I ought to do.

6. Special Obligations

I have claimed that we are excused from the demands of the prima facie duty to relieve suffering much less often than we tend to think. An adequate recognition of the badness of suffering requires us to move away from the degree of partiality permitted by commonsense morality, toward the stricter requirements of the impersonal standpoint.

This implies a potential obligation to bring greater sacrifices not only upon ourselves, but also upon those people—such as family members, friends, and compa-

---

44. "Unless such things [as deep attachments to particular persons and projects] exist, there will not be enough substance or conviction in a man's life to compel his allegiance to life itself." (Williams, "Persons, Character, and Morality," in Williams, *Moral Luck* [Cambridge: Cambridge University Press, 1981], p. 18.) The difference is that this reaction sets in earlier for Williams than it does for me.

triots—whose interests may loom larger from our own perspective than they do from the impersonal standpoint. One objection to having to sacrifice the interests of family members, friends, and others close to us is that their interests are important to us. I tried to address this objection in the last section by referring to a broad understanding of a person's "interests" that could include the well-being and success of particular other individuals, and by arguing that we are allowed much less of a bias in favor of our own interests, broadly understood, than commonsense morality permits. But another objection to having to sacrifice the interests of family members, friends, and others is that we have a *special obligation* to protect their interests. According to this objection, the duty to relieve suffering is limited not only by a prima facie permission to protect our own interests, broadly understood, but also by a *moral requirement* to protect the interests of people who are related to us in certain ways.

We need to distinguish between two different questions: First, do people have special duties to protect the interests of particular individuals (or particular classes of individuals)? Second, if there are such duties, do they place a limit on the duty to relieve suffering? One can acknowledge the existence of special duties to protect the interests of particular individuals without recognizing in those duties a limit on the duty to relieve suffering. For the attribution of special duties can be seen as a way of dividing up our collective responsibility to protect the interests of humanity at large. This is the substance of the assigned responsibility theory of special duties.[45] Special duties are necessary according to this theory, because, for various reasons, "it is simply the case that our general duties toward people are sometimes more effectively discharged by assigning special responsibility for that matter to some particular agents."[46]

Thus, for example, patients are best looked after when they are assigned to individual doctors, and doctors best discharge their collective responsibility to the sick by assuming responsibility for the patients individually assigned to them.[47] We owe special obligations to our friends inasmuch as our friends become dependent on us for particular forms of emotional support and practical assistance. Parents owe a special duty to their children because children need support, protection, socialization, and love, which under the present social arrangements, at least, parents are, in general, best suited to provide. To put it the other way, parents have a special duty to protect and support their children because children are especially vulnerable to abuse and neglect by their parents. When parents seriously abuse and neglect their children, it is well understood that other people (state bureaucrats in the last resort) must insure the fulfillment of our collective responsibility to care for

45. This theory is most fully worked out by Robert E. Goodin. See his *Protecting the Vulnerable* (Chicago: University of Chicago Press, 1985), and "What Is So Special about Our Fellow Countrymen?," *Ethics* 98 (1988): 663–86.
46. Goodin, "What Is So Special about Our Fellow Countrymen?," p. 681.
47. This paragraph draws from Goodin's work.

the children by delegating that duty to particular agents (relatives, foster parents, children's homes) who can be depended on to discharge it competently and conscientiously.

The assigned responsibility theory explains the basis of special duties, but also sets a limit to those duties. Special duties should not be honored when they defeat their underlying purpose—which is to promote the interests of humanity at large. For example, it makes sense, other things being equal, to arrange an international division of labor whereby national governments cater principally to the needs of their own citizens. But when there arises a vast disparity in the international distribution of wealth, richer nations have a responsibility to share some of their resources with poorer nations. The degree of priority that the inhabitants of wealthier nations currently give to their fellow-citizens is inconsistent with the goals of the assigned responsibility model.[48] To take another example: because parents are well-situated to provide day-to-day care for their own children, though not as a rule for other children, it makes sense to ascribe to parents a special duty to provide day-to-day care for their children.[49] However, some children may lack necessities such as food, medicine, and education—perhaps because they are orphans, or because their parents are unable or unwilling to provide for them. Well-off parents can help supply the needs of these children, through donations of time and money, without sacrificing the needs of their own children. If they neglect the needs of the deprived children in order to supply their own children with luxuries, they act contrary to the goals of the assigned responsibility theory of special duties.

A maximal duty to relieve suffering is compatible with special duties that are based on and limited by the assigned responsibility theory. In order to minimize the cumulative badness of suffering, we need some kind of division of labor, in which each of us takes responsibility for preventing the suffering of particular individuals assigned to our care. It makes sense, other things being equal, for doctors to focus on the needs of their own patients, friends to watch out for friends, and parents to guard and nurture their own children. There would be mayhem if everyone tried simultaneously to look after everyone.

Nevertheless, the maximal duty to relieve suffering requires me to sacrifice the interests of particular individuals entrusted to my care whenever doing so is necessary to prevent worse cumulative suffering in the world as a whole and the sacrifice of these individuals' interests is less bad than the suffering I could prevent. Is this a reasonable requirement? Here things are complicated by the fact that sometimes people may prevent worse cumulative suffering over the long term if they are *mo-*

48. Goodin, "What Is So Special about Our Fellow Countrymen?" Goodin's closing remark is that "in the present world system, it is often—perhaps ordinarily—wrong to give priority to the claims of our compatriots" (p. 686)

49. James Rachels, "Morality, Parents, and Children," in George Graham and Hugh LaFollette, eds., *Person to Person* (Philadelphia: Temple University Press, 1989). I am indebted to Rachels's article in what follows.

tivated to place the interests of particular individuals entrusted to their care ahead of the prevention of the worst cumulative suffering in the world as a whole.[50] For example, in order to minimize the cumulative badness of suffering, we need parents to be vigilant on behalf of the their children's interests and to give their children the psychological security of feeling loved. But it is unlikely that parents can perform these tasks unless they feel a more than impersonal regard for their children's well-being. We should therefore encourage some degree of partiality on the part of parents toward their children. Though the optimal measure of partiality will lead parents to violate the maximal duty to relieve suffering on some occasions (by making them refuse to sacrifice some interest of their child in order to prevent worse cumulative suffering in the world as a whole), it will lead them to maximum compliance with the maximal duty to relieve suffering over the long term. It must be stressed that the optimal measure of partiality means neither too little *nor* too much. We might guess that the optimal amount would cause a parent to refuse compliance with the maximal duty to relieve suffering when it required her to sacrifice her child's life, but not when it required her to deny her child luxuries.

The general point underlying the last paragraph is that sometimes it is best if people are *motivated* to do what they *ought not* to do. Derek Parfit has coined the term "blameless wrongdoing" to describe wrong actions that proceed from the most desirable motives.[51] But I shall not pursue this point. I shall leave the question of desirable motives aside and return to the question of what we are morally required to do. It may be felt by some that the maximal duty to relieve suffering does not recognize the full weight of our special duties to particular individuals such as children, friends, and compatriots. It is true that the maximal duty to relieve suffering is compatible with, and indeed calls for, special duties to protect the interests of particular individuals. But it may be felt that the special duties that are compatible with the maximal duty to relieve suffering are too weak—or, in other words, that we violate our special obligations to particular individuals when we sacrifice their interests as deeply as the maximal duty to relieve suffering may require.

If we are to uphold this objection, we need some justification for special obligations that is different from the assigned responsibility theory. Different alternative justifications have been offered. I shall mention three that appear with particular frequency. Each of these justifications seeks to establish a duty on the part of agent A to promote the interests of a particular individual or set of individuals P, where compliance with the duty sometimes leads to a worse outcome overall, because the gain to P is exceeded by the costs to other people. The first justification states that A has this duty because she herself has assumed it through a previous voluntary action (such as a promise). The second justification states that A has this duty because of benefits that she has received from P. The third justification states that A has this duty because she has benefited from other people's observance of a general

---

50. See Derek Parfit, *Reasons and Persons* (Oxford: Clarendon Press, 1984), pp. 31–35.
51. Ibid.

rule that requires one to promote the interests of individuals related to one in a certain way, and P is related to A in this way. (The other people from whose observance of the rule A has benefited need not overlap with P.)[52] These three justifications can be labeled respectively as the assumed obligation argument, the gratitude argument, and the fair play argument. They lend themselves to different sorts of special obligations. The first and the third but not the second lend themselves to the special obligations of parents toward their children. The second lends itself better than the first to the obligation of children toward parents. The first and second lend themselves to obligations between friends. The third and perhaps the first lend themselves to obligations between compatriots, and between members of the same neighborhood or village.

Can special duties supported by these alternative justifications place limits on the maximal duty to relieve suffering, and if so, to what extent? One's answer will depend on how one conceives of the strength of the prima facie duty to relieve suffering—whether one views it as no more than a kind of plea, and perhaps a distant one at that, or as a presumptive moral requirement that can only be defeated by strong contradictory requirements. The reason I say this is that the alternative, non-consequentialist justifications of special duties seem plausible only against a background that is free from strong contradictory prima facie moral requirements. This does not hold true for other moral considerations, such as the alleged deontological constraint against inflicting harm. One can acknowledge a strong prima facie requirement to reduce suffering, and nevertheless feel certain that one should not reduce the cumulative badness of suffering when doing so requires the infliction of suffering on some to prevent worse suffering to others. But I doubt that the justifications of special duties based on assumed obligation, gratitude, or fair play have this kind of power. This is perhaps easiest to show with promising. It seems most unlikely that you can duck a strong prima facie moral requirement simply by promising to do what is forbidden by the requirement. The same, I would suggest, holds true of assuming obligations in other ways. As for fair play, if I benefit from other people's observance of a particular rule, then perhaps I should observe the rule—but not, it would seem, if the rule is opposed by a strong prima facie moral requirement, and the presumption is that the rule should never have been followed in the first place. Finally, when gratitude prompts us to repay some debt to a benefactor, we generally think that the debt should not be paid in a form that violates a strong prima facie moral requirement. Because I think that the duty to relieve suffering takes the form of a strong prima facie moral requirement, I am skeptical that special duties justified on grounds of assumed obligation, gratitude, or fair play can place much of a limit on the duty to relieve suffering.[53]

52. This justification can be seen as an application of Hart's fairness principle. See H. L. A. Hart, "Are There Any Natural Rights?" *Philosophical Review* 64 (1955): 175–91, p. 185. I am indebted to Bill Talbott for help in formulating this justification.

53. Does this also imply that the duty to relieve suffering is not significantly limited by democratic constraints (that is, on the critical level of morality)? It may be thought that the duty to abide by

The alternative justifications for special duties work best when the ground has already been cleared away—that is to say, when it has been demonstrated that the special duties being defended do *not* run into strong pre-existing prima facie moral requirements. For this reason, I think that the attempt to found special duties strong enough to override the maximal duty to relieve suffering on appeals to assumed obligation, gratitude, or fair play tends to lean on the implicit assumption that, even without the special duty, the agent is already *permitted* to favor the interests of certain individuals to the full extent that the special duty would require. The idea, in other words, is that the agent has a permission sometimes to prefer the interests of particular individuals over compliance with the maximal duty to relieve suffering, and in the space cleared away by this permission, special duties based on assumed obligation, gratitude, or fair play can take root. This, however, returns us to the earlier question whether an agent may give independent moral weight to a personal point of view that accords a degree of importance to his own interests and those of other individuals that is disproportionate to the impersonal significance of those interests. I have already argued that, where other people's suffering is at stake, we must grant much less weight to the personal perspective than commonsense morality permits, and that we should move closer to the impersonal perspective. I also suggested that, where other people's suffering is at stake, we *may* be required to act from a perspective that is completely impersonal.

Before my readers rally to common sense, they should guard against possible sources of confusion. Most people think we have a strong obligation to protect the interests of individuals who are related to us in special ways—for example, our children. Most people also think that we have only a minimal obligation to relieve suffering overall. On this picture, we are required to give much greater weight to the interests of our children, say, than we are required to give to the interests of strangers. I have argued that we have a much stronger duty to relieve suffering than is generally acknowledged, and this implies that we must give much greater weight to the interests of strangers than we now do. I still hold that we have a strong obligation to protect our children and others specially related to us, only that the difference in strength between our duty toward these individuals and our duty toward strangers is not as great as we thought. Some people may believe that there remains a great difference between the strength of these two duties, without realizing that this belief depends on greatly underestimating the strength of our duty toward strangers.

---

democratic norms, even at the cost of allowing worse suffering, is based on a promise between fellow-citizens, or on certain mutual restrictions to which we are subject by the principle of fair play. However, the duty to follow democratic procedures may be founded on something more than agreement or mutual restriction alone. It may rest, at a deeper level, on a duty of respect toward the rationality of persons who hold opinions on matters of public policy that differ from our own. Such a duty of respect may require us to abide by a process that allows different people's opinions to be heard and debated and chooses laws through a reasonable selection mechanism that is blind to the content of legislative proposals, so long as constitutional restrictions are adhered to. Democratic constraints justified on these grounds may carry greater weight against the prima facie duty to relieve suffering than special duties based on assumed obligation, gratitude, or the principle of fair play.

I have suggested that, where other people's suffering is at stake, morality *may* require us to act from a perspective that accords no more than impersonal significance to our own interests and the interests of individuals specially related to us. Such a perspective would require me to sacrifice the interests of individuals specially related to me whenever doing so was necessary to prevent worse cumulative suffering and the impersonal badness of the suffering I could prevent was not matched or exceeded by the impersonal badness of the requisite sacrifice. This is a hard position to accept, especially when the required sacrifice is a large one. Suppose that in order to comply with the maximal duty to relieve suffering, I would have to accede to the loss of my child's leg. (Suppose, for example, that with the money I could use to save my child's leg, I could also save other people from a great deal of suffering that is worse, from an impersonal standpoint, than the loss of my child's leg.) Am I required to sacrifice my child's leg? That I am so required is hard to accept. Our feelings strenuously oppose the idea. Perhaps these feelings point to a good reason why, in this kind of case, special obligations override the prima facie duty to relieve suffering. (For example, I may have overlooked the best arguments for special obligations in my previous discussion.) Or perhaps the feelings lead us away from the truth. I am unsure which is the case.

7. Conclusion

In these pages I have asked what limits there are on the prima facie duty to relieve suffering. I have tried to trace the far edge of the duty's requirements, an effort that has led repeatedly to uncertainty and perplexity. But there is a wide domain over which, in my opinion, no uncertainty is called for. At a modest sacrifice, fortunate individuals can prevent an enormous amount of suffering. We can save large numbers of people from torture, starvation, and other forms of extreme suffering, provided we are willing to give up our more expensive pleasures, a portion of our leisure time, and a percentage of our bank accounts. Failure to do this is unjustifiable. Some may object that our efforts, to be most effective, need to be coordinated, and that this is hard to achieve. But the difficulty of coordination should not be exaggerated. At regular intervals millions of citizens in the United States, as in other democracies, coordinate their efforts to elect their favorite candidates to office. Moreover, we can ask our governments to coordinate our efforts to relieve suffering. Making them do so also requires coordination, yet we succeed in pushing through a host of other demands. Where there is a will, there is a way. The fact that the failure to incur modest sacrifices in order to relieve suffering is standard behavior does not indicate the warrant of a good moral reason. The failure results largely from a mixture of inattention and indifference. Partly, it results from ignorance or confusion about the meaning and moral significance of suffering. It is in the hope of dispelling some of that confusion that I have written this book.

Author's Note

The author's royalties from this book will be divided equally between Amnesty International USA, Doctors Without Borders USA, and Oxfam America. Readers who want to contribute to these organizations can do so by mailing a check or making a credit card donation over the phone. The addresses and phone numbers are as follows:

Amnesty International USA
Headquarters
322 8th Avenue
New York, NY 10016
1-800 AMNESTY
(1-800 266-3789)

Doctors Without Borders USA, Inc.
6 East 39th Street, 8th floor
New York, NY 10016
1-888 392-0392

Oxfam America
P.O. Box 1745
Boston, MA 02105-1745
1-800 OXFAM US
(1-800 693-2687)

Bibliography

Améry, Jean. *At the Mind's Limits: Contemplations by a Survivor on Auschwitz and Its Realities.* Translated by Sidney Rosenfeld and Stella P. Rosenfeld. Bloomington: Indiana University Press, 1980.

Anderson, Elizabeth. *Value in Ethics and Economics.* Cambridge, Mass.: Harvard University Press, 1993.

Anscombe, G. E. M. *The Collected Philosophical Papers of G. E. M. Anscombe.* Vol. 3. *Ethics, Religion and Politics.* Minneapolis: University of Minnesota Press, 1981.

Aristotle. *Nicomachean Ethics.* Translated by Martin Ostwald. Indianapolis: Babbs–Merrill, 1962.

Bailey, James Wood. *Utilitarianism, Institutions, and Justice.* Oxford: Oxford University Press, 1997.

Bakan, David. *Disease, Pain, and Sacrifice: Toward a Psychology of Suffering.* Chicago: University of Chicago Press, 1968.

Beecher, H. K. *Measurement of Subjective Responses.* New York: Oxford University Press, 1959.

Behr, Edward. *The Algerian Problem.* London: Hodder and Stoughton, 1961.

Bennett, Jonathan. *The Act Itself.* Oxford: Clarendon Press, 1995.

Bentham, Jeremy. *The Principles of Morals and Legislation.* Buffalo: Prometheus, 1988.

Billig, Nathan. *To Be Old and Sad: Understanding Depression in the Elderly.* Lexington, Mass.: Lexington Books, 1987.

Bok, Sissela. *Lying: Moral Choice in Public and Private Life.* New York: Vintage, 1978.

Brandt, Richard B. *A Theory of the Good and the Right.* Oxford: Clarendon Press, 1979.

Carlen, P. L., P. D. Wall, H. Nadvorna, and T. Steinbach. "Phantom Limbs and Related Phenomena in Recent Traumatic Amputations." *Neurology* 28 (1978): 211–17.

Cassell, Eric J. *The Nature of Suffering and the Goals of Medicine.* New York: Oxford University Press, 1991.

Cicero. *De Finibus Bonorum et Malorum.* Translated by H. Rackham. Loeb Classical Library. Cambridge, Massachusetts: Harvard University Press, 1983.

Cowan, J. L. *Pleasure and Pain: A Study in Philosophical Psychology*. London: MacMillan, 1968.

Cullity, Garrett. "International Aid and the Scope of Kindness." *Ethics* 105 (1994): 99–127.

Dawkins, Marian. "The Scientific Basis for Assessing Suffering in Animals." In *In Defense of Animals*, edited by Peter Singer. Oxford: Basil Blackwell, 1985.

DeGrazia, David. *Taking Animals Seriously*. Cambridge: Cambridge University Press, 1996.

Dworkin, Ronald. "What Is Equality?, Part II: Equality of Resources." *Philosophy and Public Affairs* 10 (1981): 283–345.

———. *Life's Dominion*. New York: Vintage, 1994.

Edwards, Rem B. *Pleasures and Pains: A Theory of Qualitative Hedonism*. Ithaca, N.Y.: Cornell University Press, 1979.

Elster, Jon. "Sour Grapes—Utilitarianism and the Genesis of Wants." In *Utilitarianism and Beyond*, edited by Amartya Sen and Bernard Williams. Cambridge: Cambridge University Press, 1982.

Epicurus. *Letters, Principal Doctrines, and Vatican Sayings*. Translated by Russel M. Geer. Indianapolis: Bobbs Merrill, 1964.

Fieve, Ronald R. *Moodswing*. rev. ed. New York: Bantam, 1989.

Finley, M. I. *Ancient Slavery and Modern Ideology*. New York: Viking, 1980.

Finnis, John. *Natural Law and Natural Rights*. Oxford: Clarendon Press, 1980.

Freud, Sigmund. "Mourning and Melancholia." Translated by Joan Riviere. In Freud, *Collected Papers*. Vol. 4. New York: Basic Books, 1959.

Gärdenfors, Peter, and Nils-Eric Sahlin, "Introduction: Bayesian Decision Theory—Foundations and Problems." In *Decision, Probability and Utility*, edited by Peter Gärdenfors and Nils-Eric Sahlin. Cambridge: Cambridge University Press, 1989.

Gibbard, Allan. "Interpersonal Comparisons: Preference, Good, and the Intrinsic Reward of a Life." In *Foundations of Social Choice Theory*, edited by John Elster and Aanund Hylland. Cambridge: Cambridge University Press, 1986.

Glover, Jonathan. *Causing Deaths and Saving Lives*. Harmondsworth: Penguin, 1977.

Goodin, Robert E. *Protecting the Vulnerable*. Chicago: University of Chicago Press, 1985.

———. "What Is So Special about Our Fellow Countrymen?" *Ethics* 98 (1988): 663–86.

Greist, John H., and James W. Jefferson. *Depression and Its Treatment*. New York: Warner, 1984.

Griffin, James. "Is Unhappiness Morally More Important than Happiness?" *Philosophical Quarterly* 29 (1979): 47–59.

———. *Well-being: Its Meaning, Measurement and Moral Importance*. Oxford: Clarendon Press, 1986.

———. "Against the Taste Model." In *Interpersonal Comparisons of Well- being*, edited by Jon Elster and John E. Roemer. Cambridge: Cambridge University Press, 1991.

Gutmann, Amy. "The Challenge of Multiculturalism in Political Ethics." *Philosophy and Public Affairs* 22 (1993): 171–206.

Gutmann, Amy, and Dennis Thomson. *Democracy and Disagreement*. Cambridge, Mass.: Harvard University Press, 1996.

Hampton, Jean. "The Moral Education Theory of Punishment." *Philosophy and Public Affairs* 13 (1984): 208–38. Reprinted in *Punishment*, edited by A. John Simmons, Marshall Cohen, and Charles R. Beitz. Princeton, N.J. : Princeton University Press, 1995.

Hardin, Russell. *Morality Within the Limits of Reason*. Chicago: University of Chicago Press, 1988.

Hare, R. M. "Pain and Evil." In *Moral Concepts*, edited by Joel Feinberg. Oxford: Oxford University Press, 1969.

———. *Moral Thinking: Its Levels, Method and Point*. Oxford: Clarendon Press, 1981.

———. "Ethical Theory and Utilitarianism." In *Utilitarianism and Beyond*, edited by Amartya Sen and Bernard Williams. Cambridge: Cambridge University Press, 1982.

Harris, John. "The Marxist Conception of Violence." *Philosophy and Public Affairs* 3 (1974): 192–220.

Harsanyi, John. "Cardinal Welfare, Individualistic Ethics, and Interpersonal Comparisons of Utility." *Journal of Political Economy* 63 (1955): 309–21.

———. "Morality and the Theory of Rational Behaviour." In *Utilitarianism and Beyond*, edited by Amartya Sen and Bernard Williams. Cambridge: Cambridge University Press, 1982.

Hart, H. L. A. "Are There Any Natural Rights?" *Philosophical Review* 64 (1955): 175–91.

Herman, Judith Lewis. *Trauma and Recovery*. New York: Basic Books, 1992.

Hurka, Thomas. *Perfectionism*. New York: Oxford University Press, 1993.

Jackson, Frank. "Decision-theoretic Consequentialism and the Nearest and Dearest Objection." *Ethics* 101 (1991): 461–82.

James, William. *Essays in Pragmatism*. Edited by Alburey Castell. New York: Hafner, 1958.

Jensen, Mark P., and Paul Karoly. "Self-Report Scales and Procedures for Assessing Pain in Adults." In *Handbook of Pain Assessment*, edited by Denis C. Turk and Ronald Melzack. New York: Guildford, 1992.

Jones, Ernest. *The Life and Work of Sigmund Freud*. Vol. 3. New York: Basic Books, 1957.

Kagan, Shelly. *The Limits of Morality*. Oxford: Clarendon Press, 1989.

Kahneman, Daniel, and Amos Tversky. "Prospect Theory: An Analysis of Decision under Risk." In *Decision, Probability and Utility*, edited by Peter Gardenfors and Nils-Eric Sahlin. Cambridge: Cambridge University Press, 1989.

Kamm, F. M. *Morality, Mortality*. Vol. 1. *Death and Whom To Save from It*. New York: Oxford University Press, 1993.

———. *Morality, Mortality*. Vol. 2. *Rights, Duties, and Status*. New York: Oxford University Press, 1996.

Kant, Immanuel. *Foundations of the Metaphysics of Morals*. Translated by Lewis White Beck. Indianapolis: Bobbs Merrill, 1959.

———. "On a Supposed Right To Lie from Altruistic Motives." Reprinted in Sissela Bok, *Lying: Moral Choice in Public and Private Life*. New York: Vintage, 1978.

———. *The Metaphysics of Morals*. Translated by Mary Gregor. Cambridge: Cambridge University Press, 1991.

Kateb, George. *The Inner Ocean: Individualism and Democratic Culture*. Ithaca, N.Y.: Cornell University Press, 1992.

Katz, Leonard David. "Hedonism as Metaphysics of Mind and Value." Ph.D. diss., Princeton University, 1986.

Koestler, Arthur. *Darkness at Noon*. Translated by Daphne Harty. New York: Macmillan, 1941.

Korsgaard, Christine M. "The Reasons We Can Share: An Attack on the Distinction between Agent-Relative and Agent-Neutral Values." In *Altruism*, edited by Ellen Franken Paul, Fred D. Miller, Jr., and Jeffrey Paul. Cambridge: Cambridge University Press, 1993.

———. "Personal Identity and the Unity of Agency: A Kantian Reply to Parfit." *Philosophy and Public Affairs* 18 (1989): 101–32. Reprinted in Korsgaard, *Creating the Kingdom of Ends*. Cambridge: Cambridge University Press, 1996.

Kramer, Peter D. *Listening to Prozac*. New York: Viking, 1993.

Kübler-Ross, Elizabeth. *On Death and Dying*. New York: MacMillan, 1969.

Kymlicka, Will. *Contemporary Political Philosophy*. Oxford: Clarendon Press, 1990.

Lewis, C. S. *The Problem of Pain*. New York: MacMillan, 1948.

Loeser, John D., and Wilbert E. Fordyce. "Chronic Pain." In *Behavioral Science in the Practice of Medicine*, edited by J. E. Carr and H. A. Dengerink. New York: Elsevier, 1983.

McClennen, Edward F. "Sure-thing Doubts." In *Decision, Probability, and Utility*, edited by Peter Gärdenfors and Nils-Eric Sahlin. Cambridge: Cambridge University Press, 1989.

McKerlie, Dennis. "Priority and Time." *Canadian Journal of Philosophy* 27 (1997): 287–309.

Mackie, John. *Ethics: Inventing Right and Wrong*. Harmondsworth: Penguin, 1977.

McMahan, Jeff. *Killing at the Margins of Life*. New York: Oxford University Press, forthcoming.

Melzack, Ronald, and W. S. Torgerson. "On the Language of Pain." *Anesthesiology* 34 (1971): 50–59.

Melzack, Ronald, and Patrick D. Wall. *The Challenge of Pain*. New York: Basic Books, 1983.

Middle East Watch. *Syria Unmasked: The Suppression of Human Rights by the Asad Regime*. New Haven: Yale University Press, 1991.

Mill, John Stuart. "Nature." In *Collected Works of John Stuart Mill*, Vol. 10, edited by J. M. Robson. Toronto: University of Toronto Press, 1969.

———. *Utilitarianism, On Liberty and Considerations on Representative Government*. Edited by H. B. Acton. London: Dent, 1972.

Moore, G. E. *Principia Ethica*. Cambridge: Cambridge University Press, 1903.

Mulgan, Tim. "A Non-Proportional Hybrid Moral Theory." *Utilitas* 9 (1997): 291–306.

Murphy, Liam. "The Demands of Beneficence." *Philosophy and Public Affairs* 22 (1993): 267–92.

Nagel, Thomas. *Mortal Questions*. Cambridge: Cambridge University Press, 1979.

———. *The View from Nowhere*. New York: Oxford University Press, 1986.

———. *Equality and Partiality*. New York: Oxford University Press, 1991.

Norcross, Alastair. "Comparing Harms: Headaches and Human Lives." *Philosophy and Public Affairs* 26 (1997): 135–67.

Norman, Richard. *Ethics, Killing, and War*. Cambridge: Cambridge University Press, 1995.

Nozick, Robert. *Anarchy, State, and Utopia*. New York: Basic Books, 1974.

Nussbaum, Martha. "Human Functioning and Social Justice: In Defense of Aristotelian Essentialism." *Political Theory* 20 (1992): 202–46.

O'Neill, Onora. *Faces of Hunger: An Essay on Poverty, Justice and Development*. London: Allen and Unwin, 1986.

Parfit, Derek. "Innumerate Ethics." *Philosophy and Public Affairs* 7 (1978): 285–301.

———. "Future Generations: Further Problems." *Philosophy and Public Affairs* 11 (1981): 113–72.

———. *Reasons and Persons*. Oxford: Clarendon Press, 1984.

———. "Equality or Priority?" 1991 Lindley Lecture. University of Kansas, 1995.

Peters, Edward. *Torture*. New York: Basil Blackwell, 1985.

Plato. *Apology*. In *The Trial and Death of Socrates*. Translated by G. M. A. Grube. Indianapolis: Hackett, 1975.

———. *Gorgias*. Translated by Donald J. Zeyl. Indianapolis: Hackett, 1987.

———. *Republic*. Translated by B. Jowett. New York: Modern Library, 1982.

Popper, Karl R. *The Open Society and Its Enemies*. Princeton, N.J.: Princeton University Press, 1950.

Quinn, Warren. "Putting Rationality in Its Place." In Quinn, *Morality and Action.* Cambridge: Cambridge University Press, 1993.

Rachels, James. "Killing and Starving To Death." *Philosophy* 54 (1979): 159–71.

———. "Morality, Parents, and Children." In *Person to Person,* edited by George Graham and Hugh LaFollette. Philadelphia: Temple University Press, 1989.

Rachels, Stuart. "Counterexamples to the Transitivity of Better Than." *Australasian Journal of Philosophy* 76 (1998): 71–83.

Railton, Peter. "Alienation, Consequentialism, and the Demands of Morality." *Philosophy and Public Affairs* 13 (1984): 134–71.

Rawls, John. *A Theory of Justice.* Cambridge, Mass.: Harvard University Press, 1971.

Register, Cheri. *Living with Chronic Illness: Days of Patience and Passion.* New York: Bantam, 1987.

Ross, W. D. *The Right and the Good.* Oxford. Oxford University Press, 1930.

Ruthven, Malise. *Torture: The Grand Conspiracy.* London: Weidenfeld and Nicolson, 1978.

Sacks, Oliver. *Awakenings.* New York: E. P. Dutton, 1983.

———. *The Man Who Mistook His Wife for a Hat and Other Clinical Tales.* New York: Harper and Row, 1985.

Scanlon, Thomas M. "Contractualism and Utilitarianism." In *Utilitarianism and Beyond,* edited by Amartya Sen and Bernard Williams. Cambridge: Cambridge University Press, 1982.

———. "The Moral Basis of Interpersonal Comparisons." In *Interpersonal Comparisons of Well-being,* edited by Jon Elster and John E. Roemer. Cambridge: Cambridge University Press, 1991.

———. "Value, Desire, and the Quality of Life." In *The Quality of Life,* edited by Martha Nussbaum and Amartya Sen. Oxford: Oxford University Press, 1993.

Scarre, Geoffrey. "Epicurus as a Forerunner of Utilitarianism.'" *Utilitas* 6 (1994): 219–31.

Scarry, Elaine. *The Body in Pain: The Making and Unmaking of the World.* Oxford: Oxford University Press, 1985.

Scheffler, Samuel. *The Rejection of Consequentialism.* Oxford: Clarendon Press, 1982.

———. *Human Morality.* New York: Oxford University Press, 1992.

Scheper-Hughes, Nancy. *Death Without Weeping: The Violence of Everyday Life in Brazil.* Berkeley: University of California Press, 1992.

Schopenhauer, Arthur. *The World as Will and Representation.* 2 vols. Translated by E. F. J. Payne. New York: Dover, 1958.

———. *Essays and Aphorisms.* Translated and edited by R. J. Hollingdale. Harmondsworth: Penguin, 1970.

Sen, Amartya. "Rational Fools: A Critique of the Behavioral Foundations of Economic Theory." *Philosophy and Public Affairs* 16 (1977): 317–44.

———. *Commodities and Capabilities.* Amsterdam: North-Holland, 1985.

———. *Inequality Reexamined.* New York: Russell Sage, 1992.

Sher, George. *Desert.* Princeton, N.J.: Princeton University Press, 1987.

Shue, Henry. *Basic Rights: Subsistence, Affluence, and U.S. Foreign Policy.* Princeton, N.J.: Princeton University Press, 1980.

Sidgwick, Henry. *The Methods of Ethics.* London: Macmillan, 1907.

Singer, Peter. "Famine, Affluence and Morality." *Philosophy and Public Affairs* 1 (1972): 229–43.

———. *Practical Ethics,* 2nd ed. Cambridge: Cambridge University Press, 1993.

Smith, Adam. *The Theory of Moral Sentiments.* Oxford: Oxford University Press, 1976.

Soelle, Dorothee. *Suffering*. Translated by Everett R. Kahn. Philadelphia: Fortress Press, 1975.

Steiner, George. *No Passion Spent*. London: Faber and Faber, 1996.

Sumner, L. W. *Welfare, Happiness, and Ethics*. Oxford: Clarendon Press, 1996.

Sunstein, Cass. "Preferences and Politics." *Philosophy and Public Affairs* 20 (1991): 3–34.

Tännsjö, Torbjörn. "Classical Hedonistic Utilitarianism." *Philosophical Studies* 81 (1996): 97–115.

Taurek, John. "Should the Numbers Count?" *Philosophy and Public Affairs* 6 (1977): 293–316.

Temkin, Larry S. "Intransitivity and the Mere Addition Paradox." *Philosophy and Public Affairs* 16 (1987): 138–87.

———. *Inequality*. New York: Oxford University Press, 1993.

———. "A Continuum Argument for Intransitivity." *Philosophy and Public Affairs* 25 (1996): 175–210.

Thomson, Judith Jarvis. *The Realm of Rights*. Cambridge, Mass.: Harvard University Press, 1990.

Timerman, Jacobo. *Prisoner Without a Name, Cell Without a Number*. Translated by Toby Talbot. New York: Knopf, 1981.

Trigg, Roger. *Pain and Emotion*. Oxford: Clarendon Press, 1970.

Unger, Peter. *Living High and Letting Die: Our Illusion of Innocence*. New York: Oxford University Press, 1996,

White, John. *The Masks of Melancholy: A Christian Physician Looks at Depression and Suicide*. Downers Grove, Ill.: InterVarsity Press, 1982.

Williams, Bernard. "A Critique of Utilitarianism." In J. J. C. Smart and Bernard Williams, *Utilitarianism: For and Against*. Cambridge: Cambridge University Press, 1973.

———. *Problems of the Self*. Cambridge: Cambridge University Press, 1973.

———. *Moral Luck*. Cambridge: Cambridge University Press, 1981.

———. *Ethics and the Limits of Philosophy*. Cambridge, Mass.: Harvard University Press, 1985.

Winokur, George. *Depression: The Facts*. Oxford: Oxford University Press, 1981.

Wolf, Susan. "Moral Saints." *Journal of Philosophy* 79 (1982): 419–39.

Index